THERMAL HAIRSTYLING

10

LEARNING OBJECTIVES

AFTER COMPLETING THIS CHAPTER, YOU SHOULD BE ABLE TO:

1. Define the purpose of thermal waving and curling.
2. Demonstrate proper thermal wave techniques and implements.
3. List safety measures used in thermal waving.
4. Define blow-dry styling.
5. Demonstrate the use of implements, techniques, and cosmetics in blow-dry styling.
6. Define air waving.
7. Demonstrate the use of implements and techniques in air waving.

INTRODUCTION TO THERMAL WAVING AND CURLING

✔ Completed—Learning Objective No. 1

THE PURPOSE OF THERMAL WAVING AND CURLING

The art and technique of using thermal irons for waving and curling was developed in 1875 by a Frenchman, Marcel Grateau. Thermal waving is still known as ***marcel waving.***

Thermal waving and ***curling*** is the art of waving and curling straight or pressed hair (see chapter on thermal hair straightening) with thermal irons, either electrically heated or stove-heated, using special manipulative techniques. Modern implements have contributed to the continued success of these methods of waving and curling hair. ✔

THERMAL IRONS

Thermal irons are an important implement in hairstyling. They provide an even heat that is completely controlled by the cosmetologist. Manipulative techniques are basically the same for electric irons or stove-heated irons.

The irons must be made of the best quality steel so that they hold an even temperature during the waving and curling process. The styling portion of the irons is composed of two parts: the rod (prong) and the shell (groove or bowl).

1. The ***rod*** is a perfectly round solid steel bar.
2. The ***shell*** is perfectly round with the inside grooved so that the rod can rest in it when the irons are closed.

The edge of the shell nearest the cosmetologist is called the ***inner edge;*** the one farthest from the cosmetologist is called the ***outer edge.***

Thermal irons come in a variety of styles, sizes, and weights, from small to jumbo. They come in three different classifications:

1. Conventional (regular) stove-heated. (Fig. 10.1)
2. Electric self-heated. (Fig. 10.2)
3. Electric self-heated, vaporizing.

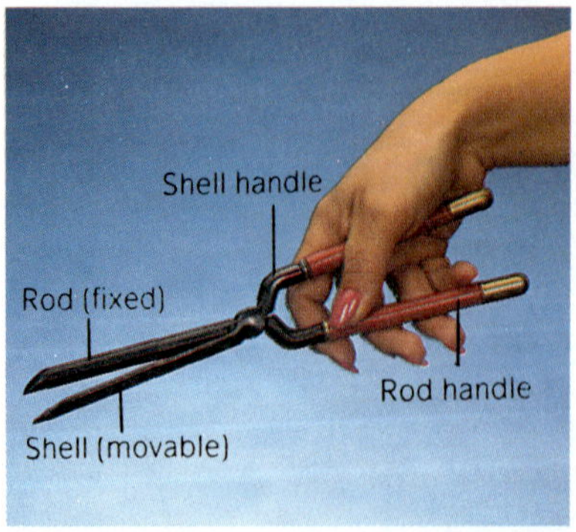

10.1—Conventional thermal (marcel) irons.

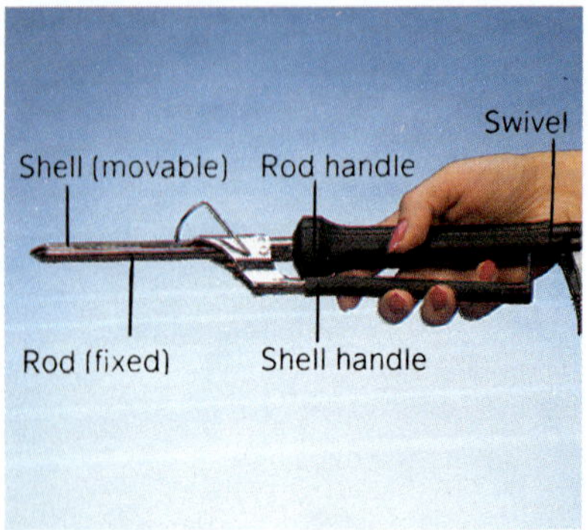

10.2—Electric thermal irons.

◆ NOTE: Do not use electric vaporizing irons on pressed hair; the moisture could cause the hair to revert to its natural overly curly state.

There is no one correct temperature used for the irons when thermal curling and waving the hair. Temperature setting for the irons depends on the texture of the hair, whether it is fine or coarse, or whether it has been lightened or tinted. Hair that has been lightened or tinted (also white hair) should be curled and waved with lukewarm irons. Coarse and gray hair, as a rule, can tolerate more heat than fine hair.

CAUTION

Do not use thermal irons on chemically treated hair; to do so could cause breakage.

Testing Thermal Irons

After heating the irons to the desired temperature, test them on a piece of tissue paper. Clamp the heated irons over the tissue and hold for 5 seconds. If the paper scorches or turns brown, the irons are too hot. Let them cool somewhat before using. Remember that fine, lightened, or badly damaged hair withstands less heat than normal hair. (Fig. 10.3)

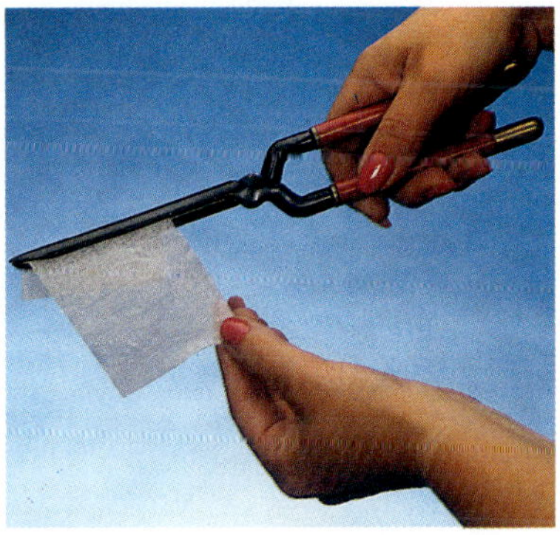

10.3—Testing the heat of thermal irons.

Care of Thermal Irons

Thermal irons should be kept clean and free from rust and carbon. To remove dirt or grease, wash the irons in a soap solution containing a few drops of ammonia. This cuts the oil and grease that usually adhere to the irons. Fine sandpaper, or steel wool with a little oil, helps to remove rust and carbon. It also polishes the irons. To permit greater facility in movement, oil the joint of the irons.

New thermal irons are ***tempered*** at the factory in order to hold heat uniformly. If you overheat the irons they usually lose their temper, and, in most cases, are ruined.

Holding the Thermal Irons

Hold the irons in a comfortable position that gives you complete control. Grasp the handles of the irons in the right hand, far enough away from the joint to avoid the heat. Place the three middle fingers on the back of the lower handle, the little finger in front of the lower handle, and the thumb in front of the upper handle.

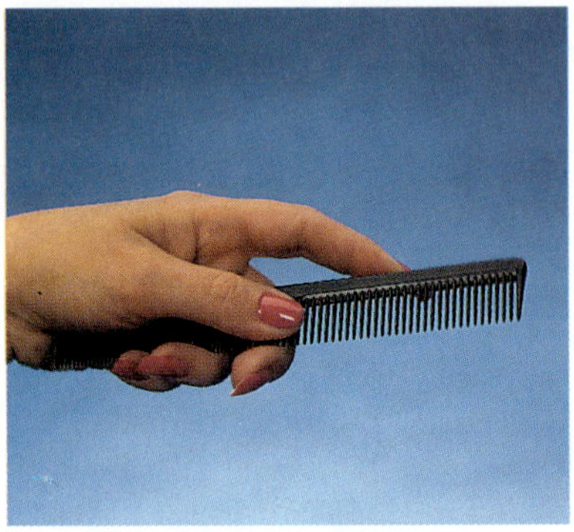

10.4—Holding the comb.

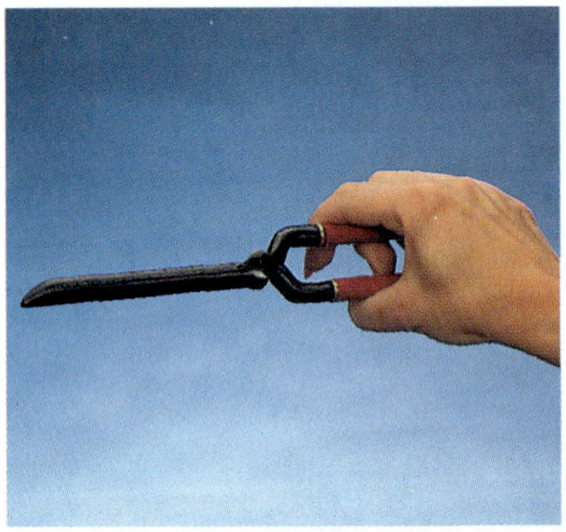

10.5—Rolling the irons.

Comb Used with Thermal Irons

The comb should be about 7" (17.5 cm) long, made of hard rubber or another nonflammable substance, and should have fine teeth; fine teeth hold the hair more firmly than coarse teeth.

Holding the Comb

Hold the comb between the thumb and all four fingers of the left hand, with the index finger resting on the backbone of the comb for better control and one end of the comb resting against the outer edge of the palm. This position assures a strong hold and a firm movement. (Fig. 10.4)

Practicing with Cold Thermal Irons

Since thermal curling and waving is a somewhat difficult operation that uses heated irons, practice with cold irons on a mannequin or hairpiece pinned to a block until you have thoroughly mastered the technique.

Rolling the Thermal Irons

Practice rolling the cold thermal irons in the hand, first forward, then backward. The rolling movement should be done without any sway or motion in the arm; only the fingers are used to roll the handles in either direction. (Fig. 10.5)

Exercises with Cold Thermal Irons

Exercise 1

At the starting position the rod of the thermal iron will be on top of the hair strand. (Fig. 10.6a) To make the curl, rotate the iron one-half turn (Fig. 10.6b) and then one full turn to complete. (Fig. 10.6c)

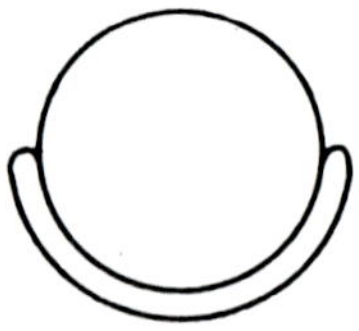

10.6a—Starting position.

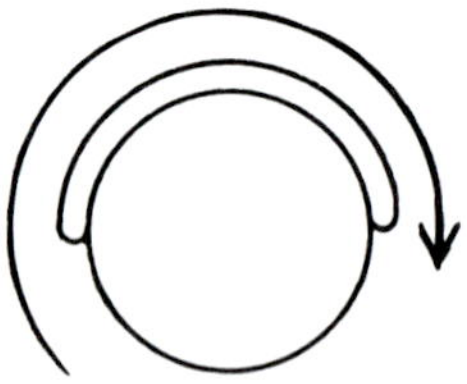

10.6b—One-half turn.

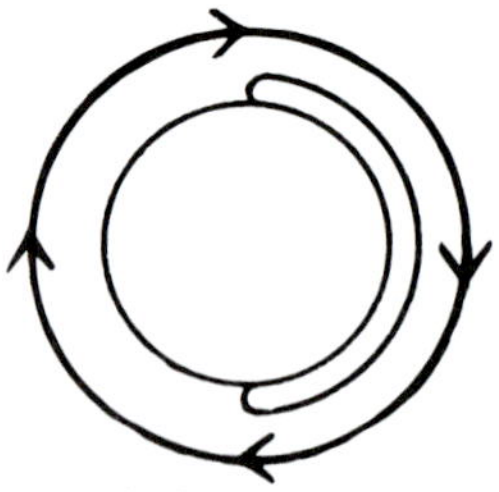

10.6c—Full turn.

Exercise 2

1. Insert hair in irons with rod on top (groove facing upward).
2. Turn irons forward for one-half turn (away from you).
3. Turn irons back to starting position.
4. Open irons slightly and slide down 1" (2.5 cm), then clamp.
5. Turn irons backward for full turn (toward you).
6. Turn irons forward to starting position.
7. Release.

THERMAL WAVING WITH CONVENTIONAL THERMAL (MARCEL) IRONS

Thermal waving is the art of waving hair using conventional marcel irons. The process requires no setting creams or lotions.

Procedure for Left-Going Wave

Comb the hair thoroughly, following its directional growth. The natural growth will determine whether or not the first wave to be formed will be a left-going wave or a right-going wave. The procedure given here is for a left-going wave.

Before the wave is begun, comb the hair in the general shape desired by the client.

1. With the comb, pick up a strand of hair about 2″ (5 cm) in width. Insert the irons in the hair with the groove facing upward. (See Fig. 10.7)

2. Close irons and turn them about one-quarter turn forward (away from you). At the same time, draw the hair with the irons about ¼″ (.625 cm) to the left, (See Fig. 10.8) and direct the hair ¼″ (.625 cm) to the right with the comb. (See Fig. 10.9)

3. Roll the irons one full turn forward (away from you). (See Fig. 10.10) (In doing this, keep the hair uniform with the comb. You will find that the hair has rolled on a slight slant on the prong of the irons.) Keep position No. 3 for a few seconds in order to allow the hair to become sufficiently heated throughout.

4. Reverse movement No. 3 by simply unrolling the hair from the irons, bringing them back into their first resting position. (See Fig. 10.11) (When this movement is completed, you will find the comb resting somewhat away from the irons.)

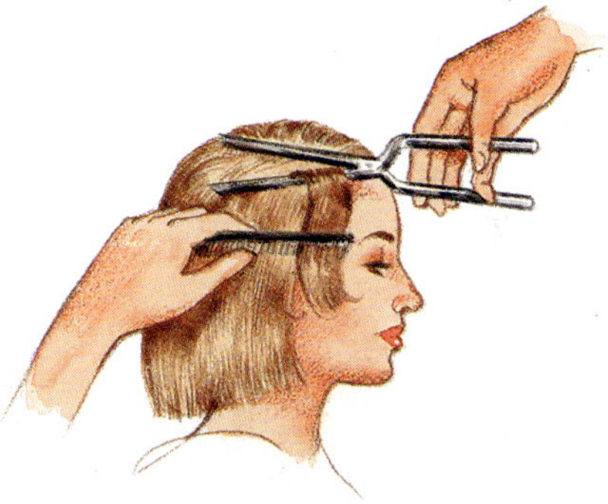

10.7—Insert irons in the hair.

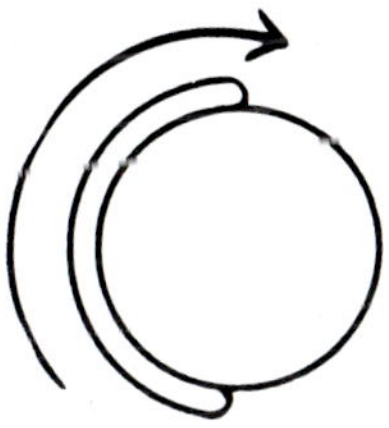

10.8—One-quarter turn.

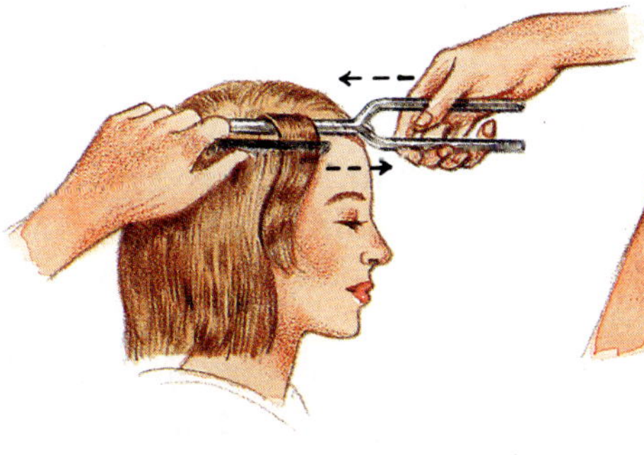

10.9—Direct hair to the right with the comb.

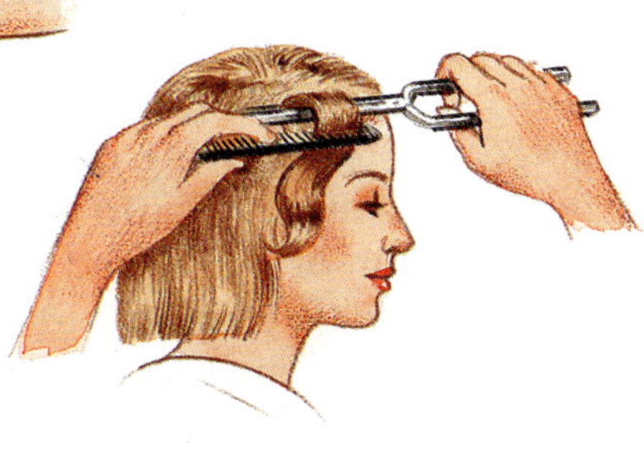

10.10—Roll irons one full turn forward.

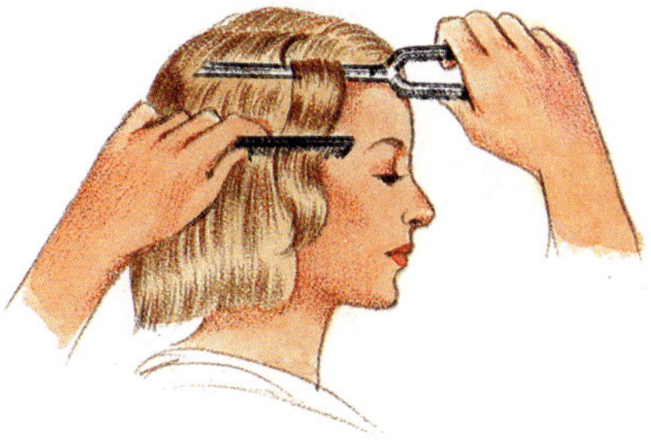

10.11—Reverse movement.

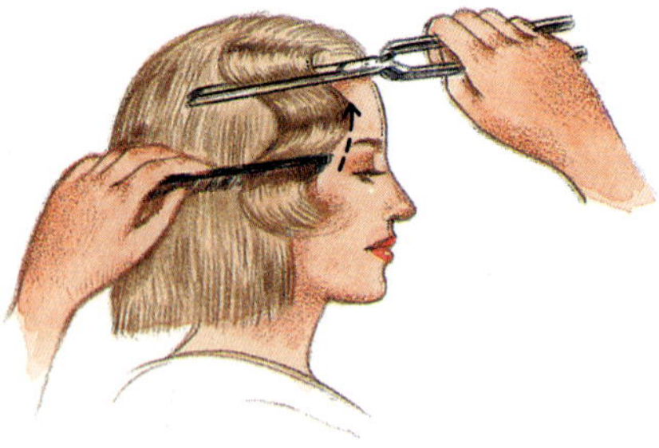
10.12—Start to form the curl.

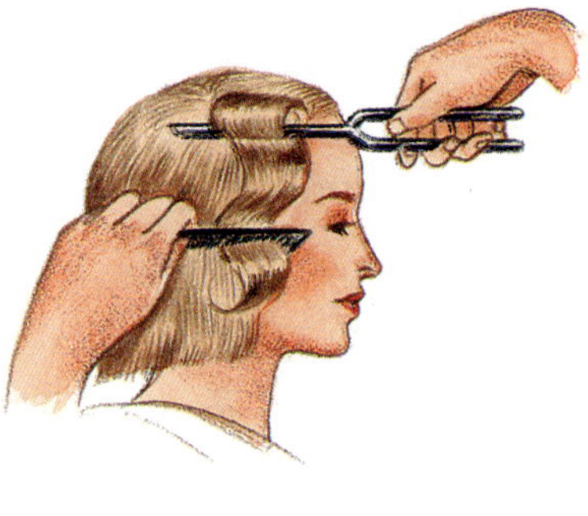
10.13—Form the hair into a half circle.

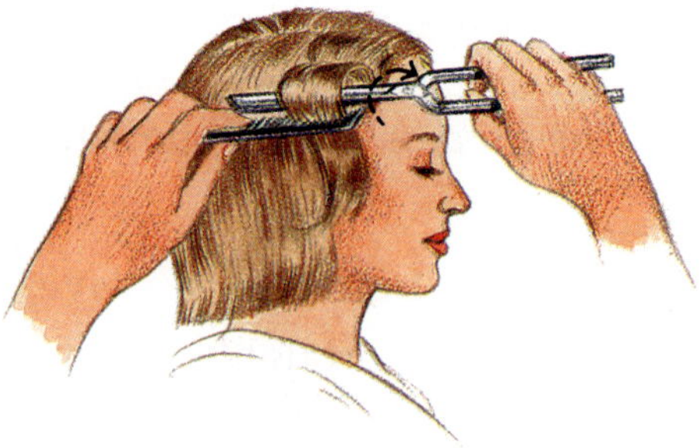
10.14—Roll irons one-half turn forward.

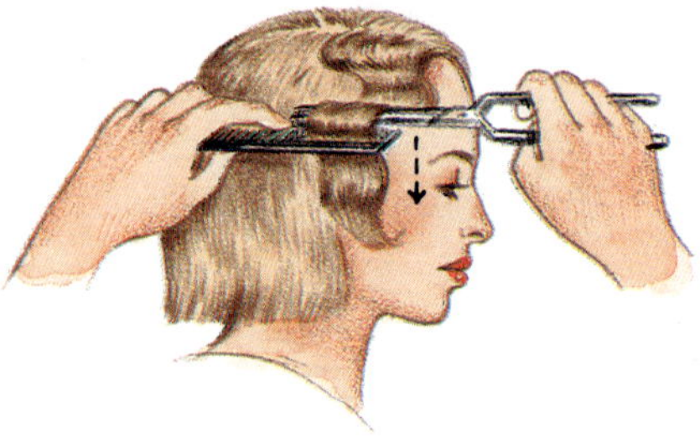
10.15—Slide irons down.

5. Open the irons with the little finger and place them just below the ridge, or crest, by swinging the rod of the irons toward you and then closing them. (See Fig. 10.12) (The outer edge of the groove should be directly underneath the ridge just produced by the inner ridge.)
6. Keep the irons perfectly still and direct the hair with the comb upward about 1″ (2.5 cm), thus forming the hair into a half circle. (See Fig. 10.13) (You must remember that, in order to perform movement No. 6 properly, you do not move the comb from the position explained in movement No. 5.)
7. Without opening the irons, roll them one-half turn forward (from you). (See Fig. 10.14) (In this movement, keep the comb perfectly still and unchanged.)
8. Slide the irons down about 1″ (2.5 cm). (See Fig. 10.15) (This movement is done by opening the irons slightly [loose grip] and then sliding them down the strand of hair.)

Right-Going Wave

After completing movement No. 8, you will find the irons and comb in a position to make the second ridge. This is the beginning of a right-going wave. As you might expect for a right-going wave, the hair is directed opposite to that of a left-going wave.

Joining or Matching the Waves

After completely waving one strand of hair, wave the next strand to match. When picking up the unwaved hair in the comb, include a small section of the waved strand as a guide to the formation of the new wave. (See Fig. 10.16)

When waving the second strand of hair, be sure that the comb and irons movements are the same as in the first strand of hair; otherwise the waves will not match.

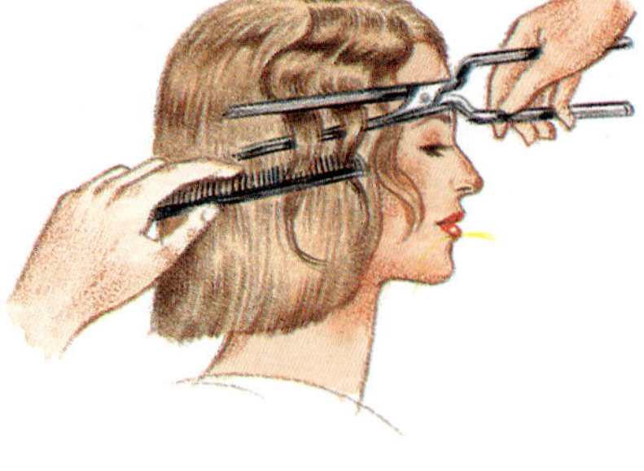
10.16—Matching the wave.

Promo Power

DIRECT MAILING

Direct mailing is probably the most advantageous of all types of advertising and marketing for a salon owner to do, especially if you mail to your existing clientele. They know and like you and are more likely to purchase what you are offering. And because your clients usually live nearby (within a five-mile radius is the norm), this is a relatively inexpensive way to advertise. Direct mail can entice first-time clients to return and keep regular clients coming back as well.

Design what you are presenting in a fashionable manner. If it is a special on permanent waves or color, use a photograph or sketch as part of the design. You will find that postcards cost less, but for a more formal or personal special, use envelopes.

If you plan to use direct mail frequently in your salon, you will save yourself a great deal of time and trouble if you purchase a computer, which can store all of your customer files and print out address labels. It is very important to keep track of the people who respond to mailings; your computer can help do this. If you don't know your rate of return, your mailing won't do you any good. And it's important to plan ahead, since having something typeset and printed takes time.

—*From* The Salon Biz: Tips for Success *by Geri Mataya*

THERMAL CURLING WITH ELECTRIC THERMAL IRONS

Thermal curling is the art of creating curls in the hair using modern thermal irons and a comb. Since thermal curling requires no setting creams or lotions, it may be used to great advantage for the following:

1. ***Straight hair***—permits quick styling. Thermal curling eliminates working with wet hair, use of rollers, and a long hair-drying process.
2. ***Pressed hair***—permits styling the hair without the danger of its reverting to its former overly curly condition. Thermal curling prepares the hair for any desired style.
3. ***Wigs*** and ***hairpieces***—presents a quick and effective method for their styling.

Curling Irons Manipulations

The following is a series of basic manipulative movements for using heated curling irons. Most other curling irons movements are variations of these basic movements.

The following illustrations show a grip with only the little finger used for opening the clamp. (See Figs. 10.17–10.23) Some cosmetologists prefer to use the little finger plus the ring finger for this purpose. Either method is correct.

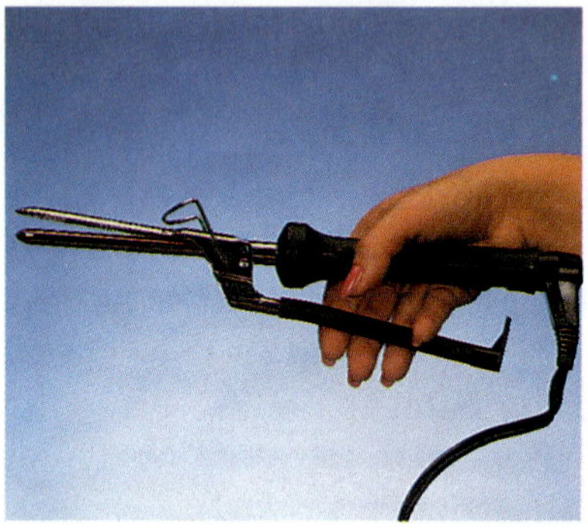

10.17—Use the little finger to open the clamp.

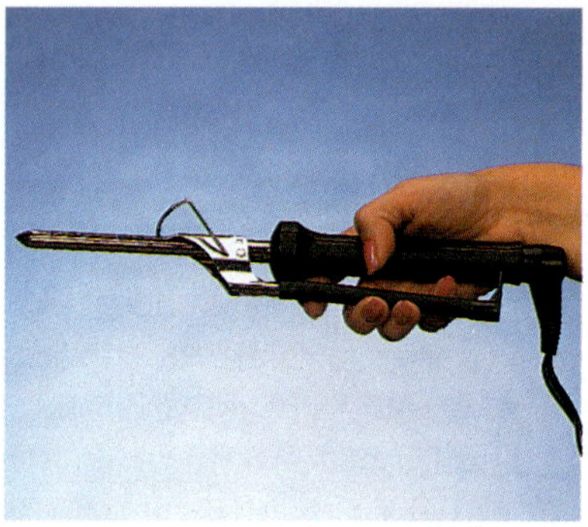

10.18—Use three middle fingers to close and manipulate irons.

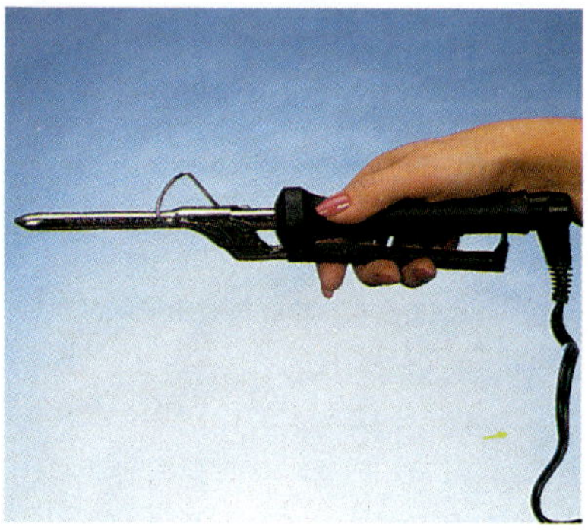

10.19—Shift the thumb when manipulating the irons.

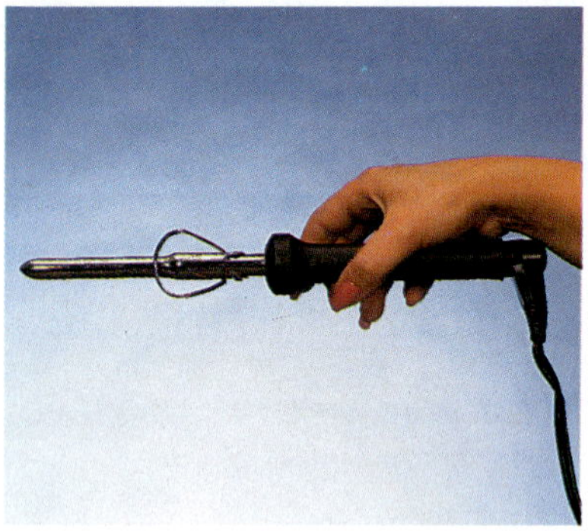

10.20—Close clamp and make a one-quarter turn downward.

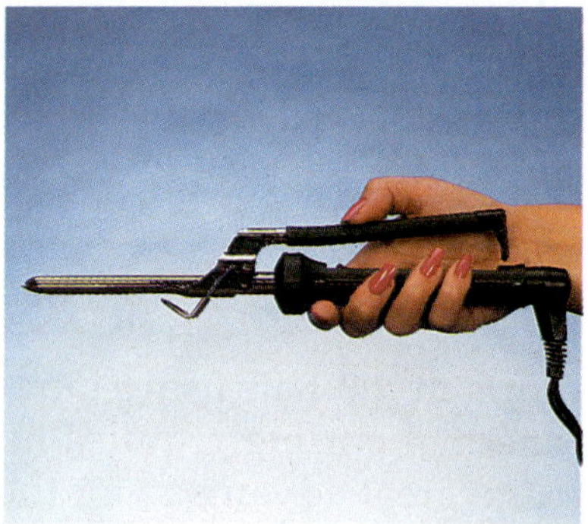

10.21—Irons have made a one-half turn. Use the thumb to open clamp and relax hair tension.

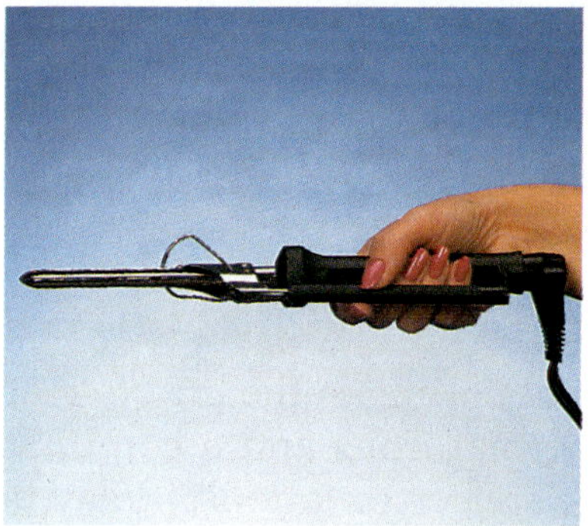

10.22—Rotate irons to three-quarters of a complete turn.

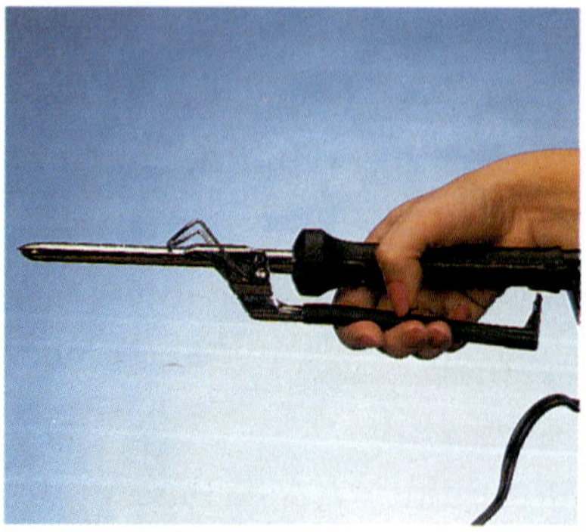

10.23—Full turn.

The method of holding the irons is a matter of personal preference. The technique used should be the one that gives you the greatest ease, comfort, and facility of movement.

Practice in manipulating the curling irons is recommended to develop proficiency in their use. Remember to practice with cold irons. The following four exercises are designed to help achieve an effective use of the irons.

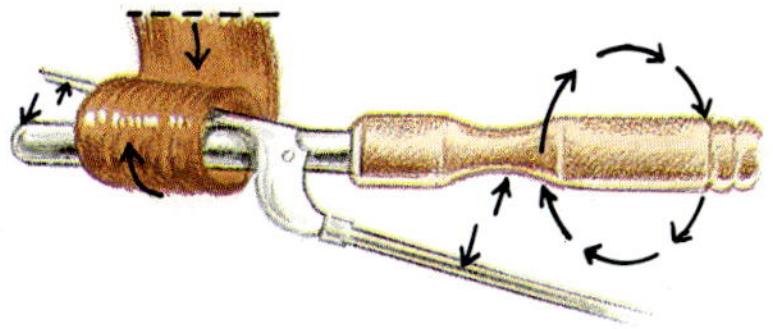

10.24—Rotating movement while opening and closing the irons.

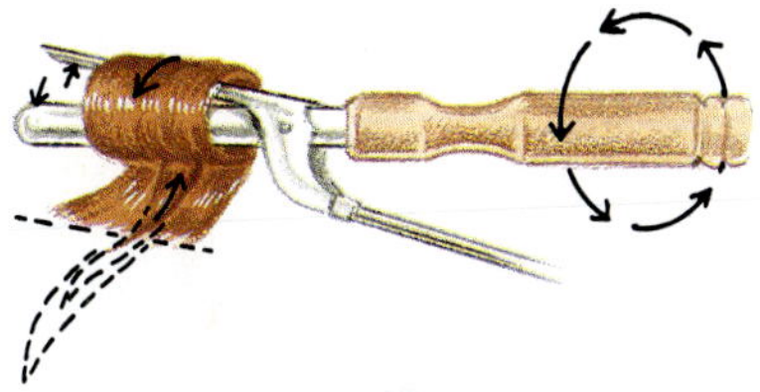

10.25—Guiding the hair strand into the center of the curl while rotating the irons.

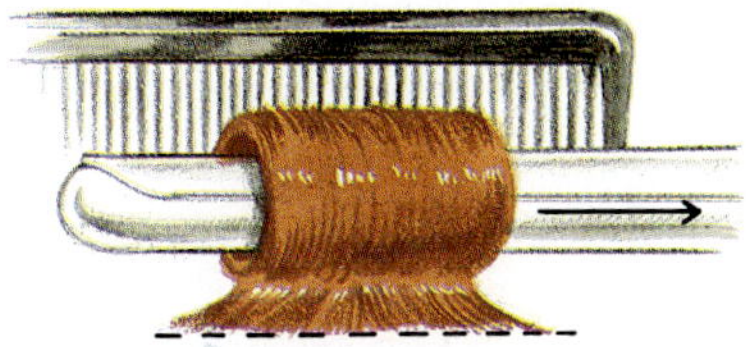

10.26—Removing the curl using comb as guide.

1. Since it is important to develop a smooth rotating movement, practice turning the irons while opening and closing them at regular intervals. Practice rotating the irons in both directions. Examples: downward (toward you) and upward (away from you). (See Fig. 10.24)
2. Practice releasing the hair by opening and closing the irons in a quick, clicking movement.
3. Practice guiding the hair strand into the center of the curl as you rotate the irons. This exercise results in the end of the strand being firmly in the center of the curl. (See Fig. 10.25)
4. Practice removing the curl from the irons by drawing the comb to the left and the rod to the right. (See Fig. 10.26) Use the comb to protect the client's scalp from burns.

THERMAL IRONS CURLING METHODS

Today's thermal irons curling methods have improved over the older techniques. The following methods may be changed or modified to conform with your instructor's procedures.

Preparation

1. Comb the hair thoroughly, removing all tangles.
2. Divide the head into five sections.
   a) First section, about 2½" (6.25 cm) wide, extends from center of forehead to nape of neck.
   b) Divide two side panels in half, from top parting to neck, to provide four additional sections.
3. Heat thermal irons (large or jumbo size).
4. Subdivide sections into ¾" by 2½" (1.875 by 6.25 cm) subsections. (Fig. 10.27) The same procedure is followed for electric irons and stove-heated irons.

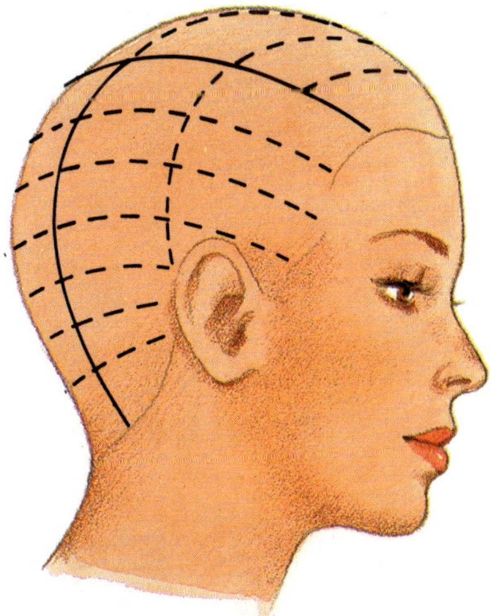

10.27—Hair sectioned and subdivided.

Curling Short Hair

The base of each curl is formed by sectioning and parting to conform with the size of the curl desired. It is important to consider hair length, density, and texture. The base is usually about 1½″ to 2″ (3.75 cm to 5 cm) in width and approximately ½″ (1.25 cm) in depth.

After sectioning off the base, comb the hair smooth and straight out from the scalp. The hair must be combed smooth in order that the heat and tension are the same for all hair in the section. Loose hairs may result in an uneven and ragged curl.

1. After the irons have been heated to the desired temperature, pick up a strand of hair and comb it up and smooth. With the groove on top, insert the irons about 1″ (2.5 cm) from the scalp and hold for a few seconds to form a base. (See Fig. 10.28)
2. Hold the ends of the hair strand with the thumb and two fingers of the left hand, using a medium degree of tension. Turn the irons downward (toward you) with the right hand. (See Fig. 10.29)
3. Open and close the irons rapidly as you turn, to prevent binding. Guide the ends of the strand into the center of the curl as you rotate the irons. (See Fig. 10.30)
4. The result of this procedure will be a smooth, finished curl, with the ends firmly fixed in the center. Remove the irons from the curl. (See Fig. 10.31)

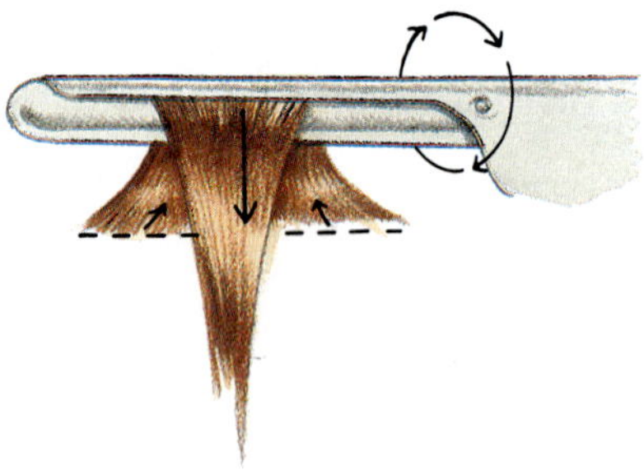

10.28—Form a base.

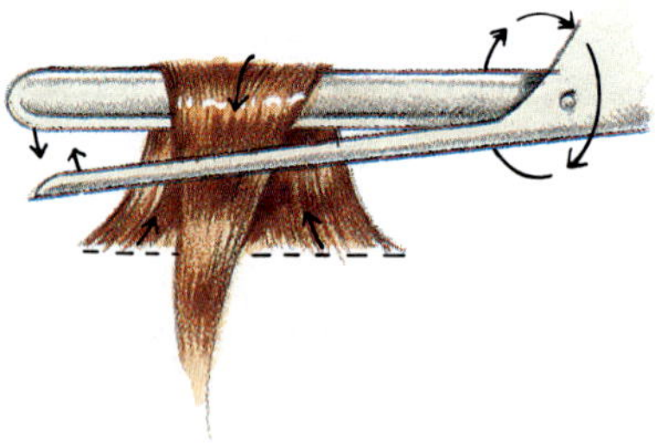

10.29—Turn irons downward.

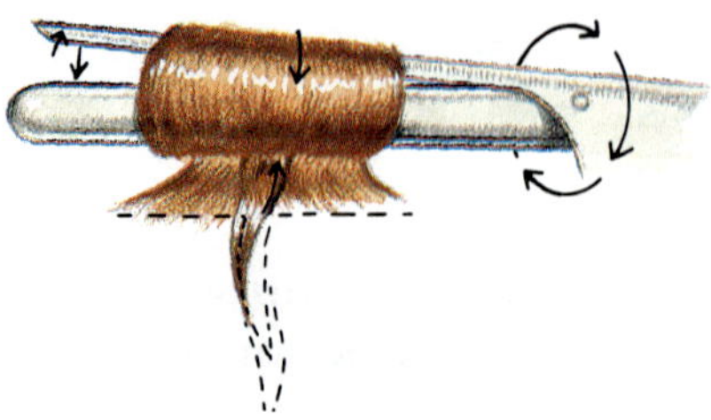

10.30—Rotate irons and guide ends of strand into center.

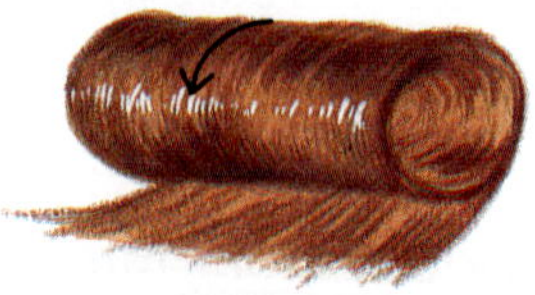

10.31—Finished curl.

Curling Medium Length Hair
(Using One Loop or "Figure 6")

Section and form the base of the curl as described for short hair.

1. Insert the hair into the open irons at the scalp. Pull the hair over the rod in the direction of the curl and close the shell. Hold irons in this position for about 5 seconds to heat the hair, and then slide irons up to 1" (2.5 cm) from the scalp. The shell must be on top. (See Fig. 10.32)
2. Turn irons downward one-half revolution; pull the end of the strand over the rod to the left and direct the strand toward the center of the curl. (See Fig. 10.33)
3. Complete the revolution of the irons, and continue directing the ends toward the center. (See Fig. 10.34)
4. Make another complete revolution of the irons. The entire strand has now been curled with the exception of the ends. Enlarge the curl by opening the shell. Insert the ends of the curl into the opening created between the shell and the rod. (See Fig. 10.35)
5. Close the shell and slide irons toward the handles. This technique will move the ends of the strand into the center of the curl. Rotate irons several times to even out the distribution of the hair in the curl. (See Fig. 10.36)

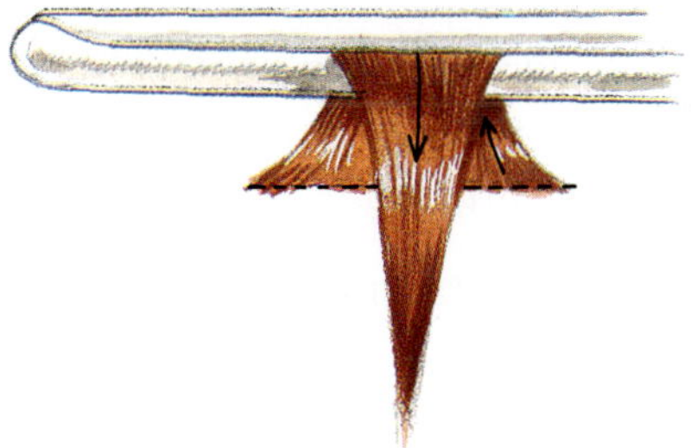

10.32—Insert the hair into open irons at the scalp.

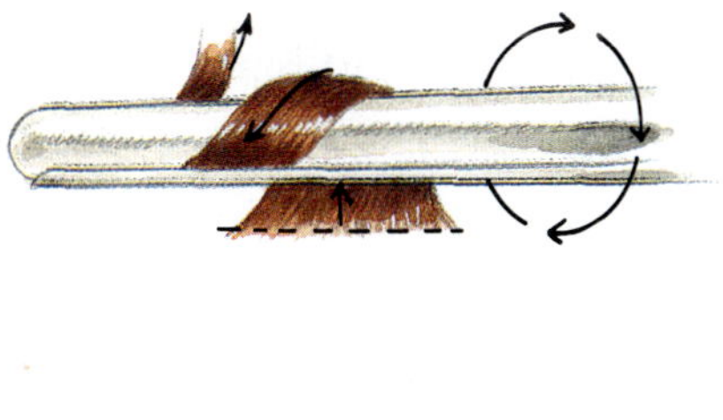

10.33—Turn irons downward one-half revolution.

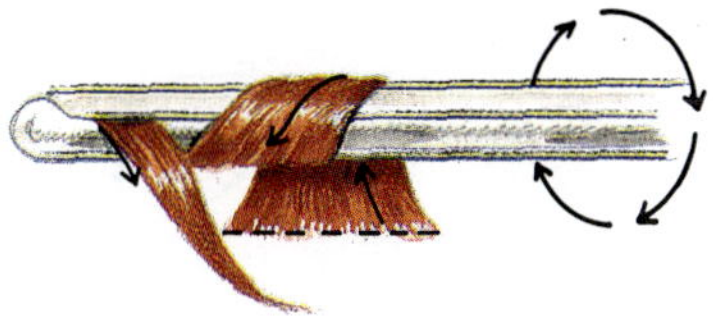

10.34—Complete the revolution of the irons.

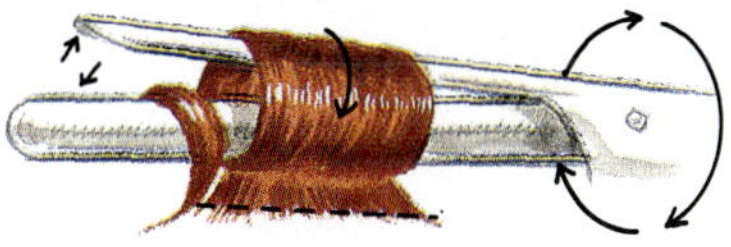

10.35—Make another complete revolution.

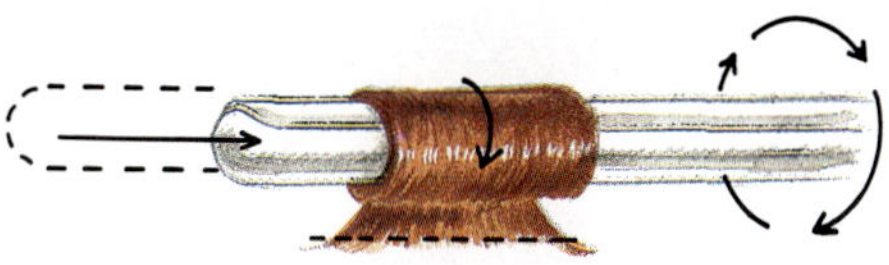

10.36—Close the shell and slide irons toward the handles.

CAUTION
To protect the client during the curling process, use the comb between the scalp and irons.

When the curl is formed and the ends are freed from between the rod and the shell, make one complete revolution of the irons inside the curl. This final revolution smoothes the ends and loosens the hair away from the irons. The comb is then used to help remove the curl from the irons. The irons are drawn slowly in one direction, while the comb draws the hair in the opposite direction. In this way the curl is removed from the irons.

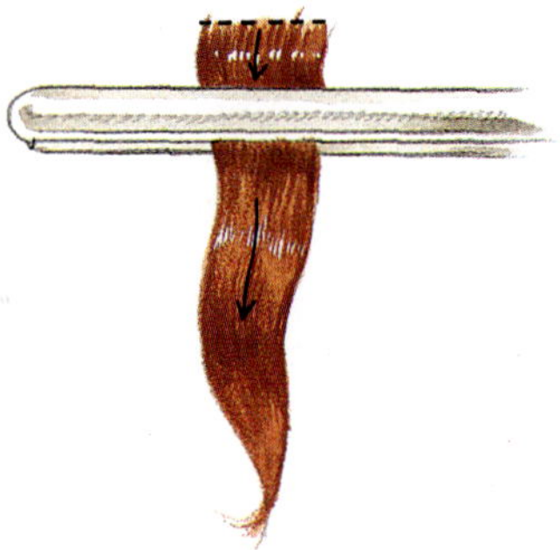

10.37—Insert hair about 1" (2.5 cm) from the scalp.

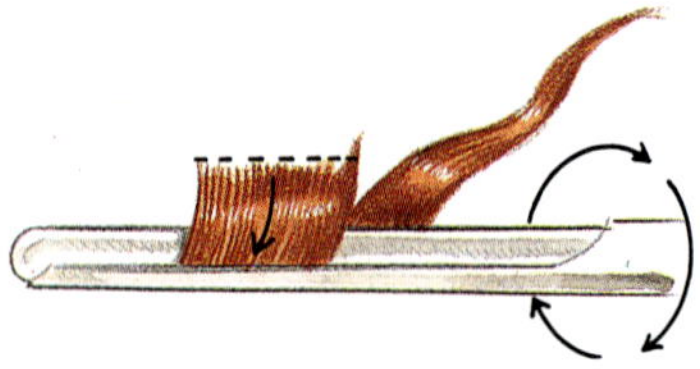

10.38—Roll irons under.

Curling Long Hair

(Using Two Loops or "Figure 8," Croquignole Technique)

Section and form the base of the curl as previously described.

1. Insert the hair into the open irons about 1" (2.5 cm) from the scalp. Pull the hair over the rod in the direction in which the curl is to move and close the shell. Hold irons in this position for about 5 seconds, in order to heat the hair. Hold the strand of hair with a medium degree of tension. (See Fig. 10.37)
2. Roll irons under. Click and roll the irons until the groove is facing you. (See Fig. 10.38)
3. With the left hand, pick up the ends of the hair. (See Fig. 10.39)
4. Continue to roll and click the irons, keeping them the same distance from the scalp. (See Fig. 10.40)
5. Draw the hair strand toward the tip of the irons. (See Fig. 10.41)

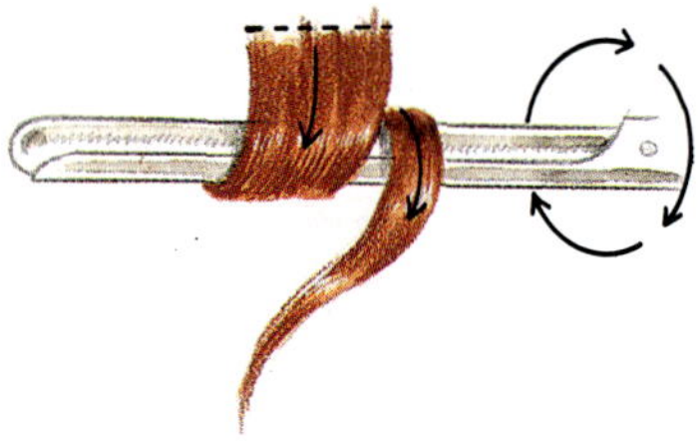

10.39—Pick up the ends of the hair.

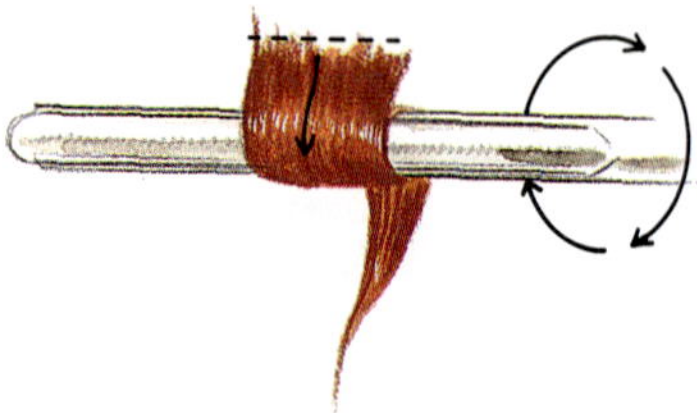

10.40—Continue to roll the irons.

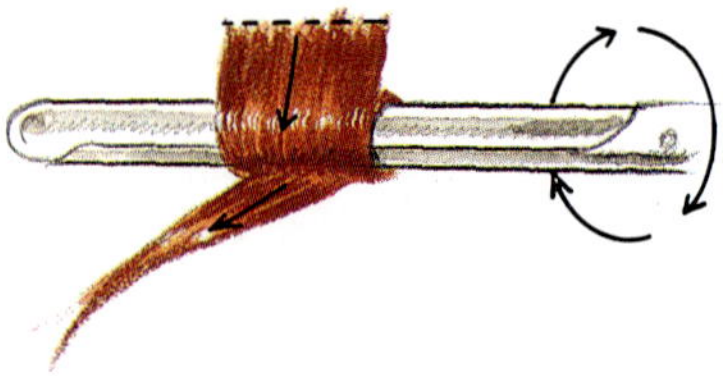

10.41—Draw hair strand toward the point of the irons.

Curling Medium Length Hair
(Using One Loop or "Figure 6")

Section and form the base of the curl as described for short hair.

1. Insert the hair into the open irons at the scalp. Pull the hair over the rod in the direction of the curl and close the shell. Hold irons in this position for about 5 seconds to heat the hair, and then slide irons up to 1" (2.5 cm) from the scalp. The shell must be on top. (See Fig. 10.32)
2. Turn irons downward one-half revolution; pull the end of the strand over the rod to the left and direct the strand toward the center of the curl. (See Fig. 10.33)
3. Complete the revolution of the irons, and continue directing the ends toward the center. (See Fig. 10.34)
4. Make another complete revolution of the irons. The entire strand has now been curled with the exception of the ends. Enlarge the curl by opening the shell. Insert the ends of the curl into the opening created between the shell and the rod. (See Fig. 10.35)
5. Close the shell and slide irons toward the handles. This technique will move the ends of the strand into the center of the curl. Rotate irons several times to even out the distribution of the hair in the curl. (See Fig. 10.36)

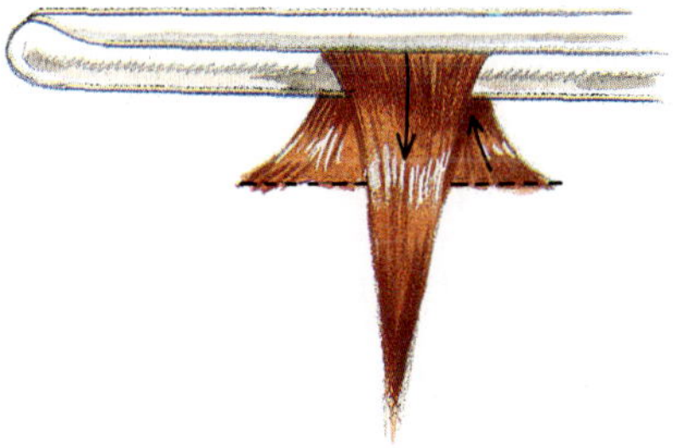

10.32—Insert the hair into open irons at the scalp.

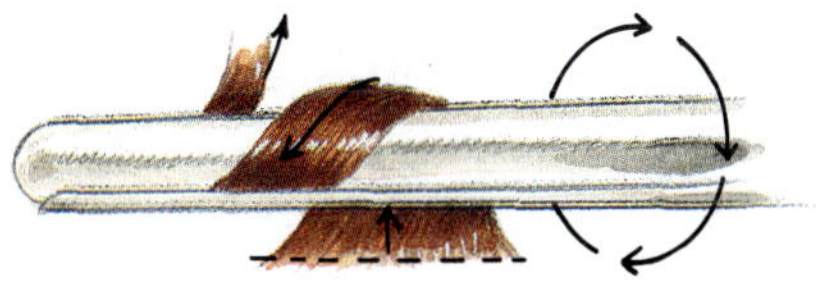

10.33—Turn irons downward one-half revolution.

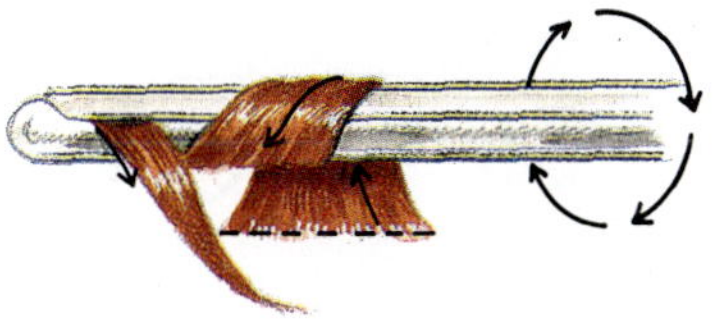

10.34—Complete the revolution of the irons.

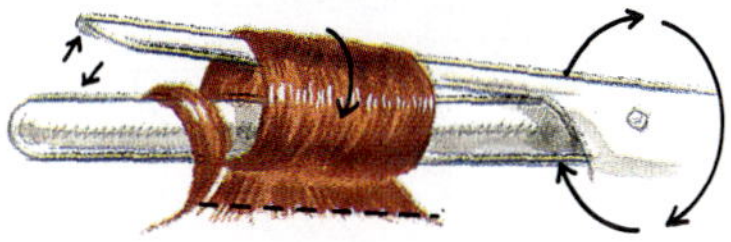

10.35—Make another complete revolution.

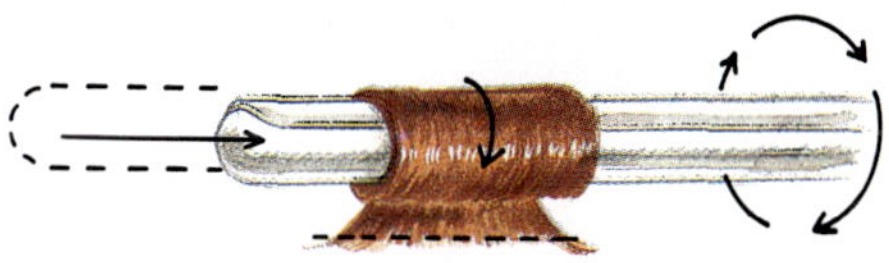

10.36—Close the shell and slide irons toward the handles.

CAUTION

To protect the client during the curling process, use the comb between the scalp and irons.

When the curl is formed and the ends are freed from between the rod and the shell, make one complete revolution of the irons inside the curl. This final revolution smoothes the ends and loosens the hair away from the irons. The comb is then used to help remove the curl from the irons. The irons are drawn slowly in one direction, while the comb draws the hair in the opposite direction. In this way the curl is removed from the irons.

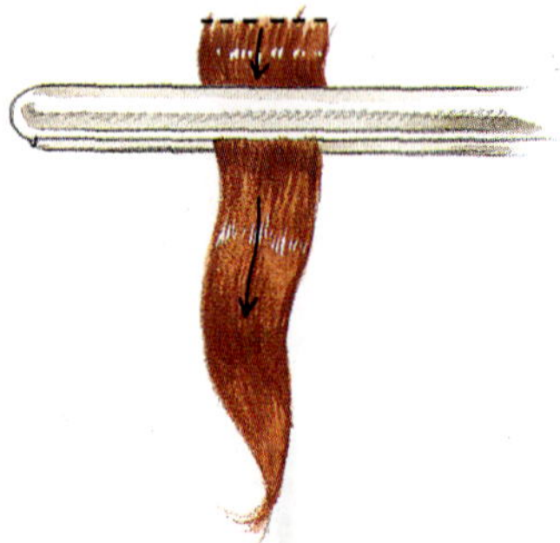

10.37—Insert hair about 1" (2.5 cm) from the scalp.

Curling Long Hair

(Using Two Loops or "Figure 8," Croquignole Technique)

Section and form the base of the curl as previously described.

1. Insert the hair into the open irons about 1" (2.5 cm) from the scalp. Pull the hair over the rod in the direction in which the curl is to move and close the shell. Hold irons in this position for about 5 seconds, in order to heat the hair. Hold the strand of hair with a medium degree of tension. (See Fig. 10.37)
2. Roll irons under. Click and roll the irons until the groove is facing you. (See Fig. 10.38)
3. With the left hand, pick up the ends of the hair. (See Fig. 10.39)
4. Continue to roll and click the irons, keeping them the same distance from the scalp. (See Fig. 10.40)
5. Draw the hair strand toward the tip of the irons. (See Fig. 10.41)

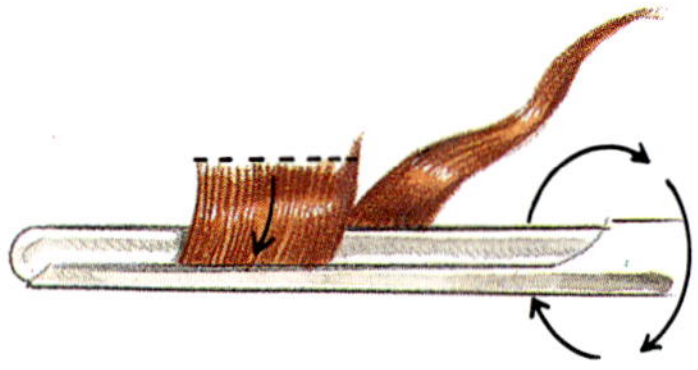

10.38—Roll irons under.

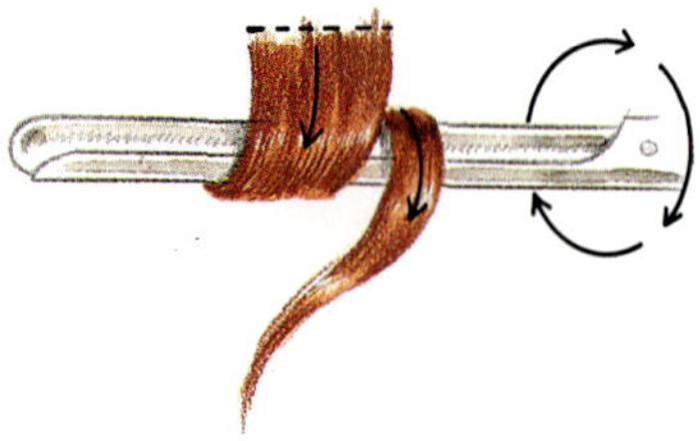

10.39—Pick up the ends of the hair.

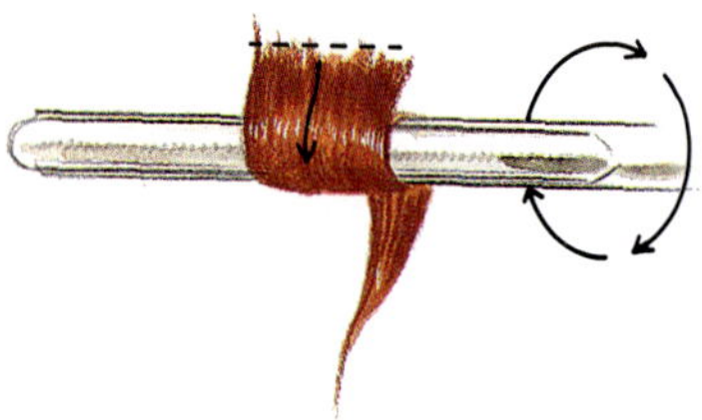

10.40—Continue to roll the irons.

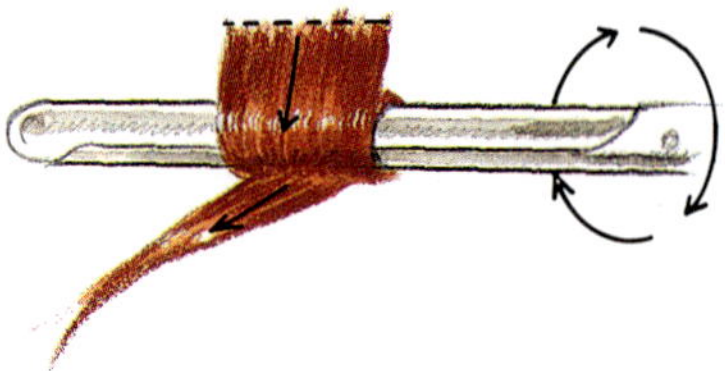

10.41—Draw hair strand toward the point of the irons.

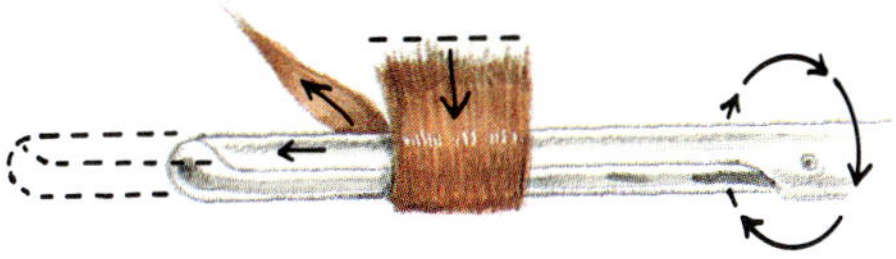

10.42—Draw strand right, push irons left.

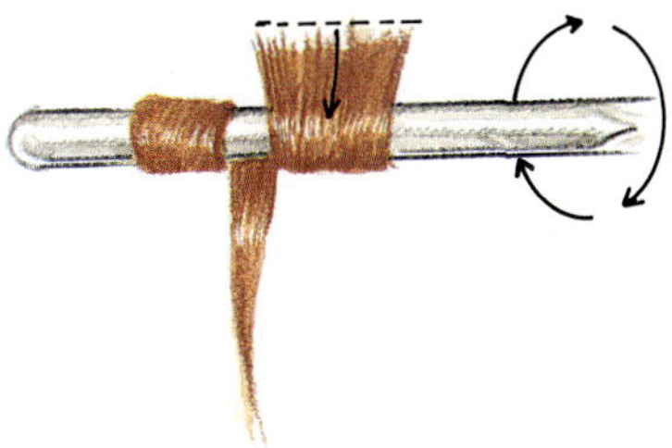

10.43—Form two loops around the closed irons.

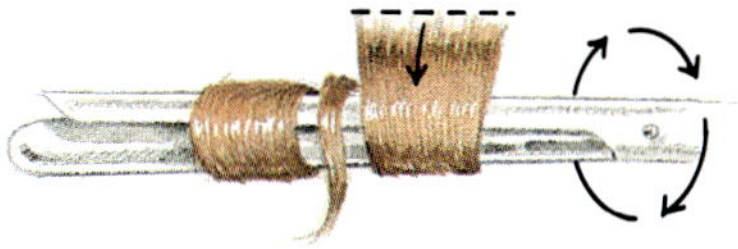

10.44—Roll irons until hair ends disappear.

6. Draw the strand a little to the right, and, at the same time, push the irons slightly to the left. (See Fig. 10.42)
7. By pushing irons forward and pushing the hair with the left hand, you form two loops around the closed irons, with the ends of the strand extending out between the loops. (See Fig. 10.43)
8. Roll under and click irons until the ends of the hair disappear. (See Fig. 10.44)
9. Rotate irons several times to even out the distribution of the hair in the curl and to facilitate the movement of the curl off the irons.

Other Types of Curls

Spiral curls are hanging curls that are suitable for long hairstyles.

Part the hair into as many sections as there will be curls and comb smooth. Insert the irons at an angle, with the bowl (groove) on top near the base of the strand, and rotate irons until all the hair is wound. Hold the curl in this position for 4 to 5 seconds, and remove the irons in the usual manner. (See Figs. 10.45–10.48)

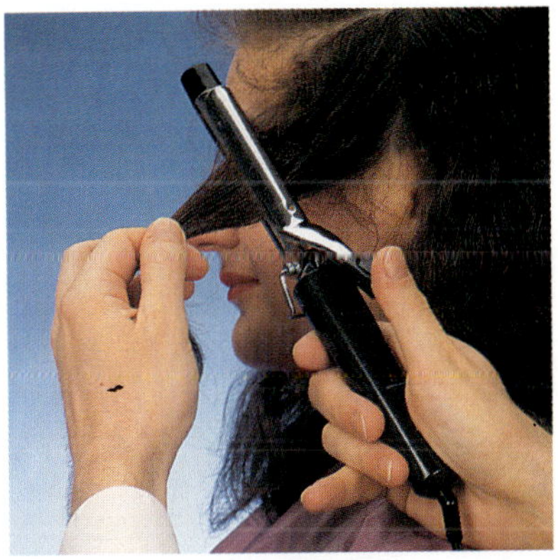

10.45—Insert irons at an angle.

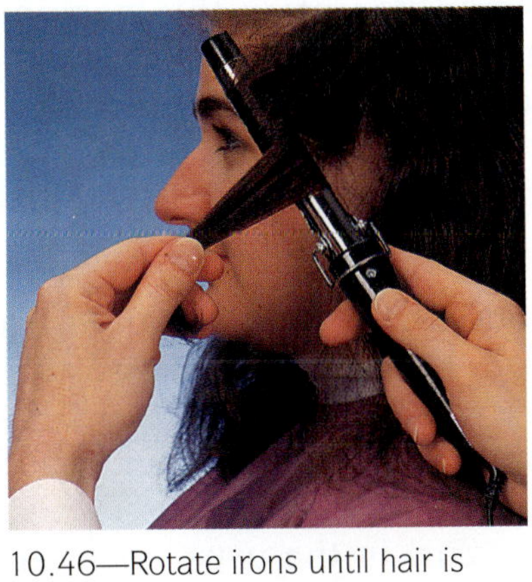

10.46—Rotate irons until hair is wound.

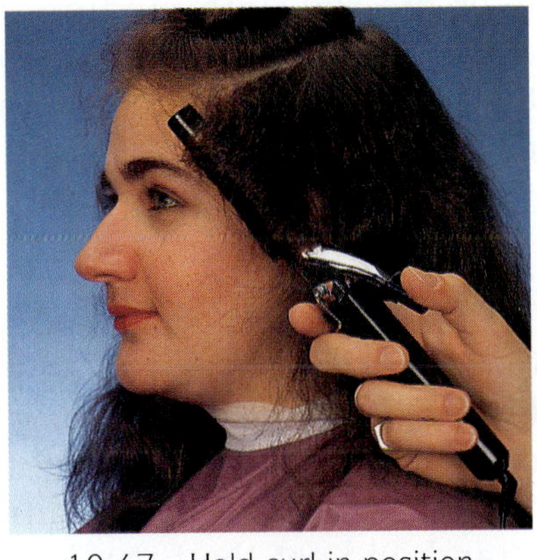

10.47—Hold curl in position.

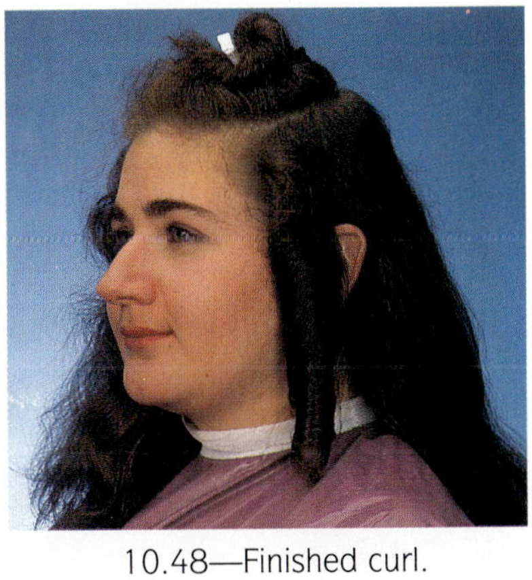

10.48—Finished curl.

End curls can be used to give a finished appearance to hair ends. Long, medium length, or short hair may be styled with end curls. The hair ends can be turned under or over, as desired.

The position of the curling irons and the direction of their movements will determine whether the end curls will turn under or over. (Figs. 10.49, 10.50)

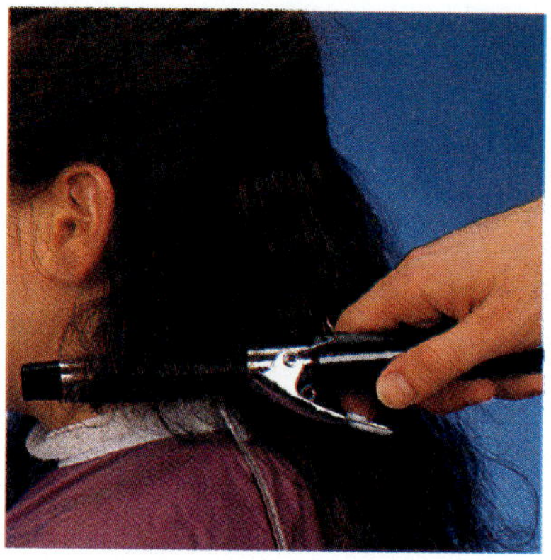

10.49—Turning irons under.

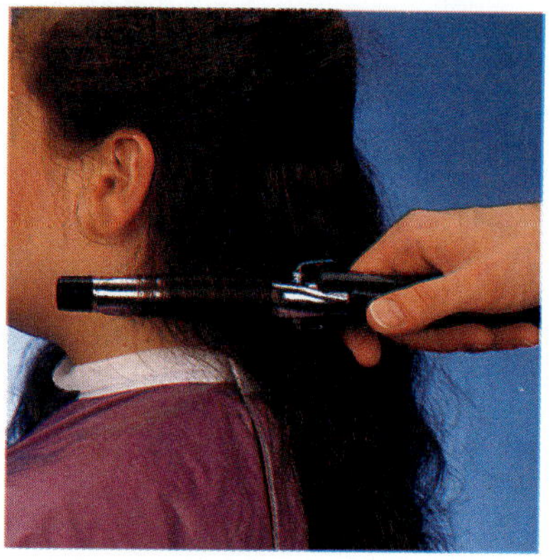

10.50—Turning irons over.

VOLUME THERMAL IRON CURLS

Volume thermal iron curls are used to create volume or lift in a finished hairstyle. The degree of lift desired determines the type of volume curls to be used.

Volume-Base Curls

Volume-base curls provide maximum lift or volume, since the curl is placed very high on its base. Section off the base as described on p. 172. Hold the curl strand at a 135° (2.36 rad.) angle. Slide irons over the strand about ½″ (1.25 cm) from the scalp. Wrap the strand over the rod with medium tension. Maintain this position for approximately 5 seconds to heat the strand and set the base. Roll the curl in the usual manner and firmly place it forward and high on its base.

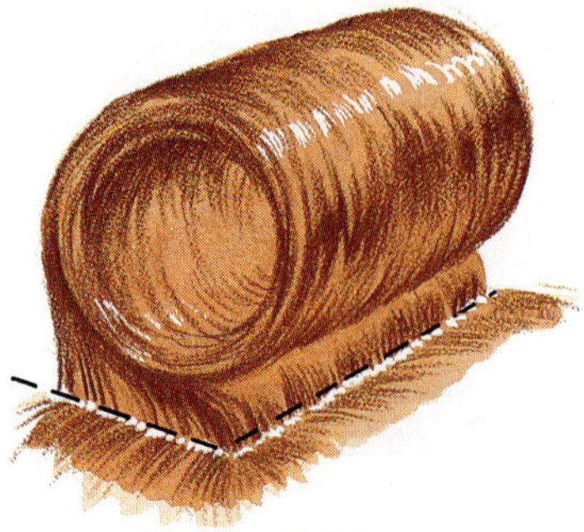

10.51—Full base.

Full-Base Curls

The full-base curl provides a strong curl with full volume. Section off the base as described on p. 172. Hold the hair strand at a 125° (2.18 rad.) angle. Slide irons over the hair strand about ½″ (1.25 cm) from the scalp. Wrap the strand over the rod with medium tension. Maintain this position for about 5 seconds to heat the strand and set the base. Roll the curl in the usual manner, and place it firmly in the center of its base. (Fig. 10.51)

Half-Base Curls

The half-base curl provides a strong curl with moderate lift or volume. Section off the base as described on p. 172. Hold the hair at a 90° (1.57 rad.) angle. Slide irons over the hair strand about ½″ (1.25 cm) from the scalp. Wrap the strand over the rod with medium tension. Maintain this position for about 5 seconds to heat the strand and set the base. Roll the curl in the usual manner, and place it half off its base. (Fig. 10.52)

Off-Base Curls

The off-base curl provides a strong curl with only slight lift or volume. Section off the base as described on p. 172. Hold the hair at a 70° (1.22 rad.) angle. Slide irons over the hair strand about ½″ (1.25 cm) from the scalp. Wrap the strand over the rod with medium tension. Maintain this position for about 5 seconds to heat the strand and set the base. Roll the curl in the usual manner, and place it completely off its base. (Fig. 10.53)

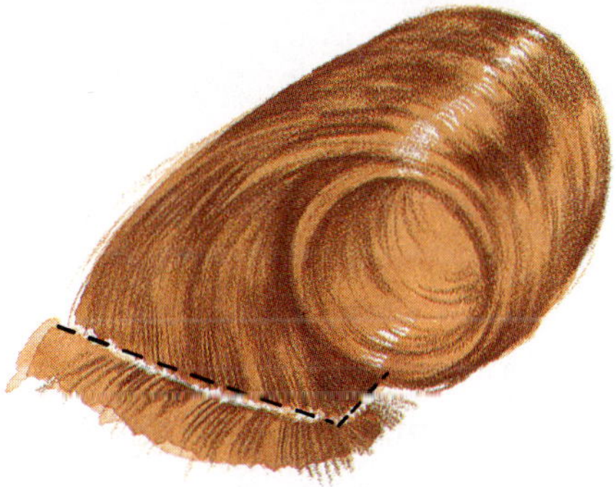

10.52—One-half off base.

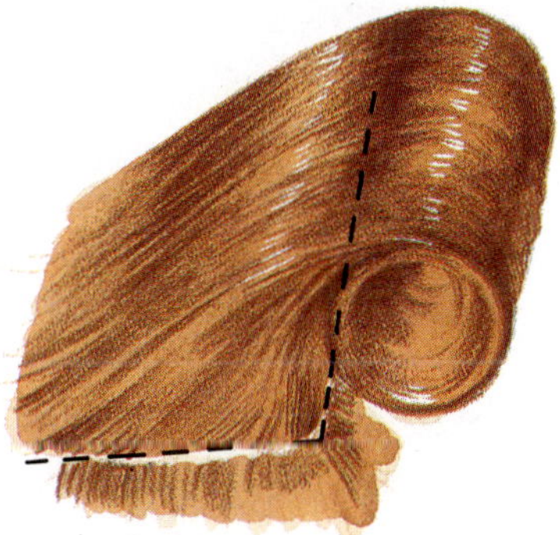

10.53—Off base.

FINISHED THERMAL CURL SETTINGS

For best results when giving a thermal setting, clip each curl in place until the whole head is complete and ready for styling. (Figs. 10.54–10.56)

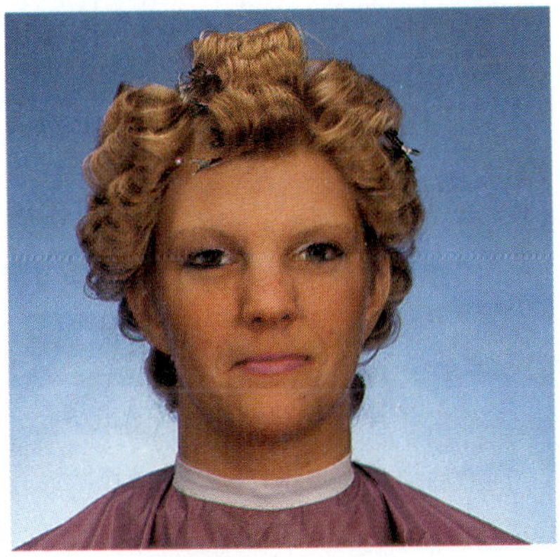

10.54—Front view completely curled.

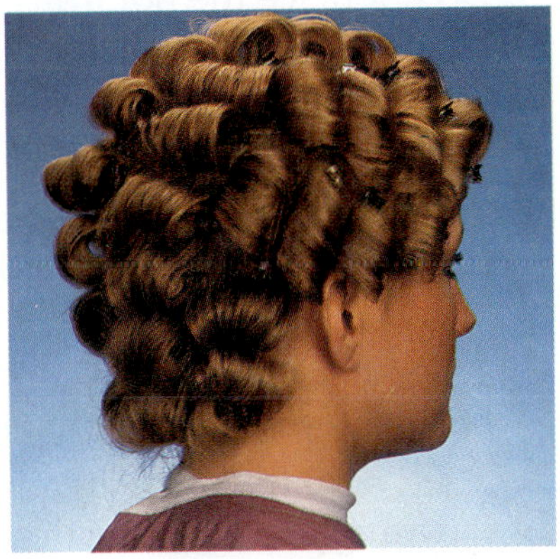

10.55—Side view.

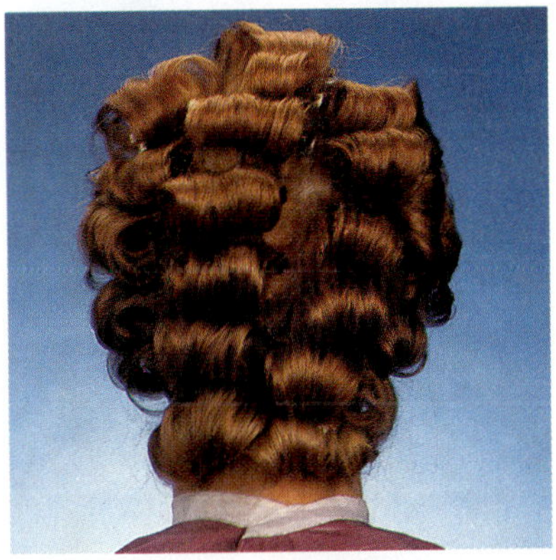

10.56—Back of head completely curled.

✔ Completed—Learning Objective No. 2

THERMAL WAVE TECHNIQUES AND IMPLEMENTS

STYLING THE HAIR AFTER A THERMAL CURL OR WAVE

After thermal waving or curling, style the hair according to the client's wishes. Brush the hair, working up from the neckline; push the waves and curls into place as you progress over the entire head. If the hairstyle is to be finished with curls, do the bottom curls last. (Figs. 10.57–10.60) ✔

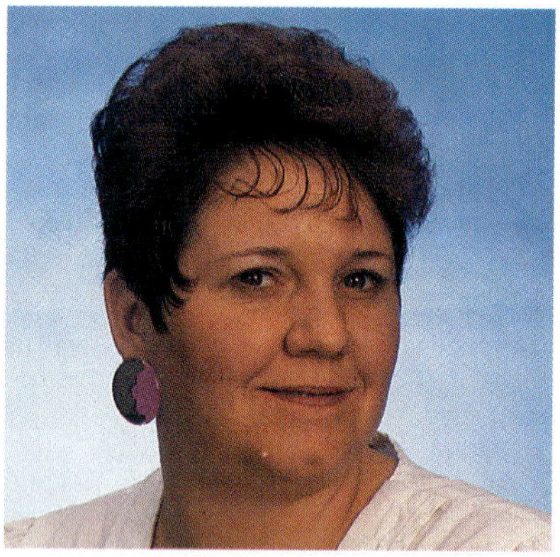

10.57—Finished thermal style for short hair.

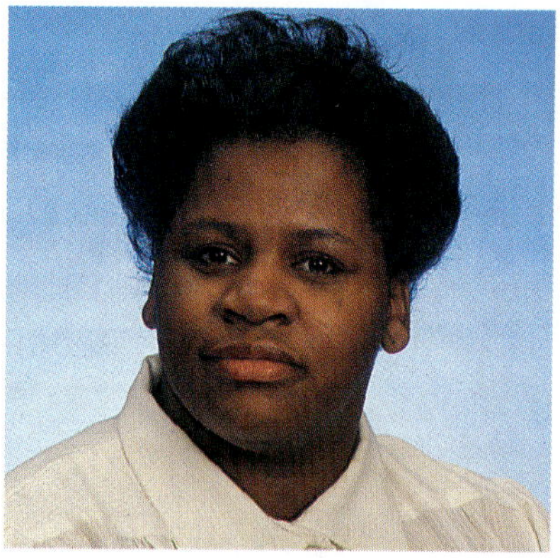

10.58—Finished thermal style for short hair.

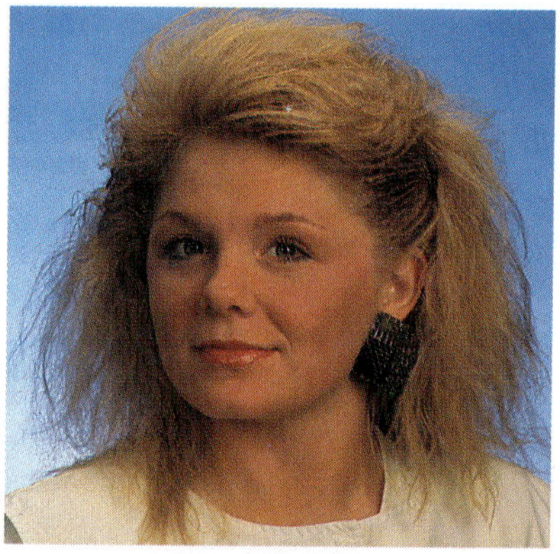

10.59—Finished thermal style for medium length hair.

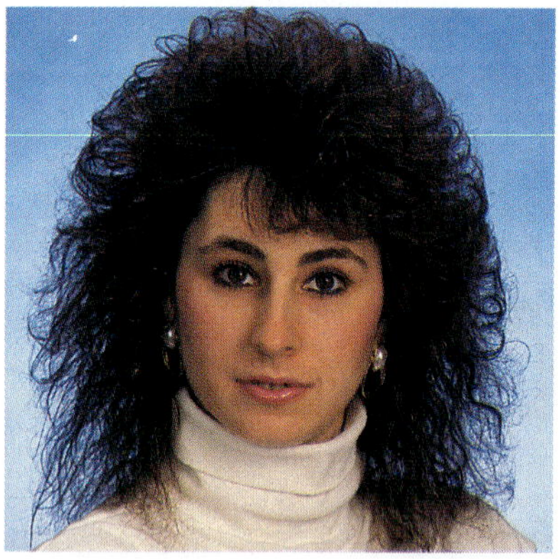

10.60—Finished thermal style for long hair.

SAFETY MEASURES

1. Keep thermal irons clean and the joint oiled.
2. Use thermal irons only after receiving instruction in their use.
3. Do not overheat the irons, because this can cause the metal to lose its temper.
4. Test the temperature of the irons on tissue paper before placing them on the hair. This will prevent the hair from being burned. Do not inhale the fumes of the irons because they are injurious to the lungs.
5. Do not place the hot irons near the face to test for temperature; a burn of the face can result.
6. Handle thermal irons carefully to avoid burning yourself or the client.
7. Place hot irons in a safe place to cool. Do not leave them where someone might accidentally come in contact with them and be burned.
8. When heating the irons, do not place handles too close to the heater. Your hand might be burned when removing the irons.
9. Make sure the irons are properly balanced in the heater, or they might fall and be damaged or injure someone.
10. Use only hard rubber or nonflammable combs. Celluloid combs must not be used in thermal curling; they are flammable.

11. Do not use metal combs; they can become hot and burn the scalp.
12. Do not use combs with broken teeth. They can break or split the hair or injure the scalp.
13. Place comb between scalp and thermal irons when curling or waving hair to prevent burning the scalp.
14. The client's hair must be clean to ensure a good thermal curl or wave.
15. If the hair is thick and bulky, thin and taper it first.
16. Never use hot pressing or thermal irons on lightened or tinted hair.
17. Do not allow the hair ends to protrude over the irons; to do so will cause fishhooks (hair that is bent or folded).
18. A first aid kit must be available in case of an accident.
19. Do not use vaporizing thermal irons on pressed hair because the hair will revert to its original overly curly state.
20. Do not use thermal irons on chemically straightened hair because they might cause damage to the hair. ✔

✔ Completed—Learning Objective No. 3

SAFETY MEASURES FOR THERMAL WAVING

Question & Answer

BLOW-DRYING LONG HAIR

Q *Drying and styling hair using a blow-dryer is considered a "quick service," yet it takes me twice as long to style the hair of some of my clients who have long hair. What can I do?*

A Towel the hair thoroughly to remove as much moisture as possible. Use your fingers to separate the hair and further dry it.

Then start at the back and throw the hair forward. First use your fingers and hand to direct the hair as the hot air is blown from back to front. When about 50 percent of the moisture has been removed start using a vent brush to direct the hair.

Only when 90 percent of the moisture has been removed (this happens rather quickly) start bringing the hair down at the nape, drying each section thoroughly before letting down the next section. Work from the nape up the back, over the crown and toward the forehead.

Finally use a round brush to shape the ends of the hair. Spin the brush through the ends, direct the warm air onto the brush, and repeat until the ends are dry and formed. Allow the hair to cool, then while the client leans forward spray the underneath sections with styling/volumizing hair spray. Work the hair back down with your fingers while you shake the form into place. All this takes very little time if you "pre-dry" the hair as suggested.

—*From* Milady's Salon Solutions *by Louise Cotter*

BLOW-DRY STYLING

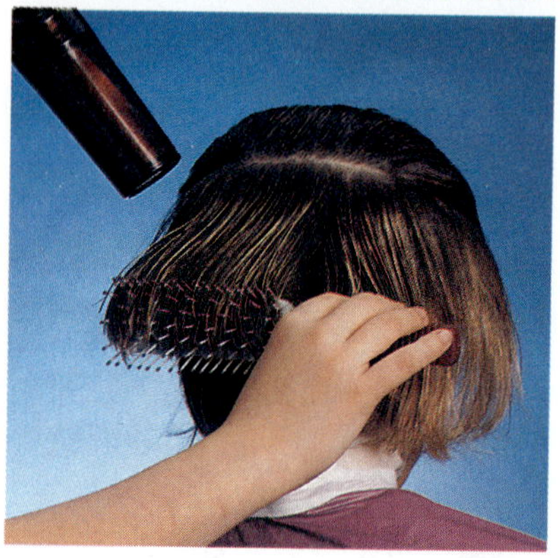

10.61—Blow-dry curling with a brush.

✔ Completed—Learning Objective No. 4

DEFINITION OF BLOW-DRY STYLING

Blow-dry styling, often referred to as a "quick salon service," is the technique of drying and styling damp hair in one operation. This technique creates the basic structure of hairstyles without time-consuming setting, drying, and combing out. It helps to develop soft, natural hairstyles with free-flowing effects. These effects can also be achieved with the use of rollers and curls. (Fig. 10.61)

There are two basic techniques used in blow-dry styling:

1. Blow-dry curling with a brush.
2. Blow-dry waving with a comb.

This section covers these two basic techniques. Many other techniques can be developed with experience and advanced training. ✔

◆ NOTE: Take special care when blow-drying curled hair that is chemically treated or damaged. This type of hair has loss of elasticity; therefore, towel-dry the hair first to remove excess moisture.

EQUIPMENT, IMPLEMENTS, AND MATERIALS

The following equipment, implements, and materials are required for blow-dry styling:

Blow-dryer (with or without attachments)
Combs (hard rubber or metal)
Shampoo
Styling lotions, gels, mousse
Conditioner
Hair spray

THE BLOW-DRYER

The blow-dryer (without attachments) is an electrical device especially designed for drying and styling the hair in a single operation. Its main parts are a handle, slotted nozzle, small fan, heating element, and controls. When in operation it produces a steady stream of temperature-controlled air. The various controls permit you to make necessary heat adjustments when operating the blow-dryer. (Fig. 10.62)

COMBS AND BRUSHES

Both hard rubber combs and those made of metal are used for blow waving and air waving. Some stylists prefer to use metal combs, since they retain and transmit heat better. With metal combs the hair can be re-styled in the shortest possible time.

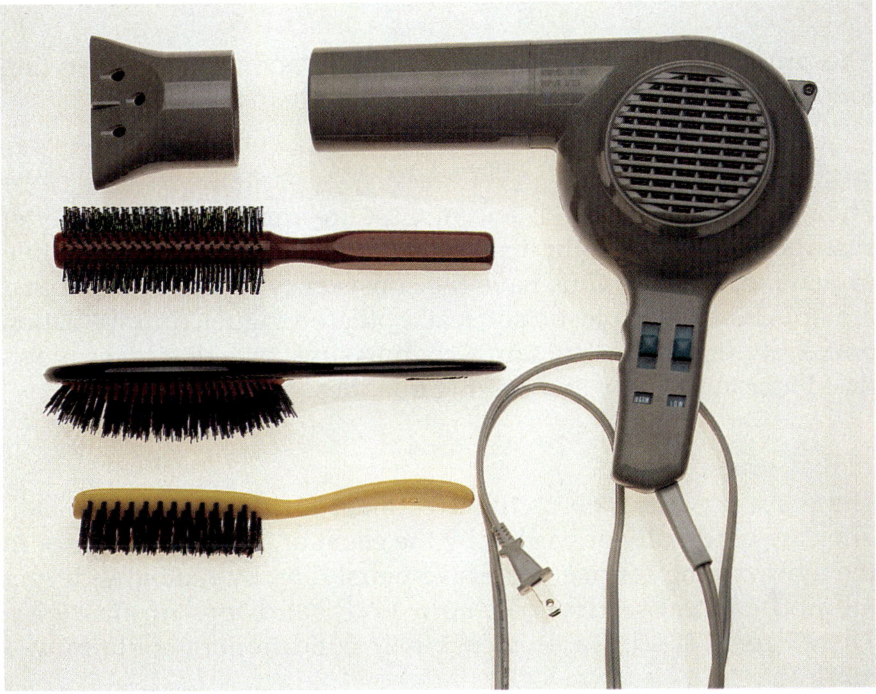

10.62—Implements for blow-dryer styling—from top to bottom: blow-dryer; large round brush; wide rounded-shoulder brush; narrow rounded-shoulder brush.

Combs are available with coarse teeth, half coarse and half fine teeth, and all fine teeth.

Special narrow synthetic bristle brushes are used in blow-dry styling. It is often easier for the stylist to brush the hair into the desired style with a narrow brush. The smaller the diameter of the brush, the tighter the curl, with better staying qualities. (Fig. 10.63)

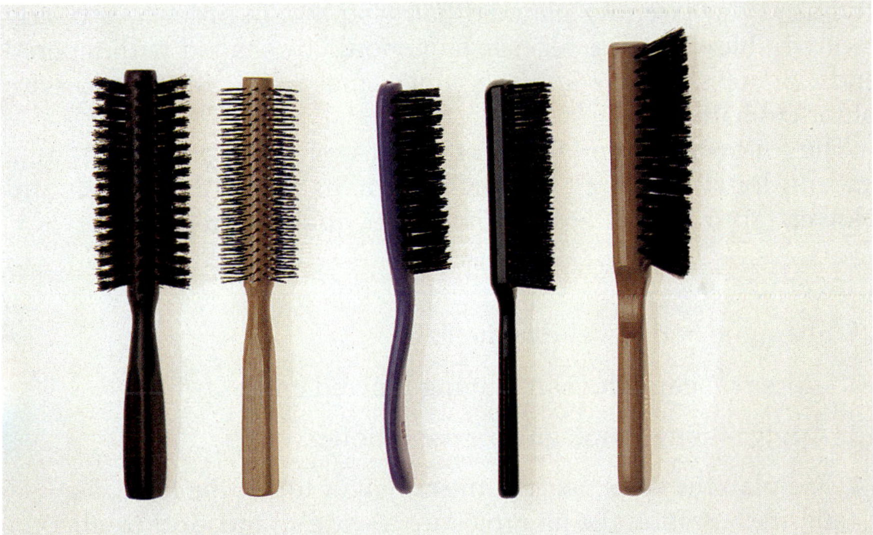

10.63—Brushes used in blow-dry styling.

COSMETICS USED IN BLOW-DRY STYLING

The principal cosmetics used in blow-dry styling include styling lotions, hair and scalp conditioners, and hair sprays.

Styling Lotions

Styling lotions such as gels and mousse are applied to the hair after shampooing to make the hair more manageable for blow curling or waving. These lotions have the consistency of dense liquid and are applied with a plastic squeeze bottle or trigger (pump) action bottle. Styling lotions contain a coating substance that gives blow-dried hair more body and staying qualities.

Hair Conditioners

These are used as a corrective treatment for dry and brittle hair. They are used daily or weekly by the client or immediately prior to the blow-drying service. Excessive hairstyling by the blow-drying method can cause dryness, split ends, and loss of elasticity. Therefore, it is advisable to use hair conditioners containing a lubricant.

Hair Sprays

These are applied to the hair to keep the finished hairstyle in place.

Be guided by the manufacturer's directions or by your instructor as to the proper usage of cosmetics on the client's hair and scalp.

BLOW CURLING WITH ROUND BRUSH

Blow curling is most successful on hair that is naturally curly or has received a permanent wave. The basis for all successful blow styling is the carefully planned hair shaping. In order to properly receive a blow-curling service, hair should be shaped with tapered ends. Successful blow curling is extremely difficult on hair with blunt-cut hair ends.

The following technique is offered as one method of creating a natural-looking, easy-to-wear, informal style with a brush and blower. (Your instructor's methods are equally correct.)

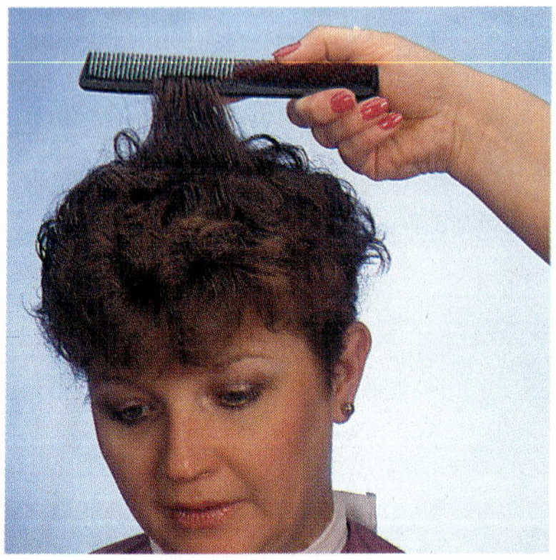

10.64—Section a wide strand and comb through.

Procedure

1. Shampoo and towel-dry the hair.
2. Properly shape the hair leaving tapered ends.
3. Apply styling lotion and/or conditioner.
4. Pre-plan the style. Start at the crown or top of the head, as desired. Section the hair, pick up a wide strand, and comb through. (See Fig. 10.64)

5. Bring the comb out to the hair ends and insert the brush. Brush through the strand, bringing the brush out to the ends.
6. Roll the hair with the brush, making a complete downward turn, away from the face, until the brush rests on the scalp. Maintain this position and start the blower. Direct the blower very slowly through the curl in a back-and-forth movement. (See Fig. 10.65) When the hair section is completely dry, release the brush with a rounded movement. Use clippies to secure each curl as it is completed and to hold it in place until it is cooled off.
7. Continue making curls in the same manner across the crown and back of the head. Clip each curl as completed.
8. Shape the neckline curls with a comb, or make pin curls on the nape for a finished, close-to-the-head look.

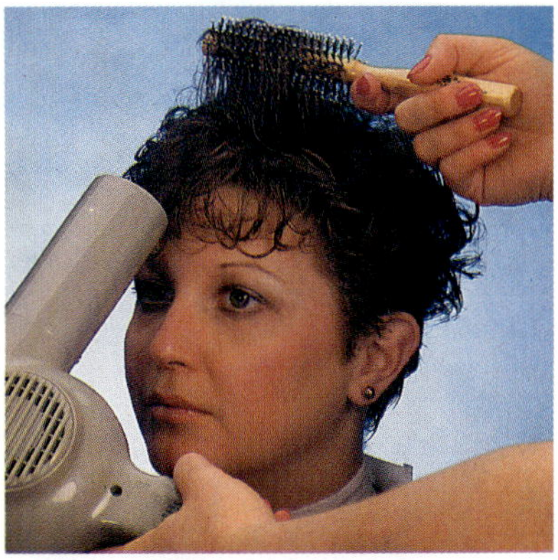

10.65—Roll the hair with brush and direct blower through the curl.

REMINDERS AND HINTS ON BLOW-DRY STYLING

In order to achieve the best results from blow-dry styling, the hair should be in good condition. Permanently waved, chemically relaxed, tinted, or lightened hair should be partially towel dried before being blow curled or waved. (The hair stretches easily and could be damaged if very wet.) The hair should be shaped with tapered ends for successful blow curling or waving.

Styling lotion or mousse is important in blow waving and curling. Comb the hair thoroughly to spread the styling lotion evenly.

BLOW-DRYING THE HAIR

Hot air is directed straight onto the head only for rough drying. For successful blow-dry styling the air should be directed from the scalp area to the hair ends. (Fig. 10.66) The flow of air is directed to the top half of the brush in a back-and-forth movement. This method acts to deflect the hot air, reduce its heat, and dry the hair nearest the scalp.

Never hold the blower too long in one place. The blower should be directed so that the hot air flows in the same direction as the hair is wound. To avoid severe scalp burns, always direct the hot air away from the client's scalp. The hair must be thoroughly cooled before it is combed out. This can be accomplished by switching the dryer to cold and cooling the hair that has been dried.

In blow styling it is essential that when the hairstyle is completed the scalp should be thoroughly dry. The hairstyle will not hold if the scalp is damp.

Complete the blow-dry styling with a light application of hair spray to give shine and holding power to the hair.

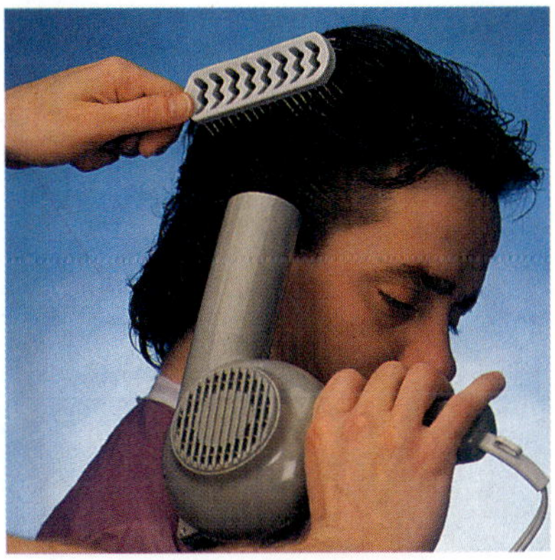

10.66—Direct air from the scalp to hair ends.

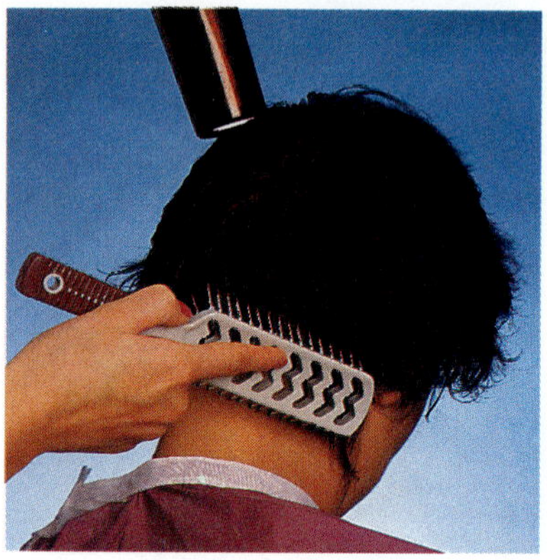

10.67—Blow-drying with a vent brush.

BRUSHES AND COMBS

The actual styling is performed with the brush or comb. The blow-dryer is an implement used for quickly drying the hair while the hair is being styled. The size of the styling brush used is determined by the style and length of the hair. As a general rule, short hair is styled with a small diameter or vent brush. (Fig. 10.67) For medium or longer hair, best results are achieved with large diameter or vent brushes. To avoid scalp burns, keep heated metal combs away from the scalp.

BLOW-DRYER

Make sure that the blow-dryer is perfectly clean and free of dirt, grease, hair, etc., before using. Dirt or hair can cause extreme heat and burn hair. The air intake at the back of the dryer must be kept clear at all times. If this intake is covered and air cannot pass through freely, the dryer element might burn out.

✔ Completed—Learning Objective No. 5

BLOW-DRY STYLING IMPLEMENTS, TECHNIQUES AND COSMETICS

BLOW-DRYING TECHNIQUES

To give the crown hair a slight lift, a vent brush is used. This vent or open-back brush allows air from the dryer to pass through it easily. The dryer is kept on the move from side to side along the curl. Secure each curl with clippies as it is completed. (See Fig. 10.68)

To create a pageboy effect, curl hair under with a brush and blow-dry. (See Fig. 10.69)

To create a smooth top with flip, the hair ends are lifted by placing a brush close to the scalp. Rotate the brush. As the brush rotates, the hot air is directed to the base within the cupped area. ✔

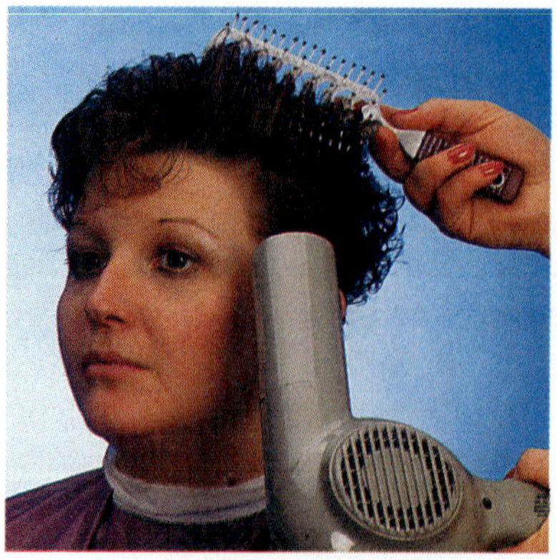

10.68—Crown hair lift.

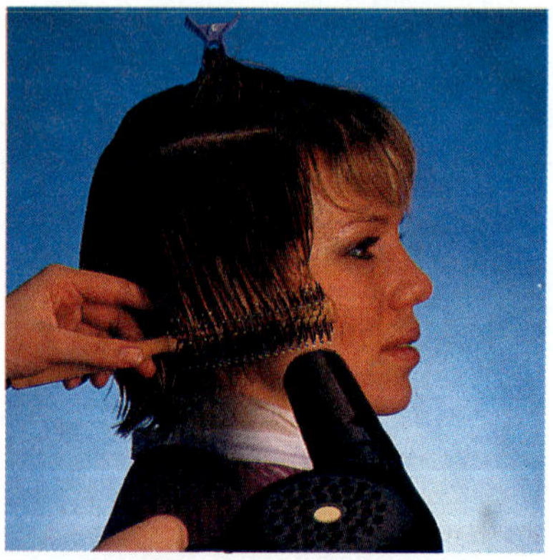

10.69—Pageboy effect.

AIR WAVING

Another technique used to create attractive hairstyles without preliminary setting and drying of the hair is by the use of the electric air waver comb and styling comb. This technique is the same as finger waving, except that you use an electric air waver comb and styling comb. (Fig. 10.70) ✔

✔ Completed—Learning Objective No. 6

DEFINITION OF AIR WAVING

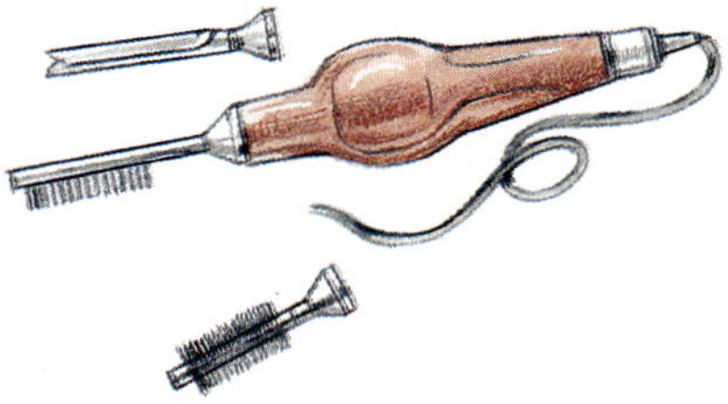

10.70—Air waver with comb attachment.

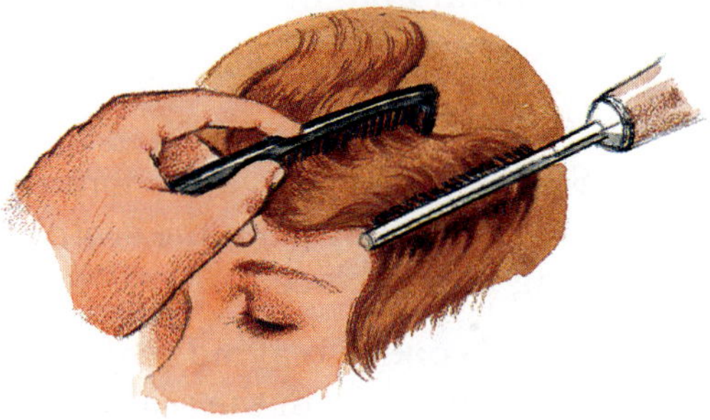

10.71—Comb hair in direction of wave desired.

The hair is styled after it has been shaped, shampooed, and towel dried. It is important to locate the natural wave formation in the hair. Comb the hair in the direction of the wave desired. This will help to establish the natural hair growth pattern. Comb the hair in the direction of the planned hairstyle. Comb the hair with the air waver until it is dry enough to hold a wave.

To achieve ridges and waves on various parts of the head, the hair must be slightly damp. Apply a light spray of styling lotion to assist in creating the desired hairstyle. Comb the hair in the desired direction. (See Fig. 10.71)

SHAPING HAIR WITH COMB

1. ***Left side part.*** Starting at the front section of the head, insert the styling comb into the hair about 1½″ (3.75 cm) from the part. Draw the styling comb toward the back. Insert the air waver under the comb and draw the air waver comb toward the face to form a ridge. Hold both combs in this position until a firm ridge has been formed. (See Fig. 10.72) Continue toward the crown until the entire length of the ridge is completed.

   Form the second ridge by starting at the crown and work toward the front. The ridge and shaping is made in reverse of the first ridge. (See Fig. 10.73) Support the completed ridgeline with the styling comb while the air waver comb lifts and designs the pattern.
2. ***Right side part.*** The procedure is exactly the same as for the left side part. The only exception is that the hand comb is held in the right hand and the air waver is controlled by the left hand. However, the waving should start at the crown and work forward toward the face.

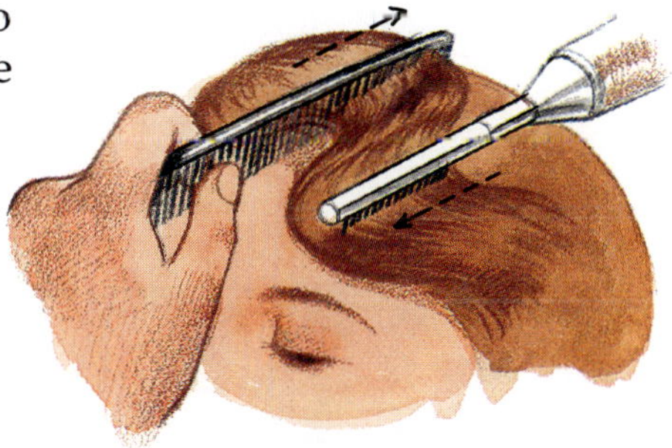

10.72—Form ridge.

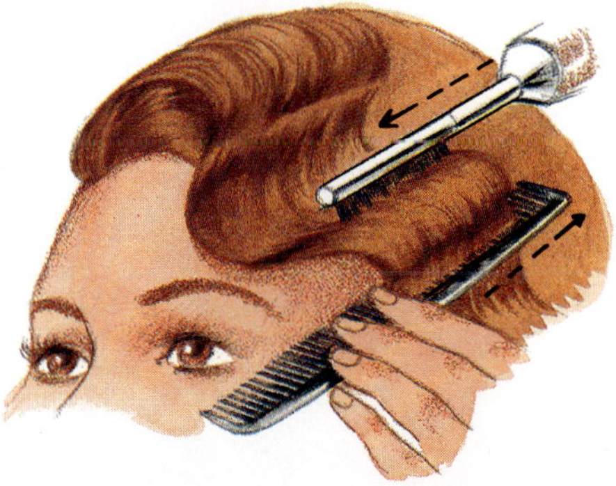

10.73—Form second ridge.

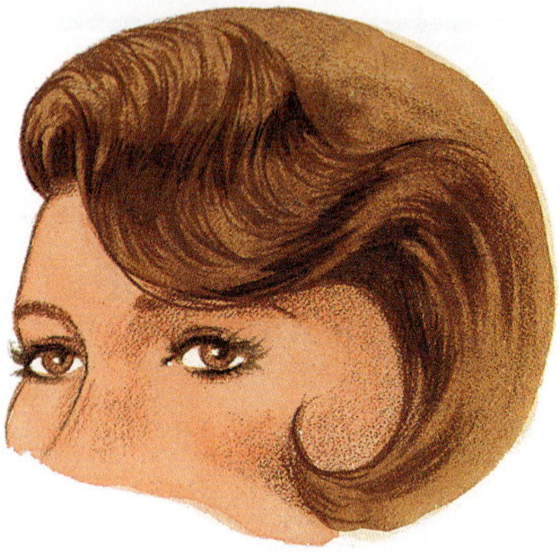

10.74—Finished style.

A finished wave is formed with the air waver comb and styling comb, taking advantage of the natural waving pattern of the hair. (See Fig. 10.74)

The air waver comb, when used in conjunction with the curling iron, presents many styling opportunities to the stylist. The number of styles and patterns that can be created with these implements working in harmony is limited only by the skill and imagination of the stylist.

SAFETY PRECAUTIONS

1. ***Styling dryer.*** Move moderately hot air back and forth on the hair and away from the scalp. Avoid holding the dryer too long in one place.
2. ***Metal comb.*** To avoid scalp burns, keep teeth of a heated metal comb away from the scalp.
3. ***In all blow-dry styling*** it is important that when the curling or waving is completed the scalp must be thoroughly dry. If the ends and the curls are dry but the scalp is damp, the hairstyle will not hold. ✔

✔ Completed—Learning Objective No. 7

AIR WAVING IMPLEMENTS AND TECHNIQUES

REVIEW QUESTIONS

THERMAL HAIRSTYLING

1. Define thermal waving or curling.
2. List the three types of irons used in thermal waving.
3. To avoid burning the scalp, what procedure should you follow?
4. Define blow-dry styling.
5. List the implements used in blow-dry styling.
6. What cosmetics are used in blow-dry styling?

PERMANENT WAVING

11

LEARNING OBJECTIVES

AFTER COMPLETING THIS CHAPTER, YOU SHOULD BE ABLE TO:

1. Define permanent waving.
2. Identify the chemistry of products used in permanent waving.
3. Describe the relationship between hair structure, perm chemistry, and perming techniques.
4. Demonstrate a client consultation and hair analysis.
5. Demonstrate proper rod selection and sectioning, parting, and wrapping procedures.
6. List safety precautions required for permanent waving.
7. Demonstrate proper perming procedures.

INTRODUCTION

Permanent waving (perming) is one of the most practical and lucrative techniques you will learn in cosmetology school. You'll use basic perming skills throughout your career as a salon stylist. The ability to create a beautiful perm style will bring you professional satisfaction and help build a loyal following of satisfied clients. A properly completed perm provides many valuable benefits to both the client and stylist:

1. Long-lasting style retention.
2. Easy manageability for the client when styling at home.
3. Additional volume and fullness for styling soft, fine hair textures.
4. Greater control in styling hair that is naturally coarse, wiry, and hard to manage.

HISTORY OF PERMANENT WAVING

Attempts to wave and curl straight hair date back to early civilization. Egyptian and Roman women were known to apply a mixture of soil and water to their hair, wrap it on crudely made wooden rollers, and then bake it in the sun. The results, of course, were not permanent.

THE MACHINE AGE OF PERMANENT WAVING

In 1905 Charles Nessler invented a heavily wired machine that supplied electrical current to metal rods around which hair strands were wrapped. These heavy units were heated during the perming process. They were kept from touching the scalp by a complex system of counterbalancing weights, suspended from an overhead chandelier mounted on a stand. (Fig. 11.1)

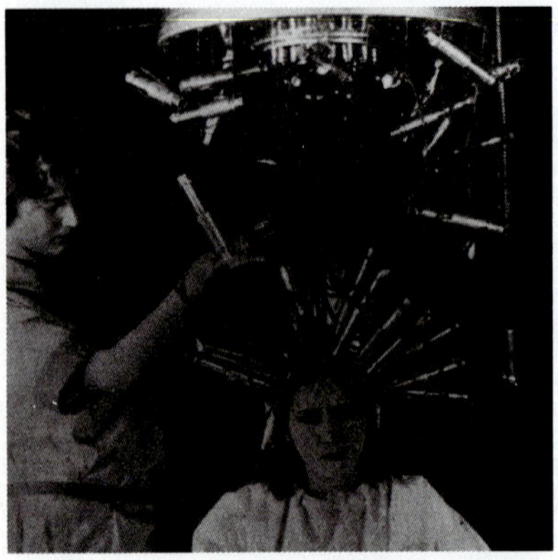

11.1—Machine permanent wave.

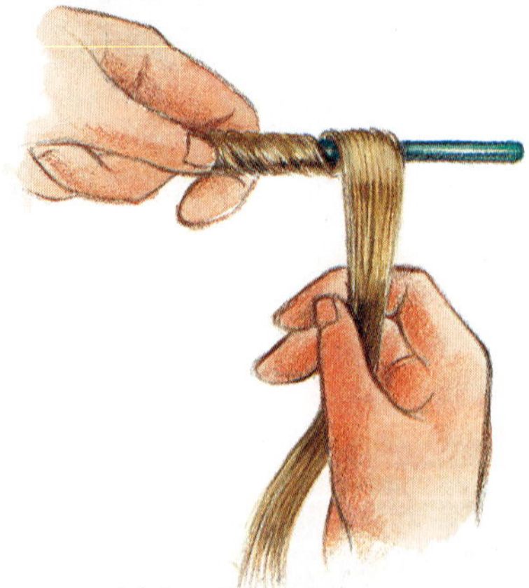

11.2—Spiral flat wave.

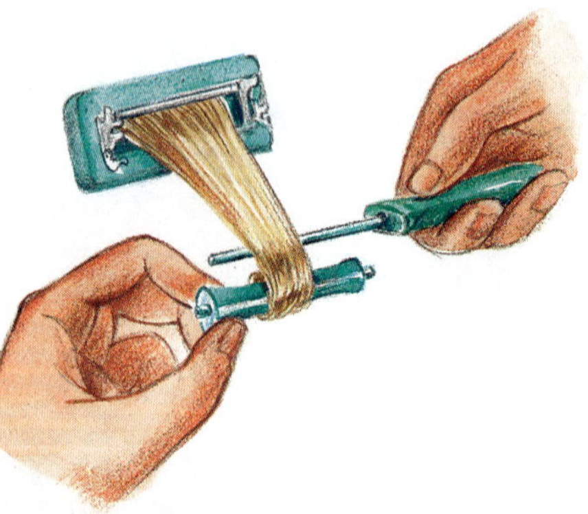

11.3—Croquignole wrap.

Two methods were used to wind hair strands around the metal units. Long hair was wound from the scalp to the ends, a technique called ***spiral wrapping.*** (Fig. 11.2) After World War I when many women cut their hair into the short bobbed style, the ***croquignole*** (**KROH**-ki-nohl) ***wrapping*** technique was introduced. Using this method, shorter hair was wound from the ends toward the scalp. The hair was then styled into deep waves with loose end curls. (Fig. 11.3)

The client's fear of being "tied" to an electrical contraption with the possibility of receiving a shock or burn led to the development of alternative methods of waving hair. In 1931, the ***pre-heat*** method of perming was introduced. Hair was wrapped using the croquignole method, and then clamps, pre-heated by a separate electrical unit, were placed over the wound curls.

THE FIRST MACHINELESS PERM

An alternative to the machine perm was introduced in 1932 when chemists Ralph L. Evans and Everett G. McDonough pioneered a method that used external heat generated by chemical reaction. Small, flexible pads containing a chemical mixture were wound around hair strands. When the pads were moistened with water, a chemical heat was released that created long-lasting curls. Thus, the first machineless permanent wave was born. Salon clients no longer were subjected to the dangers and discomforts of the Nessler machine.

COLD WAVES

In 1941 scientists discovered another method of permanent waving. They developed the waving **lotion**, a liquid that softens and expands the hair strand. After the waving lotion has done its work, another lotion called a **neutralizer** is applied. The neutralizer hardens and shrinks that hair strand, allowing it to conform to the shape of the rod around which the hair is wrapped. It also stops the action of the waving lotion.

Because this perm does not use heat, it is called a "cold wave." Cold waves replaced virtually all predecessors and competitors, and cold waving and permanent waving became almost synonymous terms. Modern versions of cold waves, usually referred to as alkaline perms, are still very popular today.

◆ NOTE: The word "perm" is now popularly used to indicate permanent waving with either an alkaline or acid-balanced solution.

NEUTRAL AND ACID-BALANCED PERMS

For many years, manufacturers sought to develop a permanent wave solution that would minimize hair damage and permit hair that had been damaged by lightening or tinting services to receive

✔ Completed—Learning Objective No. 1

DEFINITION OF PERMANENT WAVING

a perm. To achieve these goals, they developed a waving lotion that was not as highly alkaline as earlier lotions.

Neutral and acid-balanced permanent wave solutions with pH levels ranging from 4.5 to 7.9 were introduced in 1970. They did not contain strong alkalines and therefore were less damaging to the hair. Acid-balanced lotions were, however, slow to penetrate (to pass into or through; to enter by overcoming resistance) hair, and processing time was longer. To overcome this problem, the client is placed under a heated hood dryer to shorten the processing time. ✔

MODERN PERM CHEMISTRY

Perm chemistry is constantly being refined and improved. Perms are available today in many different formulas for a wide variety of hair types. Waving lotions and neutralizers for both acid-balanced and alkaline perms are being formulated with new conditioners, proteins, and natural ingredients that help protect and condition the hair during and after perming.

Stop action processing is incorporated in many waving lotions to ensure optimum curl development. The curling takes place within a fixed time without the risk of overprocessing or damaging the hair. Special prewrapping lotions have also been developed to compensate for hair that is not equally porous all over.

Virtually all permanent waves are achieved with a two-step chemical process:

1. Waving lotion, which softens or breaks the internal structure of the hair.
2. Neutralizer, which rehardens or rebonds the internal structure of the hair.

ALKALINE PERMS

The main active ingredient or ***reducing agent*** in alkaline perms, ***ammonium thioglycolate*** (a-**MOHN**-nee-um theye-oh-**GLEYE**-coh-layt), is a chemical compound made up of ammonia and thioglycolic acid. The pH of alkaline waving lotions generally falls within the range of 8.2 to 9.6, depending on the amount of ammonia. Because the lotion is more alkaline, the cuticle layers swell slightly and open, allowing the solution to penetrate more quickly than acid-balanced lotions. Some alkaline perms are wrapped with waving lotion, others with water. Some require a plastic cap for processing, others do not. Therefore, it is extremely important to read the perm directions carefully before beginning.

The benefits of alkaline perms are:

- Strong curl patterns (lotion wrapped alkaline perms are usually stronger than perms that are water wrapped).

- Fast processing time (varies from 5 minutes to 20 minutes).
- Room temperature processing.

Generally, alkaline perms should be used when:

- Perming resistant hair.
- A strong/tight curl is desired.
- The client has a history of early curl relaxation.

ACID-BALANCED PERMS

The main active ingredient in acid-balanced waving lotions is ***glyceryl monothioglycolate***, which effectively reduces the pH. This lower pH is gentler on the hair and typically gives a softer curl than alkaline cold waves. Acid-balanced perms have a pH range of approximately 4.5 to 6.5 and usually penetrate the hair more slowly. Thus, they require a longer processing time and heat for curl development. Heat is used in one of two ways:

1. The perm is activated by heat created chemically within the product. This method is called ***exothermic***.
2. The perm is activated by an outside heat source, usually a conventional hood-type hair dryer. This method is called ***endothermic.***

Recent advances in acid-balanced perm chemistry, however, have made it possible to process some acid-balanced perms at room temperature without heat. These newer acid-balanced perms usually have a slightly higher pH but still contain glyceryl monothioglycolate as the active ingredient.

All acid balanced perms are water wrapped, require a plastic cap, and may or may not require a pre-heated hood dryer for processing. Read the manufacturer's perm directions carefully before starting the perm.

The benefits of acid-balanced perms are:

- Softer curl patterns
- Slower, but more controllable processing time (usually 15 to 25 minutes)
- Gentler treatment for delicate hair types

Generally, acid-balanced perms should be used when:

- Perming delicate/fragile or color-treated hair.
- Soft, natural curl or wave pattern is desired.
- Style support, rather than strong curl, is required.

THE CHEMISTRY OF NEUTRALIZERS

Neutralizers for both acid-balanced and alkaline perms have the same important function: to permanently establish the new curl shape. Neutralizing is a very important step in the perming process. If the hair is not properly neutralized, the curl will relax or straighten within one to two shampooings. Generally, today's neutralizers are composed of a relatively small percentage of hydrogen peroxide, an oxidizing agent, at an acidic pH. As with waving lotions, there are slightly different procedures recommended for individual products. To achieve the best possible results, read the directions carefully. ✔

✔ Completed—Learning Objective No. 2

THE CHEMISTRY OF PERMANENT WAVING PRODUCTS

HAIR STRUCTURE AND PERMING

Whether using an acid-balanced or alkaline formula, all perms subject the hair to two different actions:

1. Physical action—wrapping sections of hair around a perm rod.
2. Chemical action—created first by a reducing agent (waving lotion) and second by an oxidizing agent (neutralizer).

Since both of these actions work together to create a change in the internal structure of the hair, it is important to understand the composition of hair and how it is affected during perming.

PHYSICAL STRUCTURE OF HAIR

Each strand of hair is structurally subdivided into three major components: (Fig. 11.4)

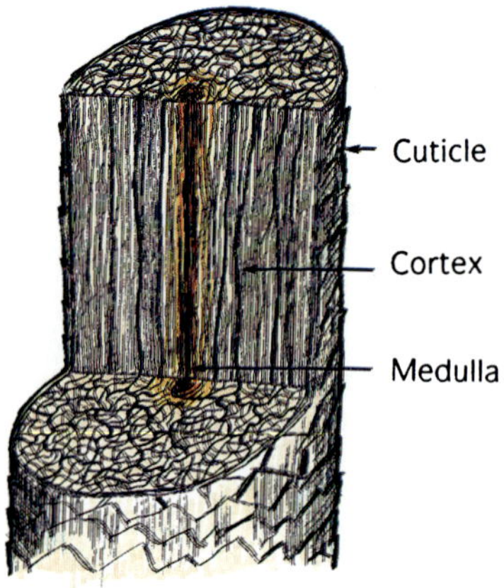

11.4—Structure of a hair.

1. The ***cuticle*** or outer covering consists of seven or more overlapping layers. Although it comprises a small percentage of the total weight of hair, the cuticle possesses unique structural properties that protect the hair. During perming, the waving lotion raises the cuticle layers and allows the active ingredients to enter the cortex.
2. The ***cortex***, the major component of the hair structure, accounts for up to 90% of its total weight. The cortex gives hair its flexibility, elasticity, strength, resilience, and color. It is in the cortex that the physical and chemical actions take place during the perming process to restructure the hair into a new curl configuration.
3. The ***medulla*** is the innermost section of the hair structure. The function of the medulla, if any, is unknown. In fact, it is not at all unusual for an otherwise normal, healthy hair to be without a medulla.

CHEMICAL COMPOSITION OF HAIR

The chemical composition of hair consists almost entirely of a protein material called ***keratin*** (**KER**-a-tin), which is made up of approximately nineteen amino acids. When many amino acids are bonded together, they form a ***polypeptide*** (pol-ee-**PEP**-teyed) ***chain***. These chains intertwine around each other in a spiral fashion to assume a helical shape very similar to a spring. Hair contains a high concentration of the amino acid ***cysteine*** (**SIS**-teen), which is joined together crosswise with ***disulfide*** (deye-**SUL**-feyed) linkages or bonds. Disulfide bonds add strength to the keratin protein, and it is these bonds that must be broken down to allow the perming process to occur.

Processing. The chemical action of a waving lotion breaks the disulfide bonds and softens the hair. When the chemical action softens the inner structure of the hair enough, it can mold to the shape of the rod around which it is wound. (Fig. 11.5a–c)

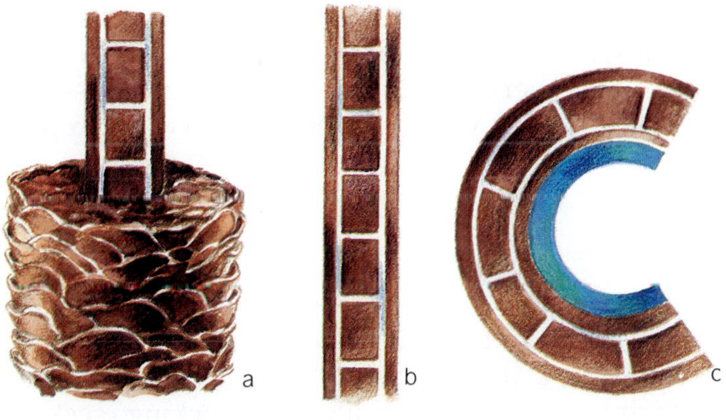

11.5a—Each hair strand is composed of many polypeptide chains. This series of illustrations shows the behavior of one such chain.

11.5b—Hair before processing. Chemical bonds (links) give hair its strength and firmness.

11.5c—Hair wound on rod. The hair bends to the curvature and size of the rod.

Neutralizing. When the hair has assumed the desired shape, the broken disulfide bonds must be chemically rebonded. Neutralizing rehardens the hair and fixes it into its new curl form. When the neutralizing action is completed, the hair is unwrapped from the rods, and you have a new curl formation. (Fig. 11.6a, b)

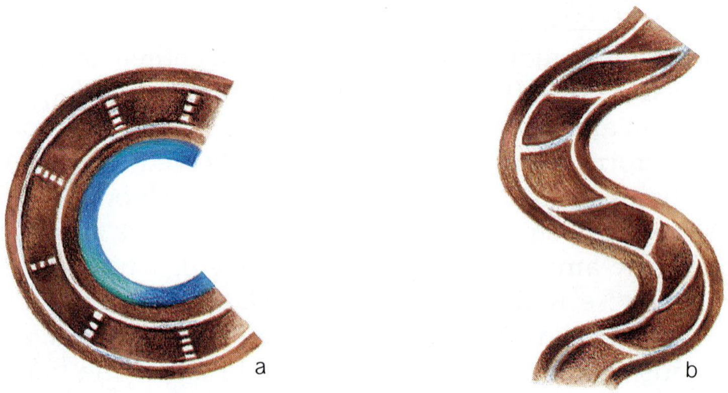

✔ Completed—Learning Objective No. 3

HAIR STRUCTURE AND PERMING

11.6a—During processing, waving lotion breaks the chemical cross-bonds (links), permitting the hair to adjust to the curvature of the rod while in this softened condition.

11.6b—The neutralizer re-forms the chemical bonds (links) to conform with the wound position of the hair, and rehardens the hair, thus creating the permanent wave. ✔

CHOOSING THE RIGHT PERMING TECHNIQUE

How do you decide which perming technique is right for your client? You must be able to evaluate and analyze your client's hair. You must consult with your client to establish what the person expects to accomplish with a perm—a tight, curly look or a loose, wavy look. This information helps you to select the correct perm product and technique.

Basic Manual Perming Skills

Successful perming requires manual dexterity. With practice, your skills in handling and manipulating hair will improve. Before actually applying a perm, you will probably spend considerable time practicing pre-perming skills like blocking, sectioning, and wrapping. Your ability to give successful perms depends on mastering these important skills.

Client Consultation

Every perm client has a different expectation for how he or she wants the perm to look. The only way to meet your client's expectations is to determine what those expectations are. Talk to your client in a friendly but professional way. Take a few minutes to discuss:

1. What hairstyle and how much curl your client wants. Photos or magazine pictures help to make this clearly understood by both of you.
2. Your client's lifestyle. Does he or she have leisure time, or a demanding schedule that requires a low-maintenance style?

3. How your client's hairstyle relates to overall personal image. Is your client concerned about current fashion trends?
4. Your client's previous experience with perming. What did he or she like or dislike about past perm services?

Once you learn what questions to ask and how to ask them, the consultation with your perm client takes only a few minutes. It is time well-spent, however, because the consultation helps establish your credibility as a professional. It inspires your client's confidence in your technical and creative abilities, and makes the perming experience more satisfactory for both of you.

Keep the vital information you learn during the client consultation as a written permanent record, along with other important data, including the client's address, home, and business phone numbers. A release form should also be filled out by the client. It releases the school or salon owner from responsibility for accidents or damages and is required for some malpractice insurance. A sample release is shown in the hair coloring chapter. Here is an example of an organized format for maintaining client records:

PERMANENT WAVE RECORD

Name .... Tel. ....

Address .... City .... State ....

DESCRIPTION OF HAIR Zip ....

Length	**Texture**	**Type**	**Porosity**	
☐ short	☐ coarse	☐ normal	☐ very porous	☐ slightly porous
☐ medium	☐ medium	☐ resistant	☐ moderately porous	☐ resistant
☐ long	☐ fine	☐ tinted	☐ normal	
		☐ highlighted		
		☐ bleached		

Condition

☐ very good ☐ good ☐ fair ☐ poor ☐ dry ☐ oily

Tinted with ....

Previously permed with ....

TYPE OF PERM

☐ alkaline ☐ acid ☐ body wave ☐ other ....

No. of rods .... Lotion .... Strength ....

Results

☐ good ☐ poor ☐ too tight ☐ too loose

Date	Perm Used	Stylist	Date	Perm Used	Stylist
....	....	....	....	....	....
....	....	....	....	....	....
....	....	....	....	....	....

Other side of Record, continue with:

Date	Perm Used	Stylist	Date	Perm Used	Stylist

Question & Answer

SUIT THE PERM TO THE CLIENT

Q *The client selected the least expensive of three perms offered by the salon. Now she is dissatisfied because the perm seems dry. What should I have done?*

A The fault lies not with the client, but with you. It is your responsibility to advise the client what type perm she should have, based on the hair analysis

The least expensive perm imaginable is formulated with the same basic ingredients as the most expensive perm imaginable. The difference lies in the additives it contains, which influence things like moisture and gentleness.

It is far better to re-do a perm than lose a client. But you can avoid having to re-do perms by starting with a consultation. Analyze the hair and inform the client of the different perms offered (by price). Explain why each one is a different price. Tell her honestly the one you would recommend and why. Then, when she has made her choice, give her the best service you know how to give.

If you follow all the correct procedures, the perm should be a good one. The hair may need a re-conditioning treatment to restore moisture and oils that may have been reduced in the process, but it will have well-formed curl. Price is never an excuse for giving a bad perm.

—*From* Milady's Salon Solutions *by Louise Cotter*

PRE-PERM ANALYSIS

After the client consultation, you must analyze the overall condition of your client's hair and scalp. This analysis is essential for you to determine:

1. If it is safe and advisable to proceed with the perm service. The hair must be in good condition and have the necessary strength to accept a chemical alteration to achieve a successful perm.
2. Which perm product should be chosen for the best results on the particular hair type.
3. Which perm technique should be used: rod and parting sizes and wrapping pattern.

First, examine the scalp for abrasions, irritations, or open sores. If any of these conditions exist, do not give the perm. Next, judge the physical characteristics of the hair with regard to these important criteria: porosity, elasticity, density, texture, length. Finally, determine the overall condition of the hair. Observe if the hair has been previously treated with chemicals: perm, tint, bleach, highlighting (frosting, dimensionally colored). This will guide you in choosing the appropriate perm.

CAUTION

If pre-perm analysis is not correct, poor curl development or hair damage can result.

Determining Porosity

Porosity (po-**ROS**-i-tee) refers to the hair's capacity to absorb liquids. There is a direct relationship between the hair's porosity, the type of perm (acid-balanced or alkaline) you will use, and the strength of waving lotion you will choose.

The processing time for any perm depends more on hair porosity than on any other factor. The more porous the hair, the less processing time it takes, and a milder waving solution is required. The degree to which hair absorbs the waving lotion is related to its porosity, regardless of texture.

Hair porosity is affected by such factors as excessive exposure to sun and wind, use of harsh shampoos, tints, and lighteners, previous perms, and use of thermal styling appliances.

Porous hair might be dry—even very dry. If hair is tinted, bleached, has been exposed to sun, or was overprocessed by a previous perm, it will absorb liquids readily. Soft, fine, thin hair usually has a thin cuticle so it will absorb liquids quickly and easily. Rough, dull-looking hair and hair that tangles easily are also signs of porous hair.

While the hair is dry, check porosity in three different areas: front hairline, in front of the ear, and in the crown area. Select a single strand of hair, hold the end securely between the thumb and forefinger of one hand, and slide the thumb and forefinger of the other hand from the end to the scalp.

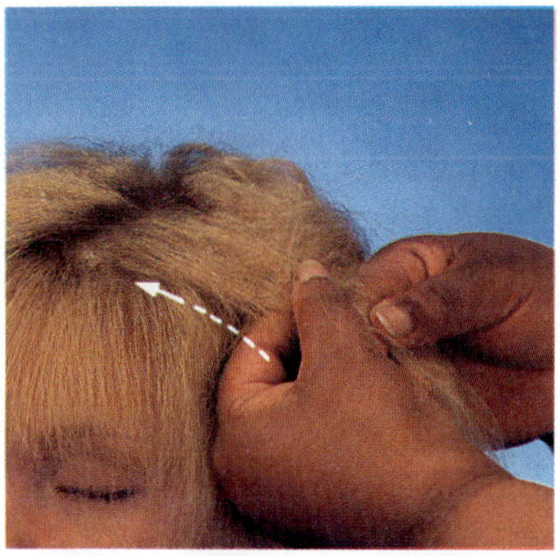

11.7—Testing for hair porosity.

If the hair feels smooth and the cuticle is dense and hard, it is considered resistant and will not absorb liquids or perm lotion easily. If you can feel a slight roughness, this tells you that the cuticle is open and that the hair is porous and will absorb liquids more readily. (Fig. 11.7)

Poor porosity (resistant hair). Hair with the cuticle layer lying close to the hair shaft. This type of hair absorbs waving lotion slowly and usually requires a longer processing time and/or a strong waving lotion.

Good porosity (normal hair). Hair with the cuticle layer slightly raised from the hair shaft. Hair of this type can absorb moisture or chemicals in an average amount of time.

Porous (tinted, lightened, or previously chemically treated hair). Hair that has been made porous by various treatments or styling. This type of hair absorbs lotion very quickly and requires the shortest processing time. Use either an acid-balanced perm or a very mild alkaline wave.

Over-porous hair (a result of overprocessing). This type of hair is very damaged, dry, fragile, and brittle. Until the hair has been reconditioned or the damaged part has been removed by cutting, it should not be permed.

If hair is unevenly porous (usually porous or over-porous at the ends with good to poor porosity near the scalp), a pre-wrap lotion, specifically designed to even out the porosity, is recommended to achieve even curl results and help prevent overprocessing porous ends. (Fig. 11.8a–d)

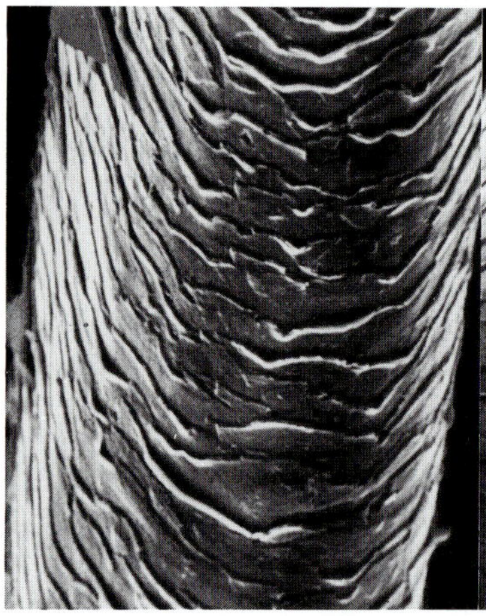

11.8a—Normal (moderate porosity).

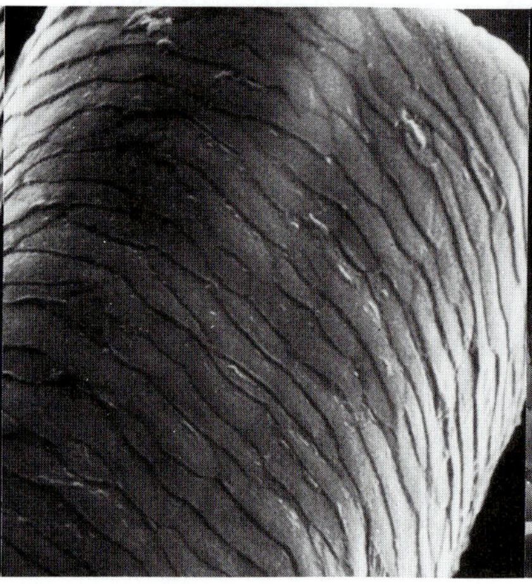

11.8b—Resistant (poor porosity).

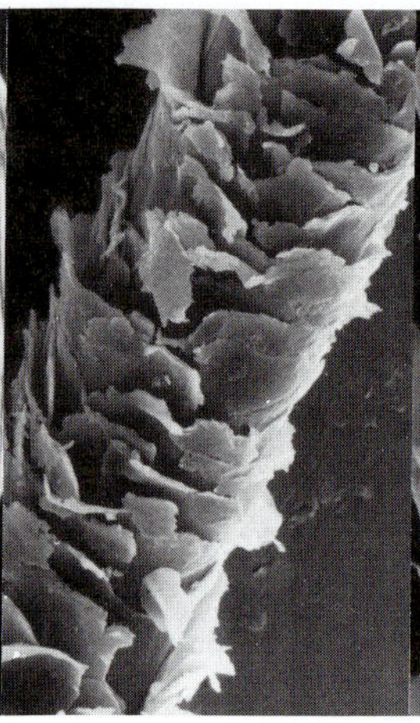

11.8c—Tinted (extreme porosity).

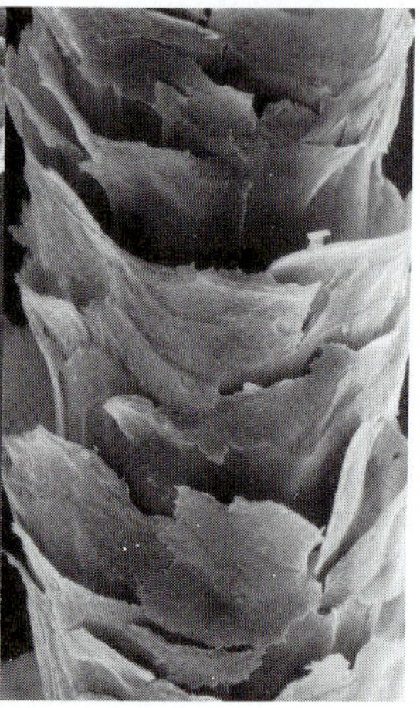

11.8d—Damaged (over-porous hair).

Determining Texture

Texture refers to how thick or thin (in diameter) each individual hair is. Fine hair has a small diameter; coarse hair has a large diameter. You can feel whether hair is fine, coarse, or medium when a single dry strand is held between the fingers.

The texture and porosity together are used to determine processing time of the waving lotion. Although porosity is the more important of the two, texture does play an important role in estimating processing time. Fine hair with a small diameter becomes saturated with waving lotion more quickly than coarse hair with a large diameter, even if both are of equal porosity. However, when coarse hair is porous, it processes faster than fine hair that is not porous.

A perm adds body to hair that appears limp, lifeless, and does not hold a style very long. For coarse, wiry hair, a perm provides greater manageability in styling. (Fig. 11.9a–c)

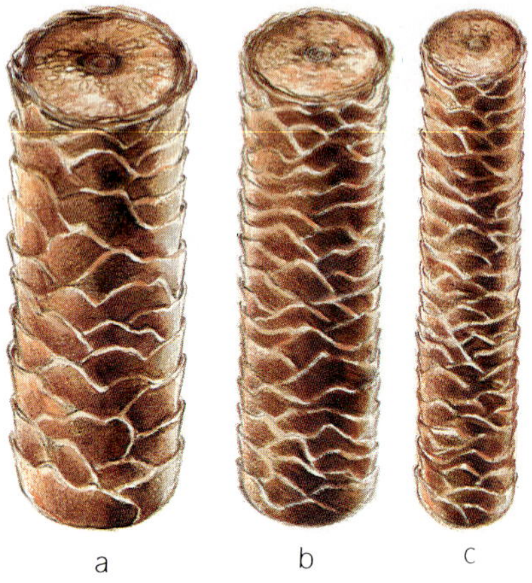

11.9a—Coarse.
11.9b—Medium.
11.9c—Fine.

Testing Elasticity

Elasticity is the ability of hair to stretch and contract. To test for elasticity, stretch a single dry hair. If the hair breaks under very slight strain, it has little or no elasticity. Other signs of poor elasticity include a spongy feel when hair is wet and/or hair that tangles easily. When hair is completely lacking in elasticity (for example, extremely damaged hair), it will not take a satisfactory permanent wave because it has lost the ability to contract after stretching. The greater the degree of elasticity, the longer the wave will remain in the hair, because less relaxation of the hair occurs. Hair with good elastic qualities can be stretched 20% of its length without breaking. (Fig. 11.10)

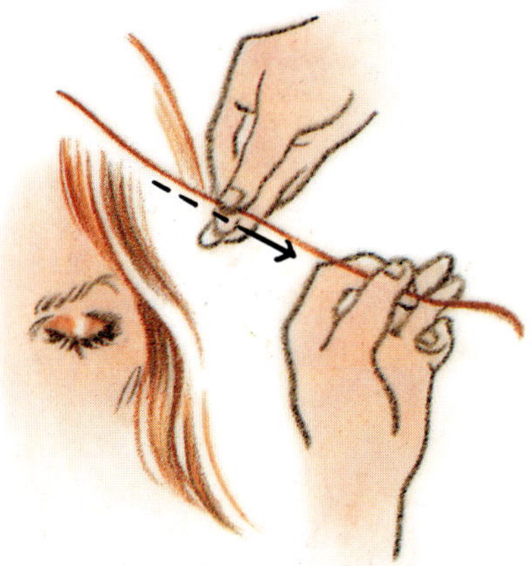
11.10—Testing for elasticity.

Assessing Density

Density, or thickness, refers to the number of hairs per square inch (6.452 sq. cm) on your client's head. Density is one characteristic that determines the size of the partings you will use. Thick hair (many hairs per square inch) will require small partings on each rod. Too much hair on the rod can result in a weak curl, especially at the scalp.

If hair is thin (fewer hairs per square inch), slightly larger partings can be used, but avoid stretching or pulling the hair toward the rod because this can cause hair breakage.

Hair Length and Perming

Hair that is 2" to 6" (5 to 15 cm) long is considered ideal for perming. Hair should be long enough to make at least 2½ turns around the rod. To perm hair longer than 6" (15 cm), smaller partings must be used to allow the waving lotion and neutralizer to penetrate more easily and thoroughly.

PERM SELECTION

The type of perm you choose depends on the total evaluation of your client's hair and wishes during the consultation and pre-perm analysis. The following is a general guide to help you decide whether to use an alkaline or an acid-balanced perm.

Hair Type	Type of Perm
Coarse, resistant	Alkaline lotion wrap or alkaline water wrap
Fine, resistant	Alkaline lotion wrap or alkaline water wrap
Normal	Alkaline water wrap or acid-balanced
Normal, porous	Alkaline water wrap or acid-balanced
Normal, delicate	Acid-balanced
Tinted, non-porous	Alkaline water wrap or acid-balanced
Tinted, porous	Acid-balanced
Highlighted/frosted/dimensionally colored	Acid-balanced
Highlighted, tinted	Acid-balanced
Bleached	Acid-balanced

Today's perm products offer a wide selection of special features and formulas for all hair types. There are alkaline formulas for bleached hair and acid-balanced formulas for resistant hair. Each formula gives excellent results if you choose the perm carefully and follow the product directions.

PRE-PERM SHAMPOOING

Today, there are shampoos specifically formulated for pre-perm cleansing that thoroughly yet gently cleanse the hair. Use of these shampoos is recommended for optimal perm results.

When analyzing a client's hair before perming, you might notice that the hair looks and feels coated. This coating might be the buildup of shampoo or conditioners, improper rinsing, resins from styling products or hair spray, or mineral deposits from hard water. This coating can prevent penetration of the waving lotion and interfere with perm results. It is very important for the hair to be free of all coatings before beginning any perm.

CAUTION

While shampooing or doing any pre-perm preparation of a client's hair, you should avoid vigorous brushing, combing, pulling, or rubbing that can cause the scalp to become sensitive to perm solutions.

Begin the process by wetting the hair, applying the shampoo, and gently working it into a lather. If the hair is extremely coated, let the shampoo remain in the hair several minutes before rinsing. Rinse thoroughly to remove all shampoo and dissolved buildup. Towel blot excess water from hair.

PRE-PERM CUTTING OR SHAPING

If the client has chosen a hairstyle that is the same or very similar to the design he or she is currently wearing, reshape the style using either a scissors or razor. If the finished style requires texturizing or thinning of the ends, wait until after giving the perm to texturize. Tapered or thinned ends are more difficult to wrap smoothly and accurately.

If the client wants a completely new style, rough cut the hair into an approximation of the final shape. After the perm is completed, you can finish shaping the style more exactly. ✔

✔ Completed—Learning Objective No. 4

CLIENT CONSULTATION AND HAIR ANALYSIS

PERM RODS

Proper selection of perm rod size is essential for successful perm results. The size of the rod controls the size of the curl created by the waving process. Perm rods are typically made of plastic and come in varying sizes. They range in diameter (distance through the center of the rod) from small to large (⅛″ to ¾″ [.3125 to 1.875 cm]). Rods are color coded to identify their size. (Fig. 11.11) Typically, the color/size designations are:

Small Rods	Medium Rods	Large Rods
Yellow	Gray	Beige
Blue	Black	Purple
Pink	White	Green
		Orange

Perm rods are also available in various lengths: short, medium, and long (1¾″ to 3½″ [4.375 to 8.75 cm]). Rods of all diameters are available in long lengths. Medium and short lengths are not always available in all diameters. These shorter rods are used for wrapping small or awkward sections.

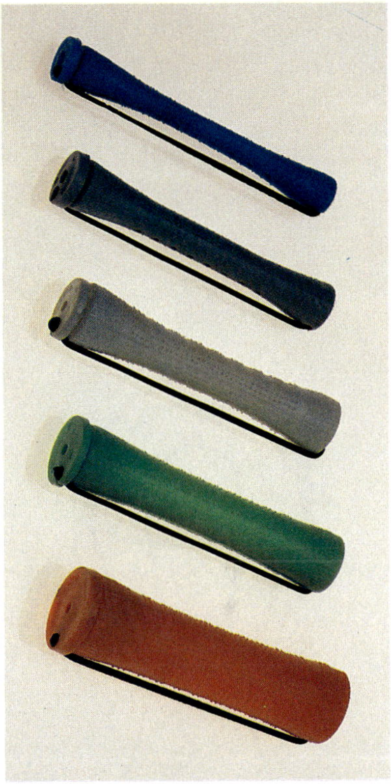

11.11—Sizes of rods—top to bottom: extra small, small, medium, large, extra large.

Types of Rods

There are two types of rods: concave and straight. Concave rods have a small diameter in the center area and gradually increase to their largest diameter at the ends, resulting in a tighter curl at the hair ends, with a looser, wider curl at the scalp. The diameter of the straight rods is the same throughout their length, creating the same size curl from end to scalp.

All rods have some means of securing the hair on the rod to prevent the curl from unwinding. Usually an elastic band, with a fastening button attached to the end, stretches across the wound hair and secures it when the button is inserted into the opposite end of the rod.

Selecting Rod Size

When selecting rod size, two things must be considered:

1. Amount of curl desired
2. Physical characteristics of the hair

Curl desired: The amount of wave, curl, or body needed is determined between you and the client during the consultation. Your success in creating a style depends primarily on the rod sizes you choose, the number of rods used, and where the rods are placed on the head.

Hair characteristics: Of the hair characteristics described earlier, three are important to rod size selection:

1. Hair length
2. Hair elasticity
3. Hair texture

Suggested Hair Parting and Rod Sizes

Although the hair length, elasticity, and texture must be considered in the choice of rods, the texture should be the determining factor.

Coarse texture, good elasticity. Requires smaller (narrower) partings and larger rods to permit better placement of rods for a definite wave pattern.

Medium texture, average elasticity. Medium or average textured hair requires average size partings and medium size rods.

Fine texture, poor elasticity. Requires smaller than average partings and small to medium size rods to prevent hair strain or breakage.

Hair in nape area. Use smaller partings and smaller rods.

Long hair. To permanently wave hair longer than 6″ (15 cm), use small partings and wrap smoothly and close to the scalp. The use of smaller partings permits the waving lotion and neutralizer to penetrate more easily and thoroughly.

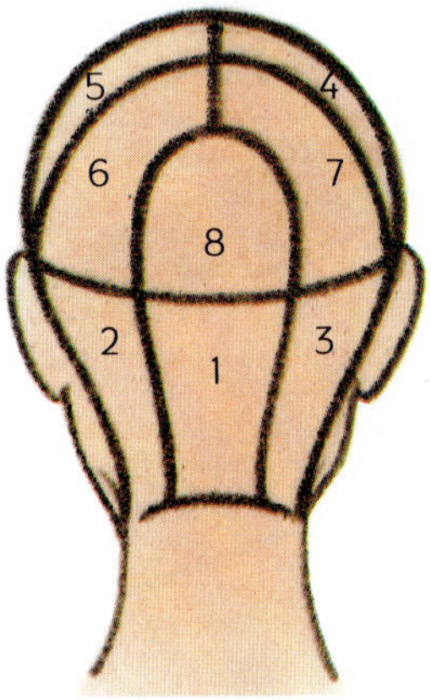

11.12—Sectioning.

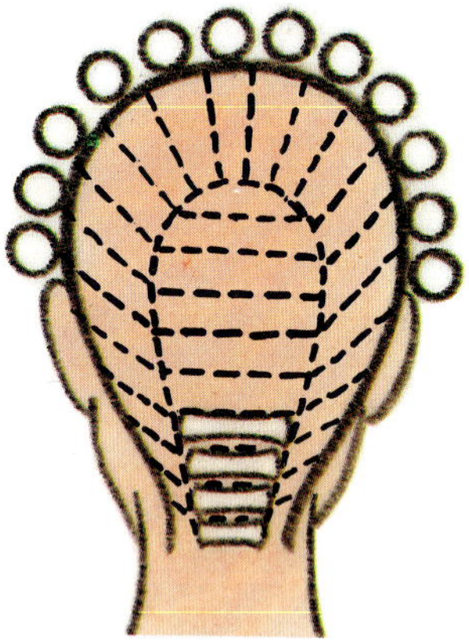
11.13—Blocking (subsections).

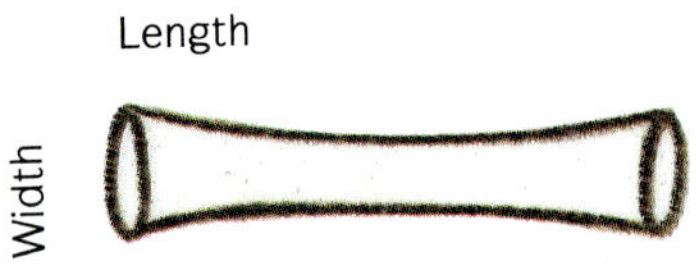

11.14—Length denotes span of blocking. Width refers to the depth of the blocking. Small or large blockings usually refer to their width.

SECTIONING AND PARTING

Sectioning is the dividing of hair into uniform working areas at the top, front, crown, sides, back, and nape. Sectioning makes your work easier because you can pin up all sections out of your way except the section you are working with.

Parting, also known as ***blocking,*** is the overall plan for rod placement. You block so that you know where to place the rods in order to give the design the support, direction, and curl pattern it needs. It is important that the blocking is done in uniform sections. You should use the following guidelines to help you:

1. Uniformly arrange sections.
2. Equally subdivide sections (blockings).
3. Create clean and uniform partings (length and width).
4. The average parting should match the diameter (size) of the rod being used.
5. The length of the blocking should be the same as or a little shorter, but never longer, than the length of the rod. (Figs. 11.12–11.14)

WRAPPING PATTERNS

Just as the rod size and parting size determine the size of the curl, the wrapping pattern determines the direction or flow of the curl.

Six popular wrapping patterns are:

1. Single halo
2. Double halo (double horseshoe)
3. Straight back
4. Dropped crown
5. Spiral wrap
6. Stack perm

These are known by other names in different areas of the country.

The following sections and partings are suggested for these wrapping patterns. Your instructor might suggest different sections, which are equally correct.

Single Halo

The single halo wrap is commonly used for average size heads to create even curls. (Figs. 11.15–11.18)

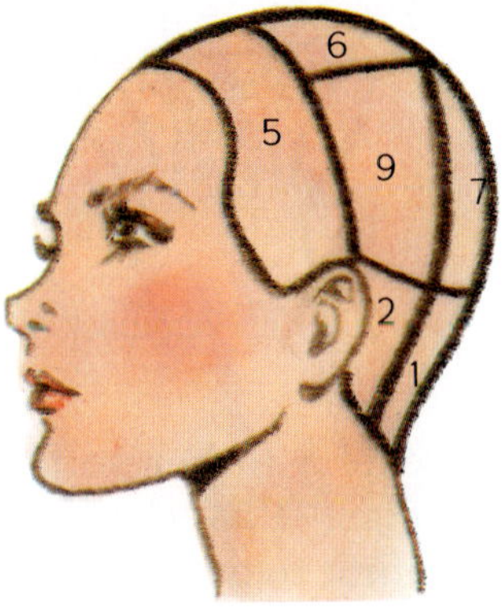

11.15—Sectioning side.

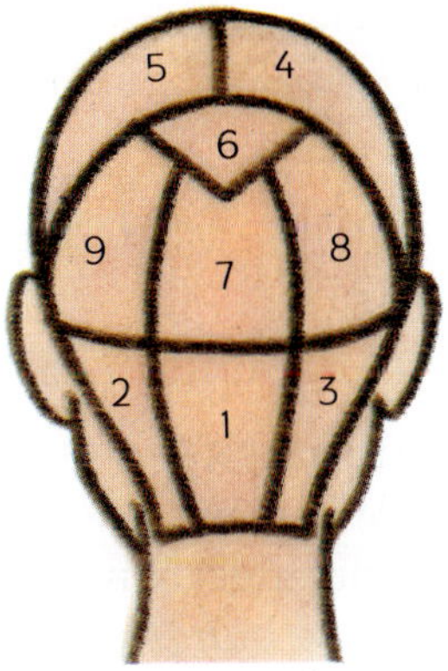

11.16—Sectioning back.

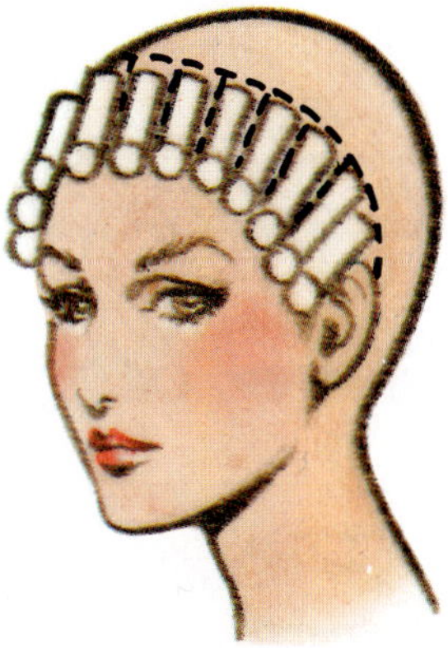
11.17—Blocking side.

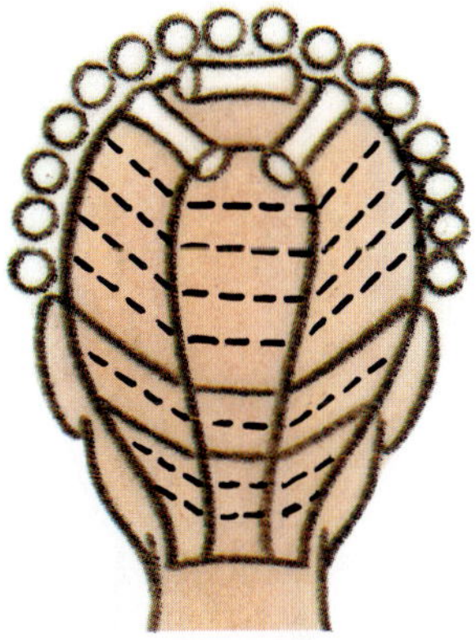
11.18—Blocking back.

Double Halo

The double halo wrap is usually used for larger size heads. (Figs. 11.19–11.22)

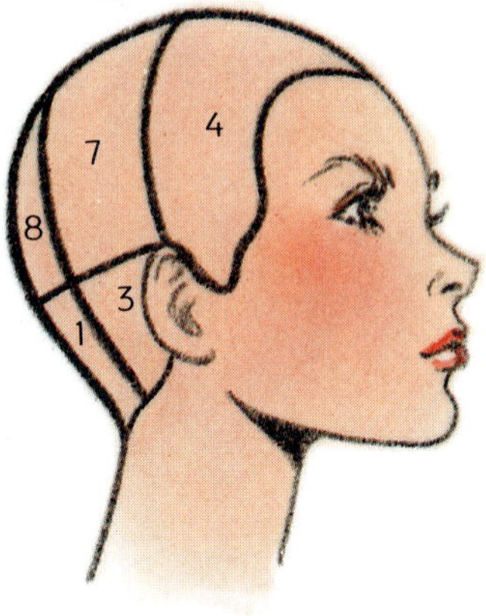

11.19—Sectioning side.

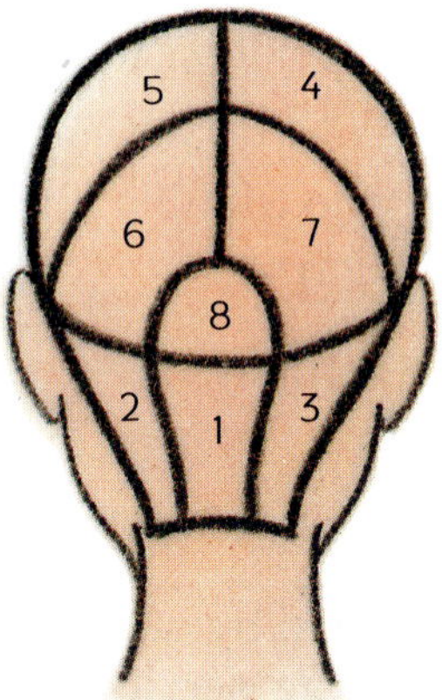

11.20—Sectioning back.

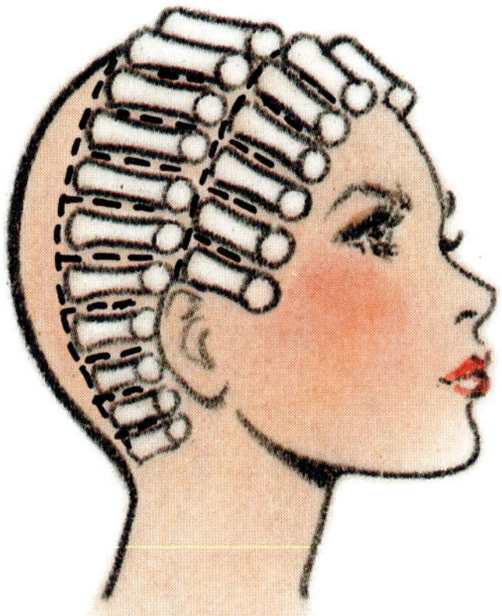

11.21—Blocking side.

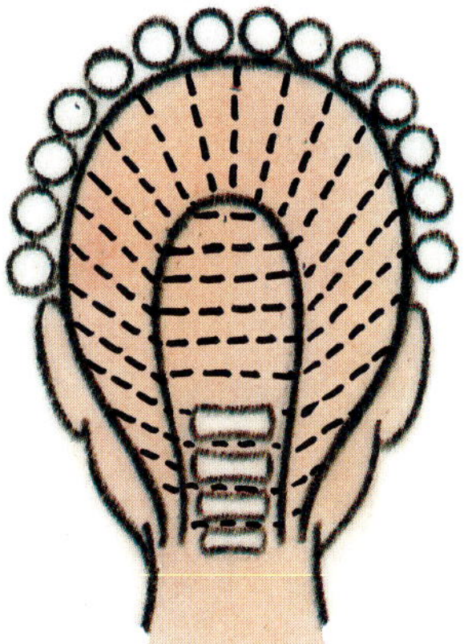

11.22—Blocking back.

Straight Back

The straight back wrap is used to create a rather soft, full, and high style effect, directed off the face. (Figs. 11.23, 11.24)

To create ***bangs*** on the forehead, the first two top front curls are wrapped in a forward direction (see directional wrapping, pages 218–220). (Fig. 11.25)

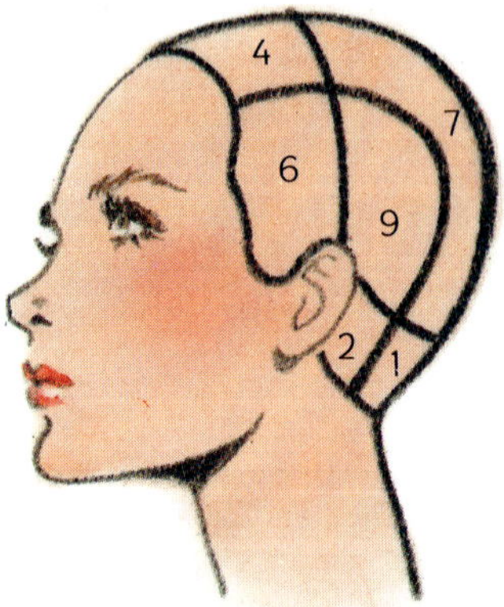

11.23—Sectioning side.

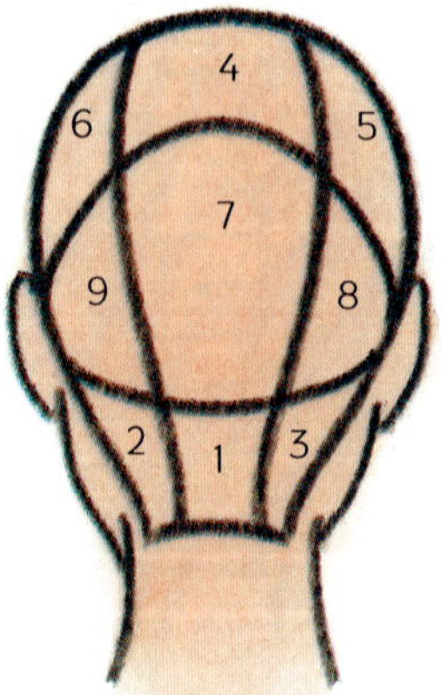

11.24—Sectioning back.

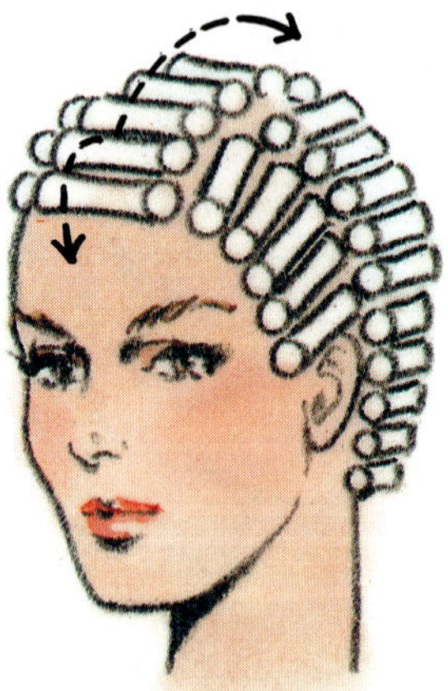

11.25—Setting for bangs.

Dropped Crown

The dropped crown wrap is usually used for longer hair and for a smooth crown effect.

The hair is sectioned in the same way as for the straight back pattern. However, in the back area that is not numbered on the illustration, larger hair sections are made, depending on the amount of hair in that section. Only the hair ends are wrapped and the rods rest on the smaller rods in the nape area (sections 2, 1, 3). Be guided by your instructor. (Figs. 11.26–11.29)

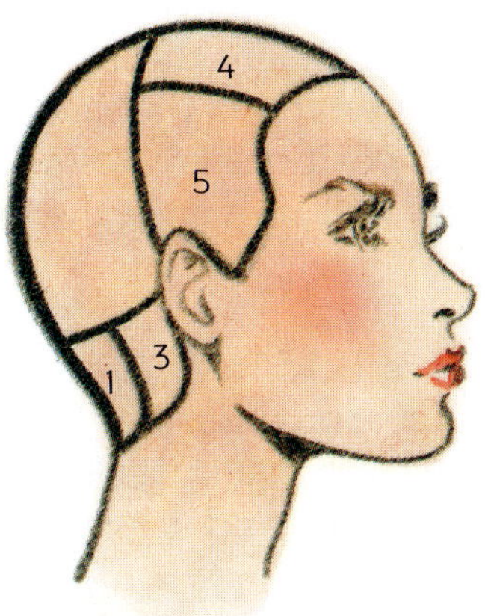

11.26—Sectioning side.

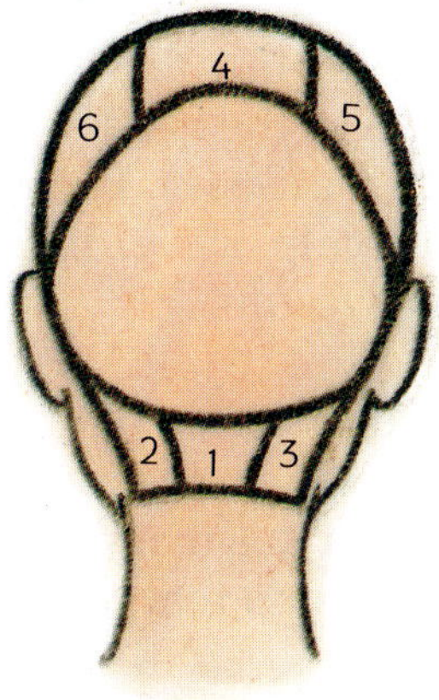

11.27—Sectioning back.

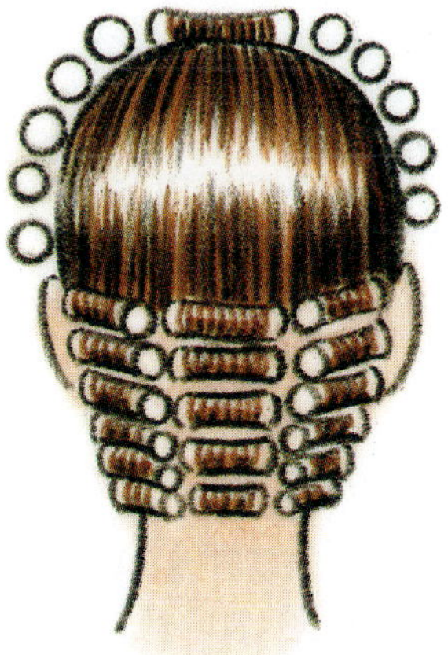

11.28—Blocking (subsectioning) pattern.

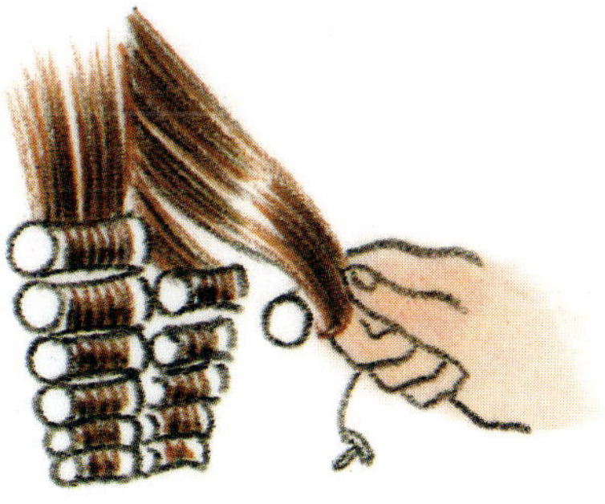

11.29—Wrapping hair ends of crown area.

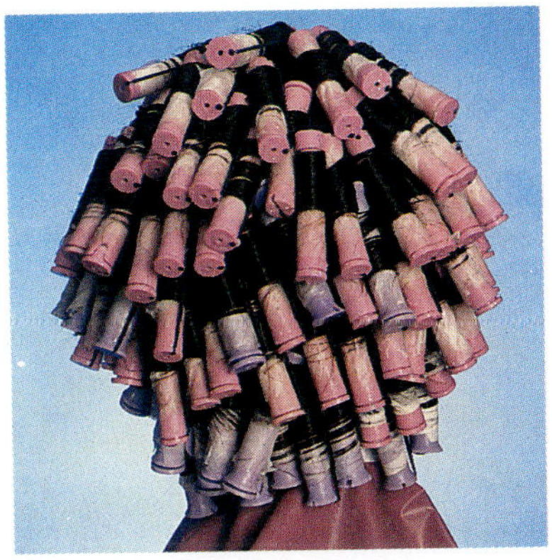

11.30—Spiral wrap.

Spiral Wrap

The spiral wrap is used for long hair to create tight, springy curls. (Fig. 11.30)

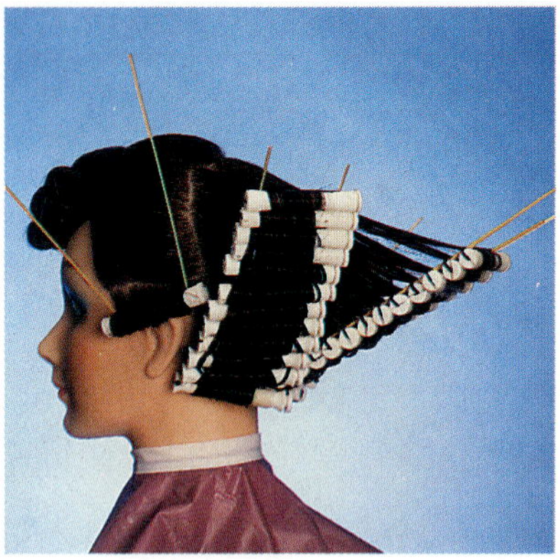

11.31—Stack perm.

Stack Perm

The stack technique is usually used for greater curl at the nape. (Fig. 11.31)

WRAPPING THE HAIR

To create a uniform wave or curl pattern, the hair must be wrapped smoothly and neatly on each perm rod *without stretching*. As noted earlier, the action of the waving lotion expands the hair. Hair that is tightly wrapped interferes with this action and prevents penetration of the waving lotion and neutralizer.

Hair Strand Parting in Relation to the Head

Base refers to the head or scalp and where the rod is placed in relation to the head. The rods can be wrapped on-base, off-base, or one-half off-base. Each of these rod positions creates a slightly different scalp wave direction, which will influence the overall curl pattern results.

Curl on-base. When the strand is held in an upward position and wound on the rod, the curl will rest on-base. (See Fig. 11.32) Hair wound in this manner will produce curls that start close to the scalp for hairstyles that require fullness, height, and upward movement.

Curl off-base. When the strand is held in a downward position and wound on a rod, the curl will rest off-base. (See Fig. 11.33) Hair wound in this manner will produce a curl that starts farther away from the scalp than hair wound on base. Off-base winding produces close-to-the-head hairstyles that do not require fullness or height.

Curl one-half off-base. When the strand is held straight out from the head and wound on a rod, the curl will rest one-half off-base. (See Fig. 11.34) Hair wound in this manner is adaptable to many hairstyles.

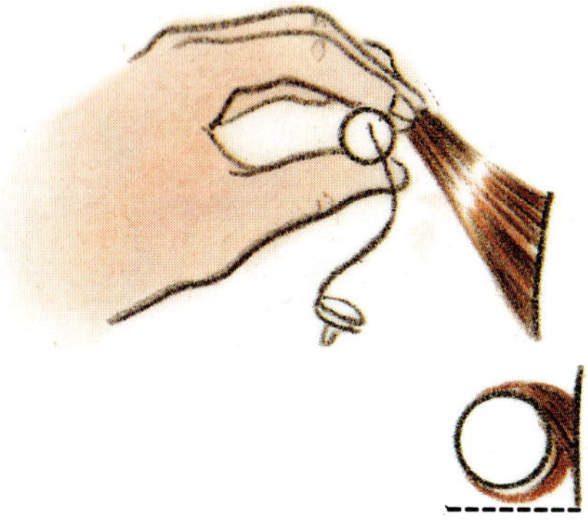

11.32—Curl on-base.

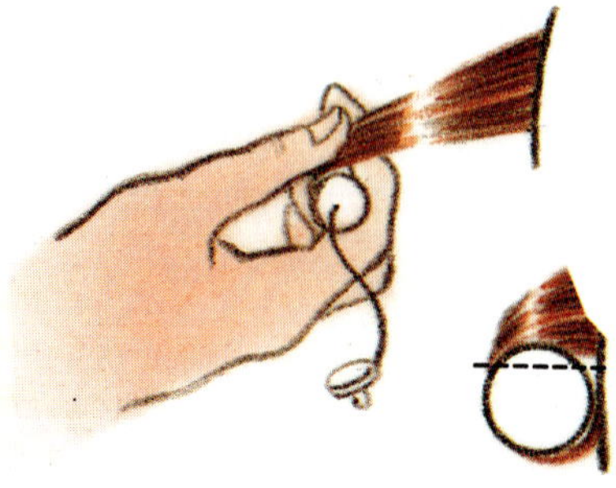

11.33—Curl off-base.

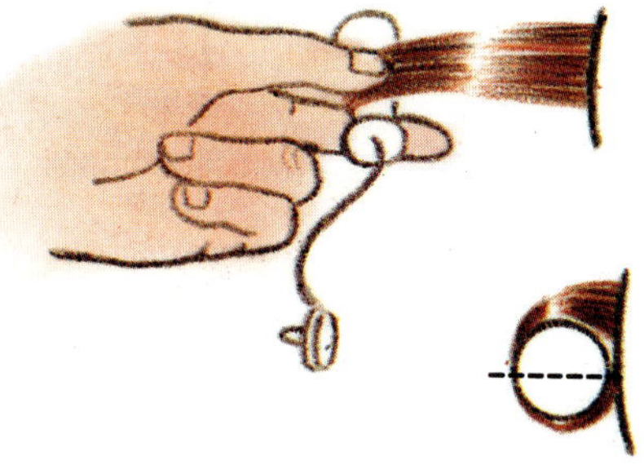

11.34—Curl one-half off-base.

End Wraps

End wraps or end papers are porous papers used to cover the ends of the hair to ensure smooth, even wrapping. End wraps minimize the danger of hair breakage and help to form smooth, even curls and waves. They are especially important in helping to wrap uneven hair lengths smoothly.

There are three methods of end wrap application in general use today. Each method is equally effective, if properly used.

1. Double end paper wrap
2. Single end paper wrap
3. Book end wrap

◆ NOTE: Hair should be shampooed and left moist (not saturated) for wrapping. Section hair, then begin by making your first parting. Remember, each parting should be no longer than the length of the rod. If the parting is too long, the hair will not wave evenly. If the hair should become dry while you are wrapping, mist the hair lightly with water.

Double End Paper Wrap

1. Part off and comb the parting up and out until all hair is smooth and evenly distributed. (See Fig. 11.35)
2. Place one end wrap under the hair strand so that it extends below the ends of the hair. Place the other end wrap on top. (See Fig. 11.36)
3. With your right hand, place the rod under the double end wraps, parallel with the parting at the scalp. (See Fig. 11.37)

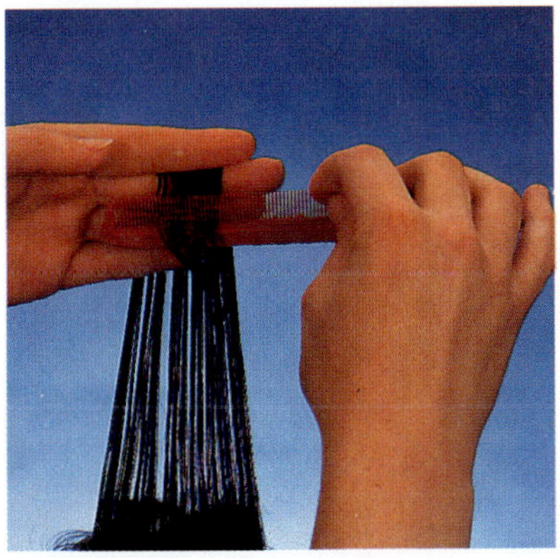

11.35—Comb and distribute strand evenly.

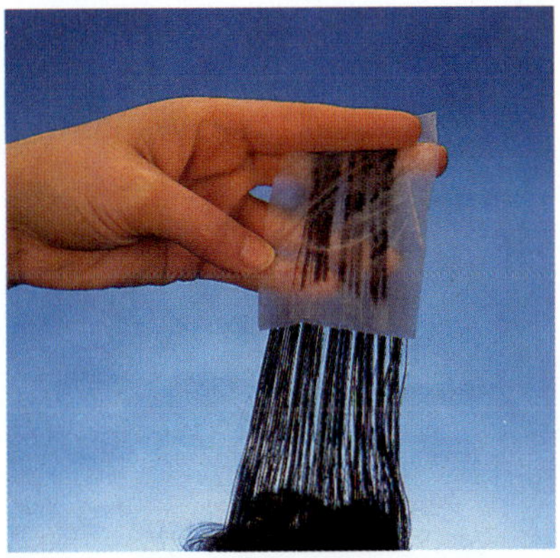

11.36—Position end papers.

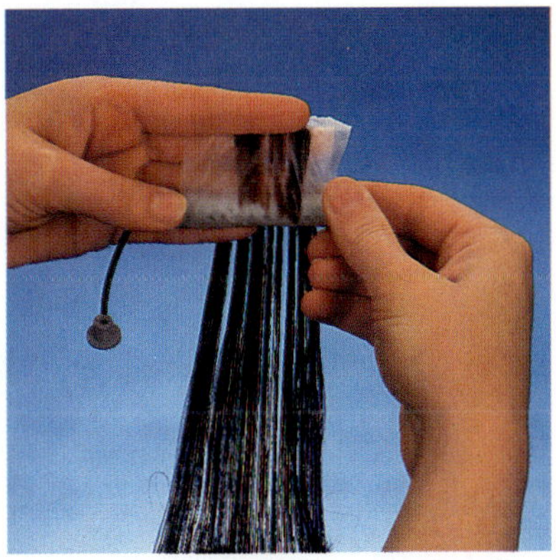

11.37—Position rod.

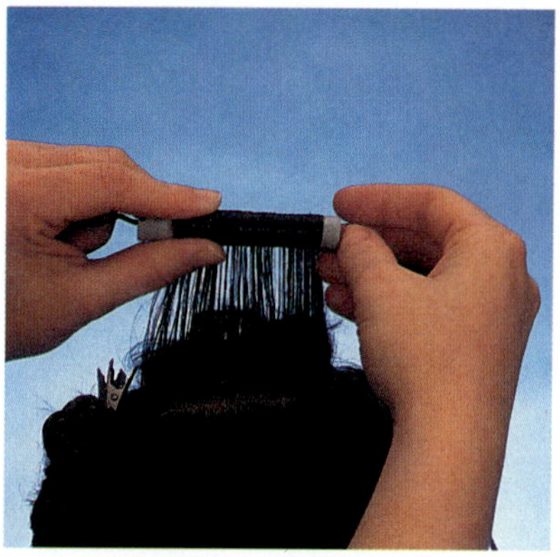

11.38—Wind the strand.

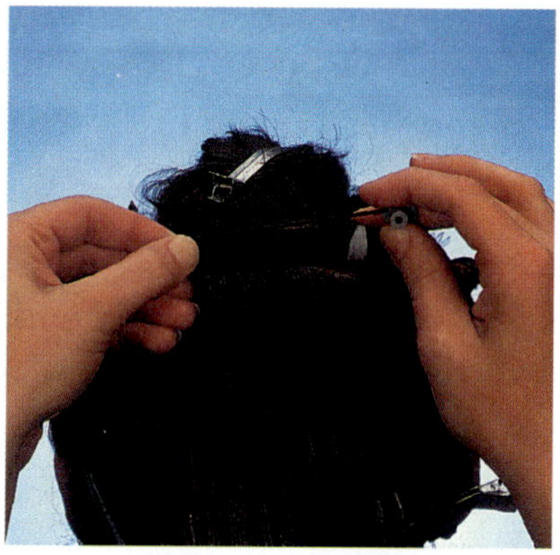

11.39—Fasten band.

4. Wind the strand smoothly on the rod to the scalp without tension. (See Fig. 11.38)
5. Fasten band at top of rod. (See Fig. 11.39)

CAUTION

To prevent breakage, the band should not press into the hair near the scalp or be twisted against the wound hair.

The preparation and winding of curls for the single end paper wrap and book end wrap are the same as the double end paper wrap, with the following exceptions:

Single end paper wrap. Place only one end wrap on top of the hair strand and hold it flat between the index and middle fingers to prevent bunching. (See Fig. 11.40) The hair is wound in the same manner as the double end paper wrap.

Book end wrap. Hold the strand between the index and middle fingers; fold and place an end paper over the strand, forming an envelope. Wind the curl as in the double end paper wrap. (See Fig. 11.41)

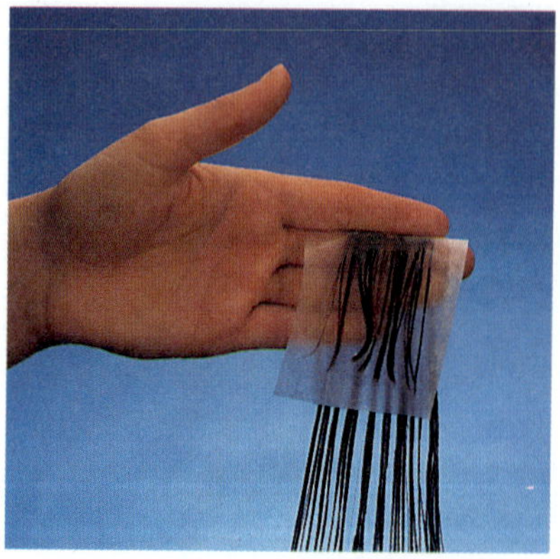

11.40—Single end paper wrap.

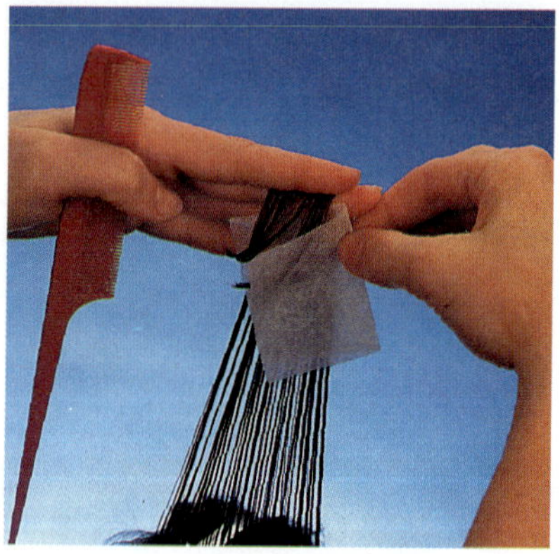

11.41—Book end wrap.

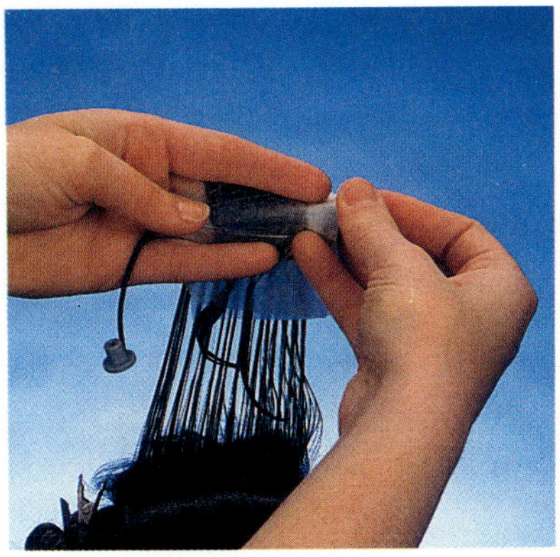

11.42—Position porous end papers.

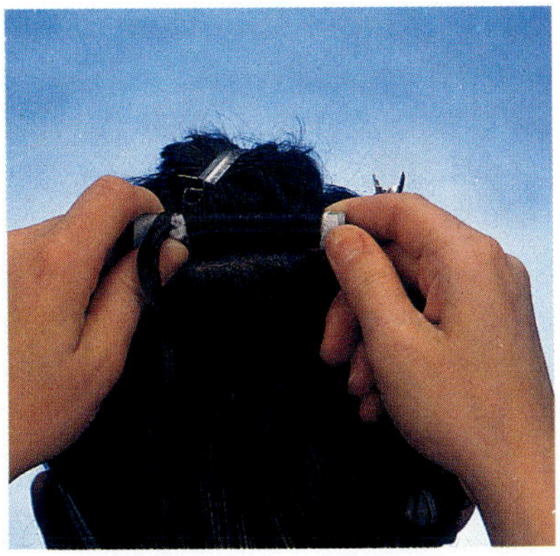

11.43—Start wrapping.

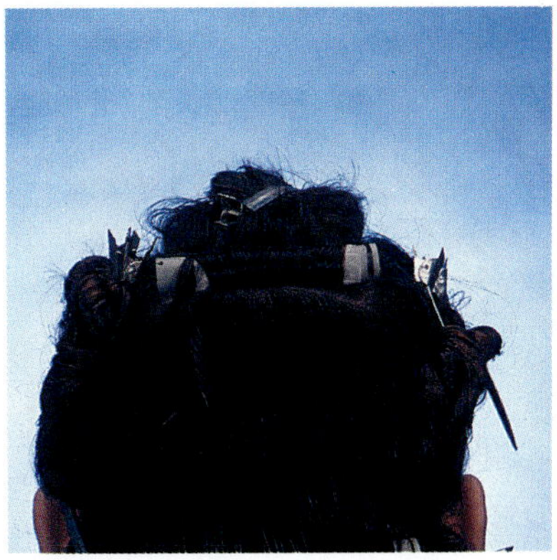

11.44—Secure the wrapped rod.

The Piggyback (Double Rod) Wrap

The piggyback (double rod) method of wrapping is especially suitable for extra long hair. This wrapping technique permits maximum control of the size and tightness of the curl from the scalp to the hair ends. Control of the amount of curl can be exercised by the size of the rods selected. Thus, the use of larger rods will result in a loose, wide wave; while small, or medium rods will give tighter curls. The following is the procedure for wrapping in the piggyback (double rod) method:

1. Section the head in the usual manner (9 sections).
2. Select the desired size rods. The rods used in the midpoint to the scalp area should be at least one size larger than those used for the hair ends.
3. About halfway up the strand, place porous end papers one on top and one underneath. (See Fig. 11.42)
4. Start at the midpoint part of the strand. Place the larger rod underneath the hair strand and start wrapping. (See Fig. 11.43)
5. Roll the rod toward the scalp and, at the same time, control the hair ends by holding them to the left away from the rod.
6. Secure the wrapped rod at the scalp, leaving the hair ends dangling free from the rod. (See Fig. 11.44)
7. Place an end paper on the hair strand covering the ends. Using the smaller size rod, wrap the hair ends up to the above larger rod. (See Fig. 11.45)
8. Secure the second rod to rest against the first one in piggyback fashion. (See Fig. 11.46)
9. To maintain better control over the wrapping and processing, it is advisable to complete the wrapping of each hair strand before proceeding to the next one.

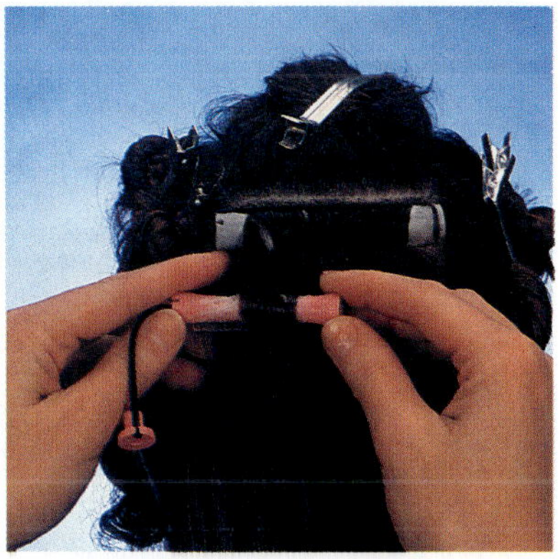

11.45—Wrap the remaining hair ends.

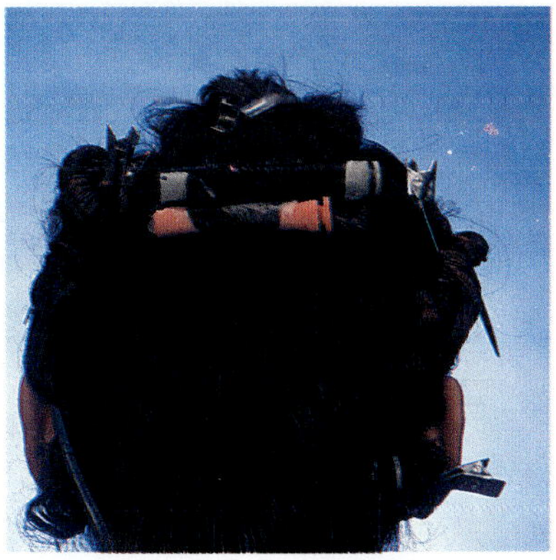

11.46—Secure the second rod beneath the first rod.

10. Test curls should be taken from the rods closer to the scalp because the hair in this area is more resistant and might require additional processing.

◆ NOTE: When wrapping hair, always avoid bulkiness on the rod. Bulkiness prevents the formation of a good curl because the hair cannot conform to the shape of the rod, and the waving lotion and neutralizer cannot penetrate evenly and thoroughly. To ensure a smooth wave formation and avoid fishhook ends, the first turn on the rod should be the end wraps without any of the hair ends between them.

Question & Answer

PERMING FINE HAIR

Q *How do you deal with hair so fine and limp it will not take a perm?*

A The hair may not have sufficient salt bonds to respond favorably to chemical re-formation. Synthetic salt bonds can be temporarily added to the hair. They will immediately make the hair bouncier, but the effect is not permanent.

Wrap the perm, apply perm solution and process. When the test curl shows sufficient response, towel blot the solution from each perm rod.

Dissolve 1 teaspoon Epsom salts in 2 oz. of water and 2 oz. liquid protein re-conditioner. Use an applicator bottle with a very fine nozzle, and apply the solution to each rod. Leave it on for 5 minutes.

Blot the solution from the hair (do not rinse), and proceed with the neutralizing (re-bonding step).

The magnesium content in the Epsom salts creates a synthetic bond similar to salt-bonds in natural hair.

This formula may be applied to fine, limp hair after each shampoo and left on for a period of 15 minutes, as often as necessary. When using after a shampoo, omit water from the formula. Use only liquid protein and Epsom salts.

—From Milady's Salon Solutions *by Louise Cotter*

PRELIMINARY TEST CURLS

Preliminary test curls help determine how your client's hair will react to a perm. It is advisable to do a test on hair that is tinted, bleached, over-porous, or shows any signs of damage.

Also, before applying waving lotion, be sure to check with your instructor or state board to find out if you are required to wear protective gloves during application.

Preliminary testing gives you the following additional information:

- Actual processing time needed to achieve optimum curl results
- Curl results based on the rod size and perm product you have selected

Procedure

1. Shampoo the hair and towel dry.
2. Following the perm directions, wrap two or three rods in the most delicate areas of the hair.
3. Wrap a coil of cotton around the rod.
4. Apply waving lotion to wrapped curls, being very careful not to allow the waving lotion to come in contact with unwrapped hair.
5. Set a timer and process the hair according to the perm directions.
6. Check the hair frequently.

To check a test curl, unfasten a rod and carefully (remember—hair is in a softened state) unwind the curl about 1½ turns of the rod. Do not permit the hair to become loose or unwound from the rod completely. Hold the hair firmly by placing a thumb at each end of the rod. Move the rod gently toward the scalp so that the hair falls loosely into the wave pattern. Continue checking the rods until a firm and definite "S" is formed. The "S" reflects the size of the rod used. (Fig. 11.47) Be guided by the manufacturer's direction.

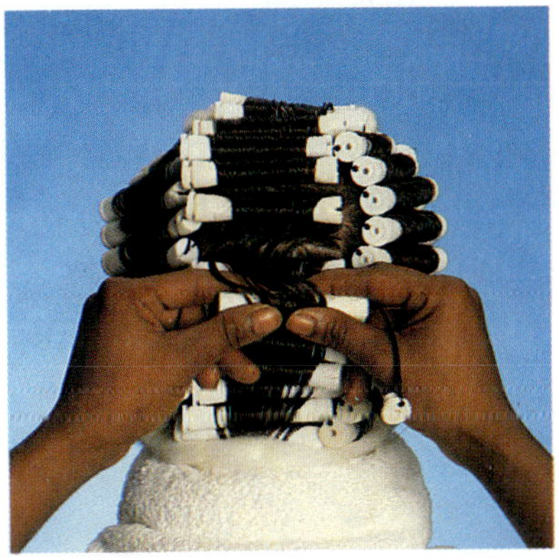
11.47—Unwinding hair carefully, without pulling or pushing.

◆ NOTE: When judging test curls, different hair textures with varying degrees of elasticity will have slightly different "S" formations. Fine, thin hair is generally softer and has less bulk. The wave ridge might be less defined and more difficult to read. Coarse, thick hair has better elasticity and seems to reinforce itself, falling into the wave pattern more readily. The wave ridge will be stronger and better defined. Long hair may produce a wider scalp wave than short hair, because larger rods are used and the diameter of the wave widens toward the scalp.

When the optimum curl has been formed, rinse the curls with warm water, blot the curls thoroughly, apply, process and rinse the neutralizer according to the perm directions and gently dry these test curls. Evaluate the curl results. If the hair is overprocessed, do not perm the rest of the hair until it is in better condition. If the test curl results are good, proceed with the perm, but ***do not re-perm these preliminary test curls.***

Overprocessing

Any lotion that can properly process the hair also can overprocess it, causing dryness, frizziness, or hair damage. Overprocessed hair is easily detected. It is very curly when wet, but frizzy when dry. It cannot be combed into a suitable wave pattern, because the elasticity of the hair has been excessively damaged, and the hair feels harsh after being dried. Reconditioning treatments should begin immediately.

Causes of overprocessing are:

1. Lotion left on too long.
2. Improperly judged pre-perm hair analysis and/or waving lotion that was too strong.
3. Test curls were not made frequently enough or were judged improperly.

✔ Completed—Learning Objective No. 5

ROD SELECTION AND SECTIONING, PARTING, AND WRAPPING PROCEDURES

Underprocessing

Underprocessing is caused by insufficient processing time of the waving lotion. After perming, underprocessed hair has a limp or weak wave formation. The ridges are not well defined, and the hair retains little or no wave formation. Typically, after a few shampooings, the hair will have no curl pattern at all. (Fig. 11.48a–e) ✔

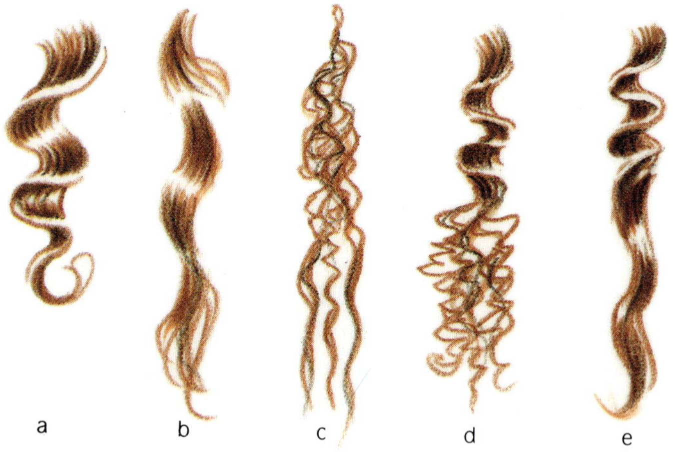

11.48a—Good results.
11.48b—Underprocessed curl.
11.48c—Overprocessed curl.
11.48d—Porous ends.
11.48e—Improper winding.

CAUTION

Underprocessed hair, even if there is no curl, has been chemically treated. If, in your professional judgment, you decide the hair can be re-permed, condition it first, choose a milder waving lotion, and test the curls frequently.

Important Safety Precautions

Remember that the lotions used for perming contain chemically active ingredients and therefore must be used carefully to avoid injury to you and your client. The following precautions should always be taken:

1. Protect the client's clothing with a plastic shampoo cape, or ask the client to change into a smock.
2. Ask the client to remove glasses, earrings, and necklaces to prevent damage.
3. Do not give a perm to a client who has experienced an allergic reaction to a previous perm.
4. Do not save any opened, unused waving lotion or neutralizer. These lotions can change in strength and effectiveness if not used within a few hours after opening the container.
5. Do not dilute or add anything to the waving lotion or neutralizer unless the product directions tell you to do so.
6. Keep waving lotion out of eyes and away from the skin. If waving lotion should contact these areas, rinse *thoroughly* with cool water.
7. Do not perm and apply hair color to a client on the same day. Perm the hair first, wait one week, then apply hair color. ✔

✔ Completed—Learning Objective No. 6

SAFETY PRECAUTIONS

PERMING TECHNIQUES

Before you begin perming, make sure you have all the necessary supplies at hand. Good organization and planning will help you develop precision and speed in completing a perm. At your station, the following equipment should be laid out in an organized, easily accessible fashion:

- The perm product
- Rods (organized by size)
- End wraps
- Cotton coil
- Towels
- Plastic hair clips and pins
- Tail comb
- Protective gloves

Always Read and Follow the Product Directions Carefully. Some alkaline perm product directions call for water wrapping, some are lotion wrapped, and others require pre-wrap lotions. Some wave lotions come in two parts that must be mixed just prior to use. Some need dryer heat. (***Note:*** Dryer should be pre-heated.) Some perms require that a plastic cap be placed over the rods during the processing, others do not. Considering all the variables, it is not a good idea to trust your memory. Make it a practice to check the printed directions that accompany every perm *each time you give a perm.*

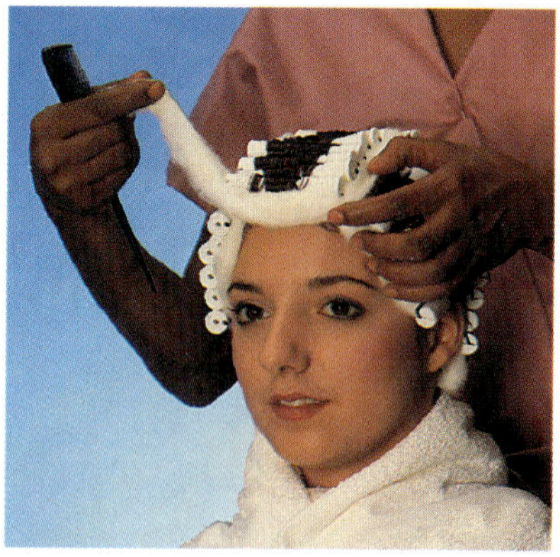

11.49—Hairline protected by cotton strips or neutralizing band.

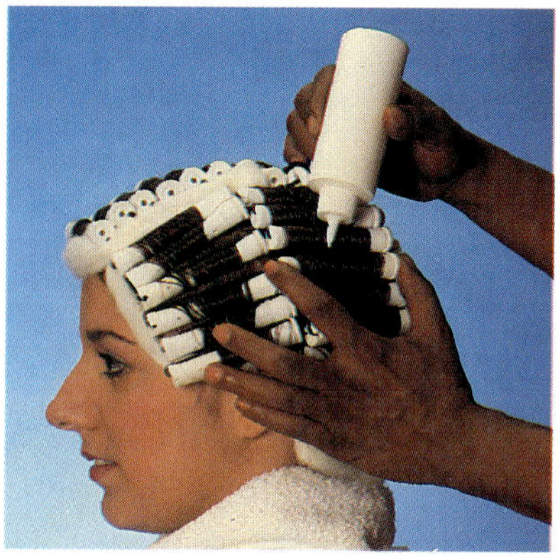

11.50—Applying waving lotion.

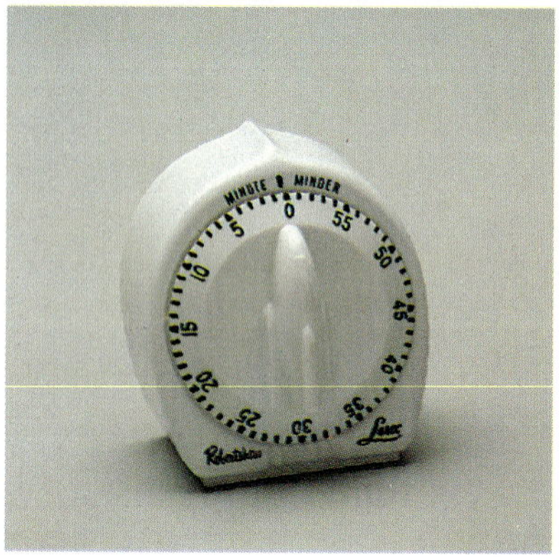

11.51—Processing timer.

APPLYING WAVING LOTION

After shampooing, shaping, and wrapping the hair, place a coil or band of cotton around the entire hairline. To prevent skin irritation and for added protection, apply a barrier cream to skin around hairline before applying cotton band. This safety precaution prevents waving lotion from coming into contact with the skin and possibly causing irritation. If lotion is applied accurately there should be a minimum of dripping, but the cotton is assurance of your client's comfort and safety. After the waving lotion has been applied, remove the cotton, gently pat the skin with water-soaked cotton, and replace with dry cotton. (Fig. 11.49)

Unless otherwise specified in the product instructions, apply waving lotion liberally to the top and underside of each wound rod. Start at the crown area and progress systematically down each section. Be sure that the surface area of the wound curls is wet with lotion so penetration is even. (Fig. 11.50)

Processing Time

Processing time is the length of time required for the hair strands to absorb the waving lotion (softening) and for the hair to re-curl (rearrangement of chemical bonds). It depends on the hair type (porosity, elasticity, length, density, texture, and overall condition) and the specific perm you are using. Again, follow the manufacturer's directions explicitly. It is usually safe to anticipate the processing time to be less than suggested by the manufacturer or a client's previous record card. Some perms have stop-action processing so that all you have to do is set a timer. (Fig. 11.51) Some perms give you a general timetable to follow and require that you do a test curl during processing. It is very important to accurately time the perm process to help prevent over- or underprocessing.

The ability of the hair to absorb moisture may vary from time to time in the same individual, even when the same lotions and procedures are used. A record of the previous processing time is desirable, but should be used only as a guide.

Often, it is necessary to resaturate all the rods a second time during the processing time. This might be due to:

1. Evaporation of the lotion or dryness of the hair.
2. Hair poorly saturated by the cosmetologist.
3. No wave development after the maximum time indicated by the manufacturer.
4. Improper selection of solution strength for the client's hair.
5. Failure to follow the manufacturer's directions for a specific formula.

A reapplication of the lotion will hasten processing. Watch the wave development closely. ***Negligence can result in hair damage.***

Most manufacturers provide instructions with their product. Here are some you will encounter:

1. ***Place a plastic cap over the wrapped rods.*** Be sure that the plastic cap covers all the rods and that the cap is airtight. Secure the cap with a plastic clip. The cap holds in heat. If it is too loose or if all the rods are not covered, processing might take longer. (Fig. 11.52)

2. ***Pre-heated dryer.*** Turn the hood dryer to the high setting and medium airflow. Allow the dryer to warm up for approximately 5 minutes before placing your client under the dryer. (***Note:*** Dryer filters should be cleaned frequently so that optimum heat and airflow will remain constant.) (Fig. 11.53)

3. ***Process at room temperature.*** Make sure the client is not sitting in a draft or too close to an air conditioner. A room that is too cool slows the processing time.

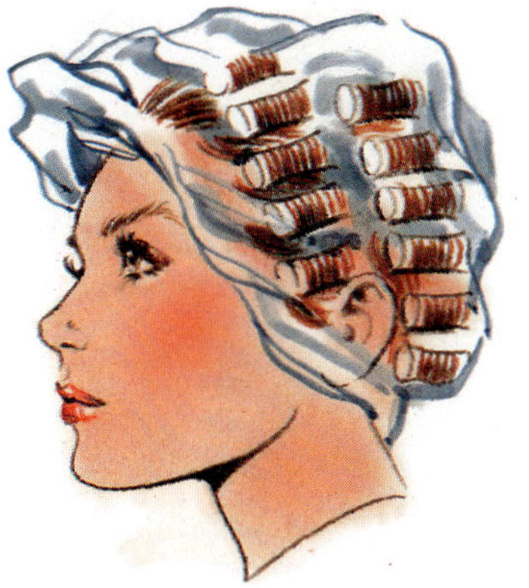

11.52—Applying processing cap.

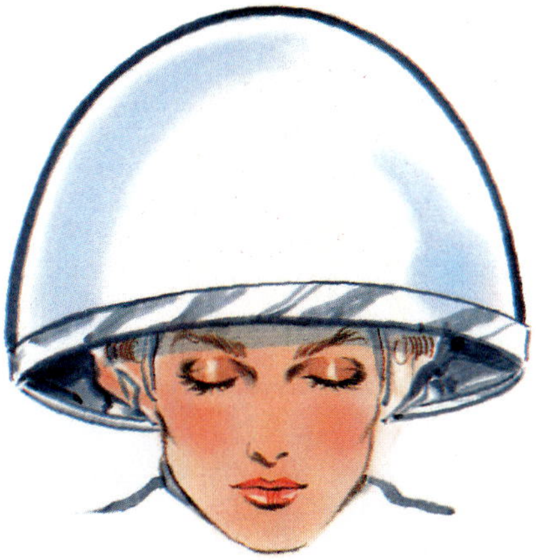

11.53 Putting client under pre-heated dryer.

Testing Curls during Processing

Optimum curl development occurs only once during the processing time. The ability to read a test curl "S" formation and recognize proper wave development will help you avoid two of the most common problems in perming: overprocessing and underprocessing. Three test curls should be taken: in the crown, on top of the head, and on the side of the head. These three locations will allow you to judge the progress of curl development on the most resistant and the least resistant areas of the head. Follow the procedure for unwinding the rod and checking the "S" pattern formation described in the preliminary test curl section (pages 210–211). (Fig. 11.54)

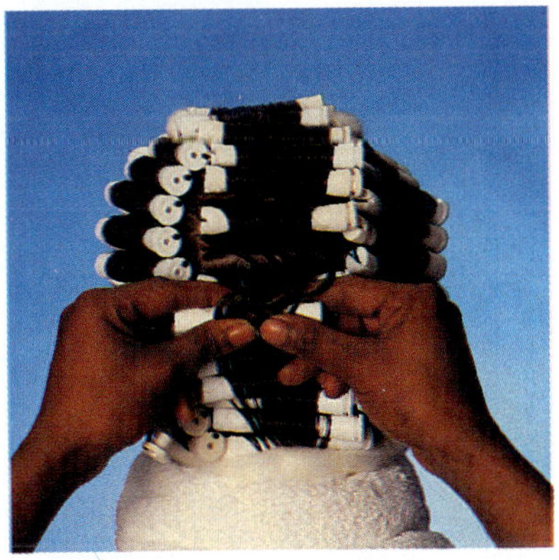

11.54—Properly processed strand opens up into "S" formation.

Water Rinsing

Rinsing the waving lotion from the hair is extremely important. Any lotion left in the hair can cause poor perm results. When your test curl indicates that optimum curl has been achieved, remove the cotton from around the hairline. Rinse the hair thoroughly with a moderate force of warm water. The manufacturer's perm directions will indicate how long you should rinse—usually 3 to 5 minutes. Always set your timer for the exact time. Remember, you are rinsing the lotion *out* of the internal hair structure, not merely off the surface. Make sure that all rods are thoroughly rinsed. Pay special attention to the rods at the nape of the neck. They are a little difficult to reach, but they must be rinsed as well as all the other rods.

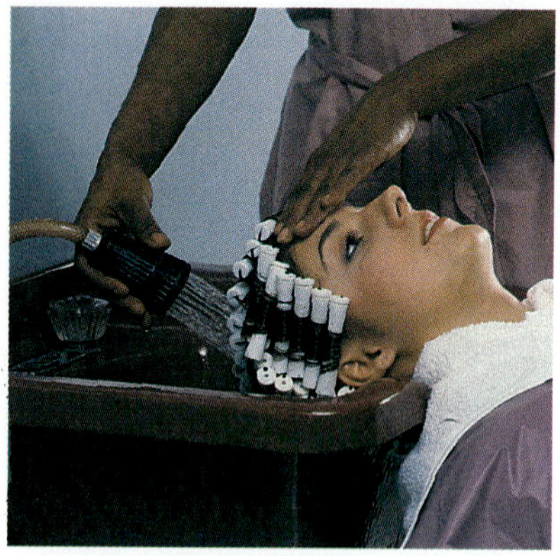

11.55—Rinsing waving lotion from the hair.

Long hair and thick hair usually require the maximum rinsing time (5 minutes) to make sure that the lotion has been removed from all the hair wrapped around the rods. (Fig. 11.55)

Undesirable effects of improper or incomplete rinsing include:

1. ***Early curl relaxation.*** Even if the perm has been processed correctly, any waving lotion left in the hair can interfere with the action of the neutralizer. If the neutralizer is not able to properly rebond the hair, the curl will be weak or will not last very long.
2. ***Lightening of hair color (natural or tint).*** Rinsing helps reduce the pH of the hair and helps to close the cuticle layer. If the hair is not rinsed properly, the hydrogen peroxide in the neutralizer can react with waving lotion left in the hair and cause the hair color to lighten. This lightening effect is usually seen on the hair ends.
3. ***Residual perm odor.*** If any waving lotion is left in the hair, it will become trapped inside the hair when the neutralizer is applied. This is especially true of acid-balanced perms. Unpleasant odors may be evident each time the hair gets wet or damp.

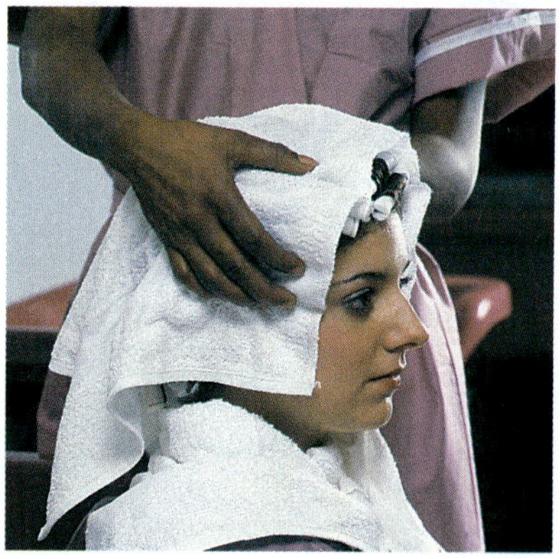

11.56—Towel blotting.

Blotting after Water Rinsing

Careful blotting assures that the neutralizer will penetrate the hair immediately and completely: Do not omit this important step. To obtain the best results from towel blotting, carefully press a towel between each curl, using your fingers. Do not rock or roll the rods while blotting. When the hair is in a softened state, any such movement can cause hair breakage. Change to dry towels frequently in order to remove as much excess water as possible. Excess water left in the hair can dilute or weaken the action of the neutralizer. If this happens the curl can be either weak or relaxed. (Fig. 11.56)

After rinsing and blotting has been completed, place a fresh, clean band of cotton around the hairline before applying neutralizer.

NEUTRALIZING

Neutralizing procedures can vary according to the perm product you are using. Again, follow the manufacturer's directions explicitly. In general, the following procedure is the accepted method for neutralizing:

1. Apply neutralizer to the top and underside of all rods. Apply to the top of the rod, then gently turn the rod up and apply to the underside of the rod in the same manner you applied the waving lotion.
2. Repeat the entire application a second time.

3. Wait 5 minutes to allow for optimum rebonding. Set a timer for accuracy. (Figs. 11.57, 11.58)
4. Remove the rods carefully and gently.
5. Work any remaining neutralizer through the hair gently with the palms of your hands.
6. Remove cotton from hairline and rinse the hair thoroughly with warm water.
7. Towel blot the hair.

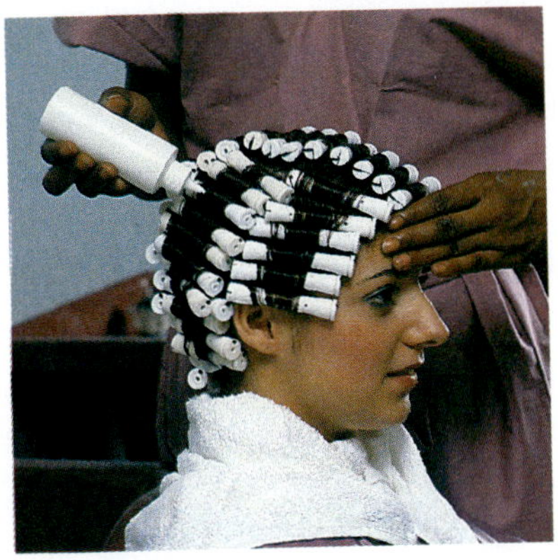
11.57—Neutralizing—direct or on-the-rod method.

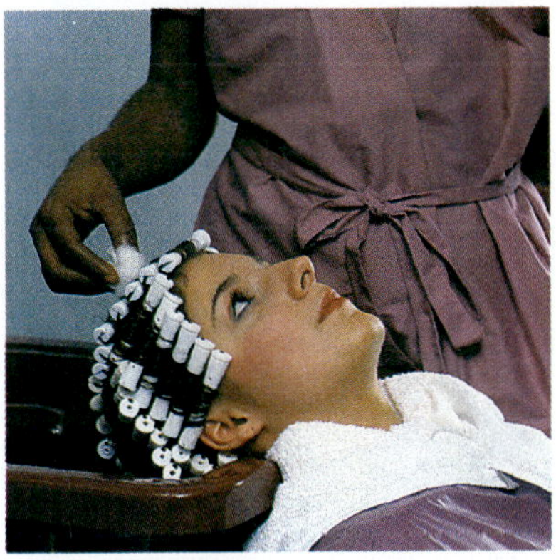
11.58—Neutralizing—splash-on method.

Post-Perm Precautions

After blotting, your new perm is ready for final shaping and styling. It is important to avoid shampooing, conditioning, stretching, or excessive manipulations of freshly permed hair. When styling, do not pull on the hair or use intense heat that could result in curl relaxation. Generally, hair should not be shampooed, conditioned, or treated harshly for 48 hours after perming. This special care will help ensure that the perm does not relax.

TEN POINTERS FOR A PERFECT PERM

1. Consult with the client.
2. Analyze the hair and scalp carefully.
3. Select the correct rod size for the desired style.
4. Choose the appropriate perm product for the hair type and final design. Follow the manufacturer's directions carefully.
5. Section and make accurate partings for each rod. Wrap specifically for the style chosen.
6. Apply waving lotion to the top and underside of all wound rods. Saturate thoroughly.
7. If the perm product requires a test curl, be sure the result is a firmly formed "S" shape.
8. Water rinse for at least 3 to 5 minutes and carefully towel blot each rod.
9. Apply neutralizer to the top and underside of all rods. Saturate thoroughly.
10. Wait 5 minutes, remove the rods carefully, apply any remaining neutralizer, and gently work through the hair. Rinse with warm water.

CLEANUP

1. Discard all used supplies.
2. Clean up the work area.
3. Thoroughly clean and sanitize the rods and implements.
4. Wash and sanitize your hands.
5. Complete the client record card.

SPECIAL PERMING TECHNIQUES

DIRECTIONAL WRAPPING

Directional wrapping refers to the angle of the partings, placement of the rods, and the wrapping pattern you choose to create specific direction or movement in the final design. There are six basic directions in which hair can be wrapped. (Figs. 11.59–11.70)

By using a combination of these basic wrapping directions you will be able to create very specific designs. Directional wrapping allows for lamp or natural drying and easier styling, particularly for the client. Use the following method for directional wrapping:

1. While the hair is wet, comb it in the direction that you want in your final design, including a part if one is required.
2. Use your fingers and a comb to mold a wave pattern as if you were finger waving.
3. Wrap the hair based on the direction of the design pattern.

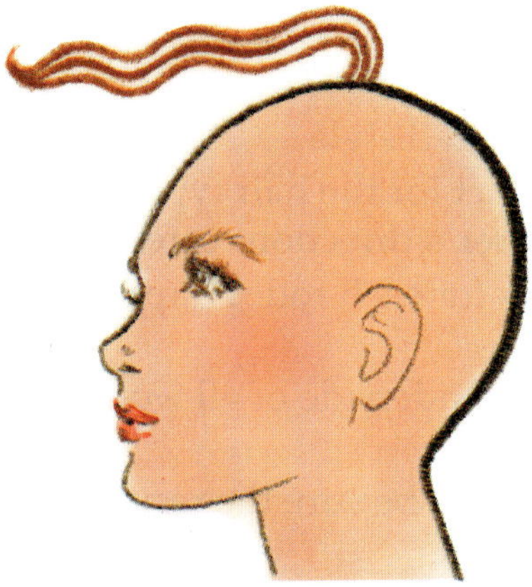

11.59—Vertical direction (forward).

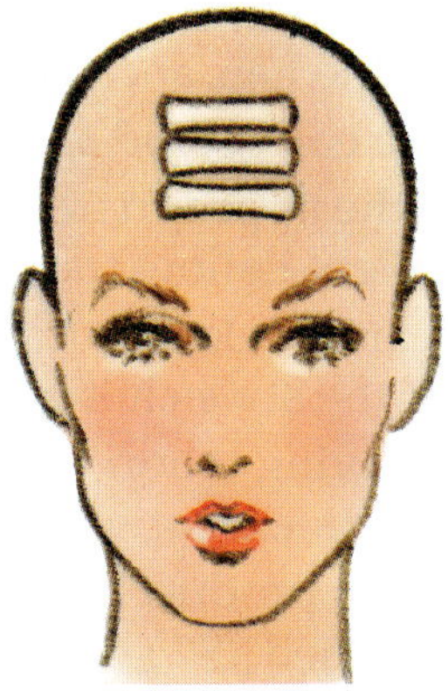

11.60—Forward blocking.

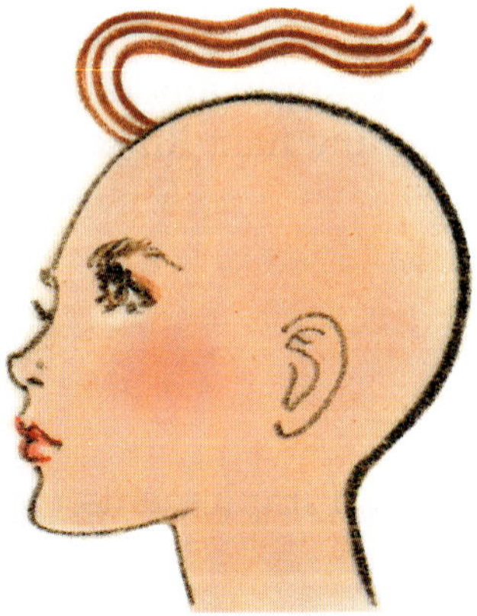

11.61—Vertical direction (back).

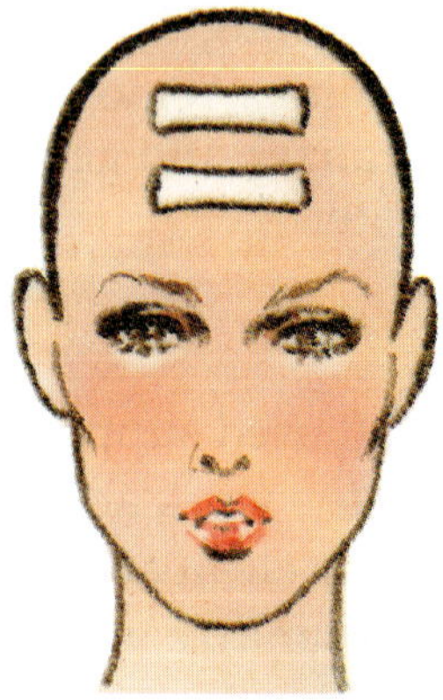

11.62—Back blocking.

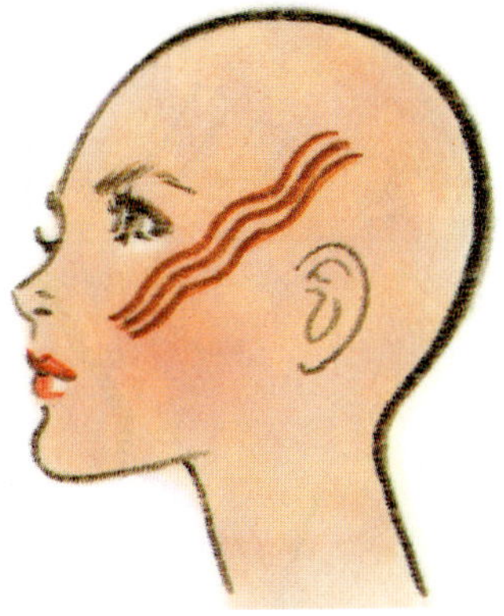

11.63—Horizontal direction (forward).

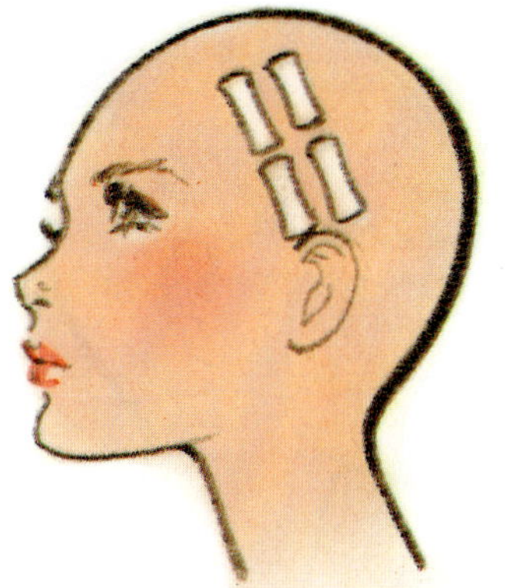

11.64—Forward blocking.

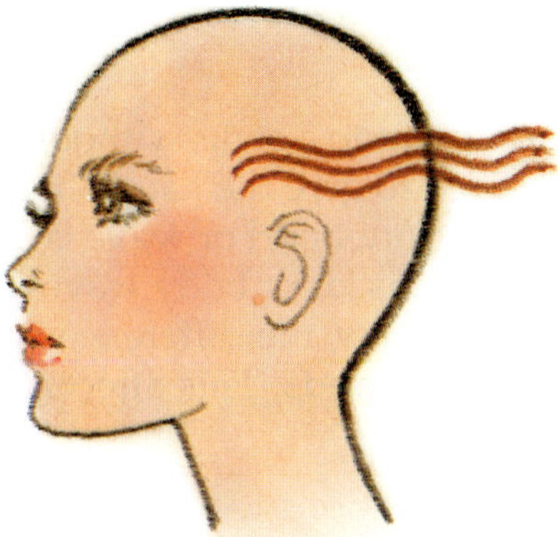

11.65—Horizontal direction (back).

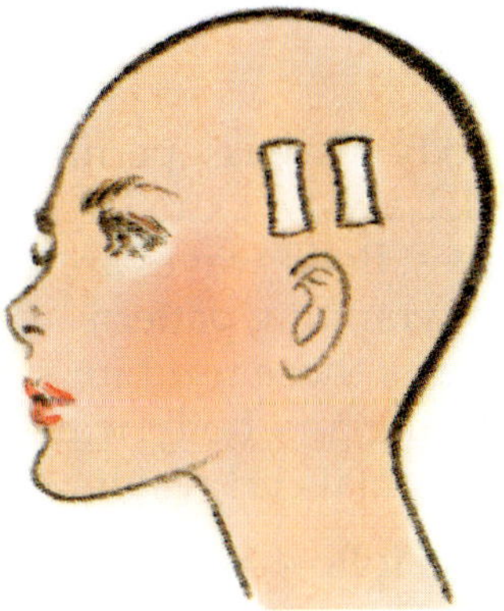

11.66—Back blocking.

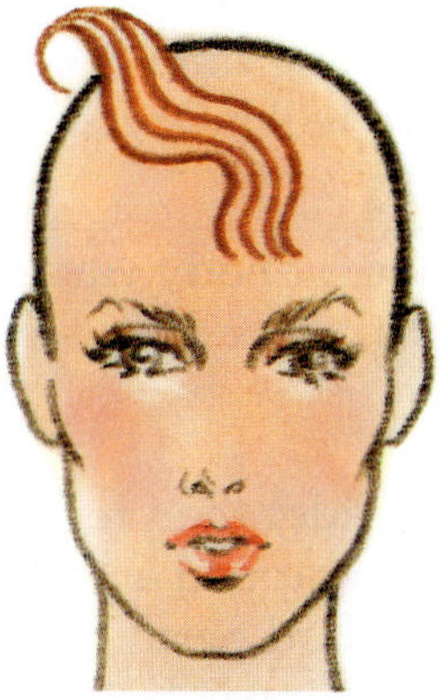

11.67—Diagonal direction (down).

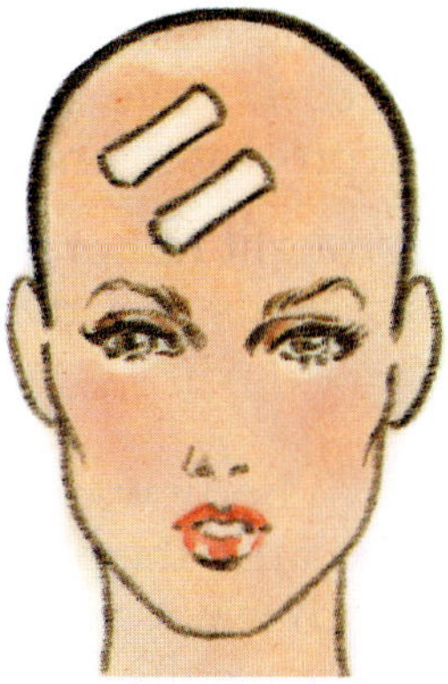

11.68—Diagonal blocking (down).

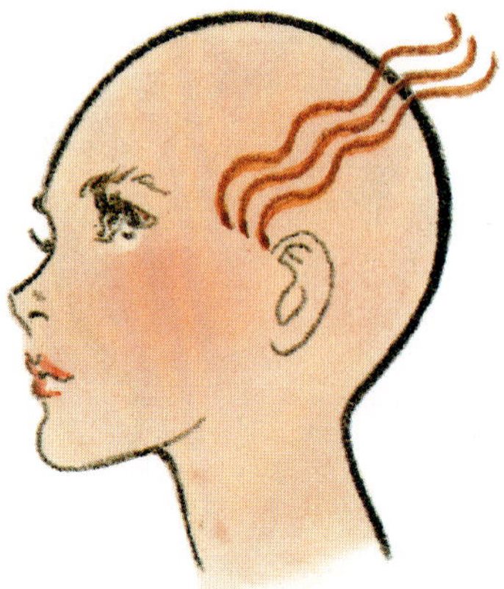

11.69—Diagonal direction (up).

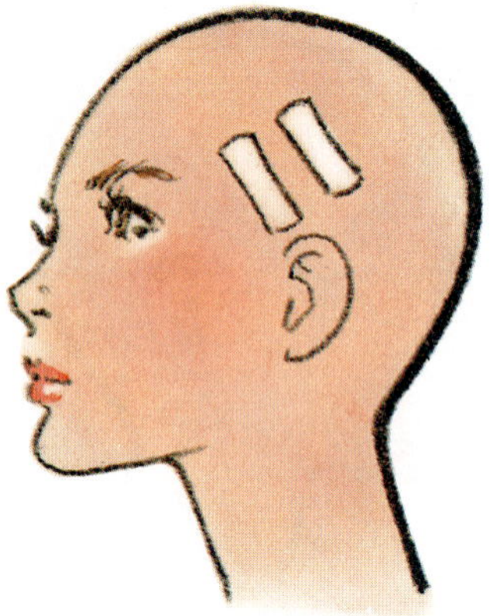

11.70—Diagonal blocking (up).

BODY WAVES

A body wave is a perm that gives support to a style, without definite curl. Large or extra large rods are used to give the hair softer, wider waves. Body waves are given when a softer curl or wave is desired. The wrapping patterns and techniques used for body waves are the same as those used for perming. Generally, the difference between perming and body waving is the size of rods. This affects the size of the final curl results.

The following are important considerations when giving a body wave:

1. Use large to extra large rods and make slightly larger partings. Do not take extra large partings or the waving lotion and neutralizer will not be able to penetrate all of the hair on the rod to properly form the curl/wave.
2. Follow perm directions regarding procedure, especially the processing time. Never reduce processing time to produce a softer curl/wave. Although the wave will be softer, it will be underprocessed and will not last very long.
3. Use straight rather than concave rods for body waving. The straight rods will give a more uniform wave from scalp to ends.

◆ NOTE: Body waves are softer and wider than regular perm curls because the physical force (hair wrapped around a very large rod) is not as great as in the standard perming method. The wave results from body waving will relax faster than a curl.

PARTIAL PERMING

Perming only a section of a whole head of hair is called ***partial perming.*** Partial perming can be used on:

1. Clients (male and female) who have long hair on the top and crown and very short, tapered sides and nape.
2. Clients who need volume and lift only in certain areas.
3. Designs that require curl support in the nape area but a smooth, sleek surface.

Partial perming uses the same techniques and wrapping patterns that you have already learned. There are a few extra considerations:

1. When you are wrapping the hair and reach the area that will be left unpermed, go to the next larger rod size so that the curl pattern of the permed hair will blend into the unpermed hair.
2. After wrapping the area to be permed, place a coil of cotton around the wrapped rods as well as around the entire hairline.
3. Before applying the waving lotion, apply a heavy, creamy conditioner to the sections that *will not* be permed to protect this hair from the effects of the waving lotion (waving lotion softens and straightens unwrapped hair).

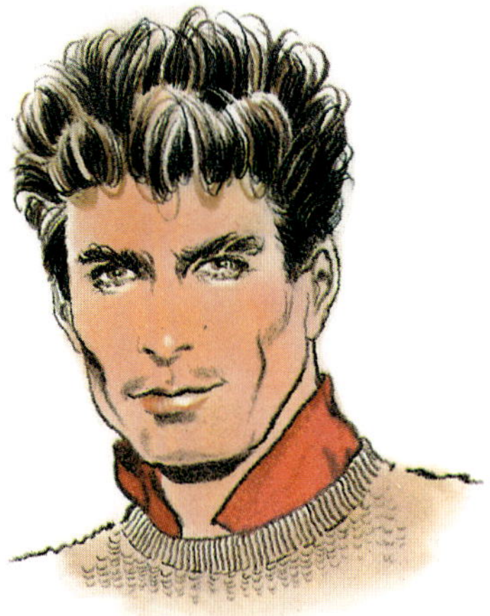

11.71—Man's short, curly style.

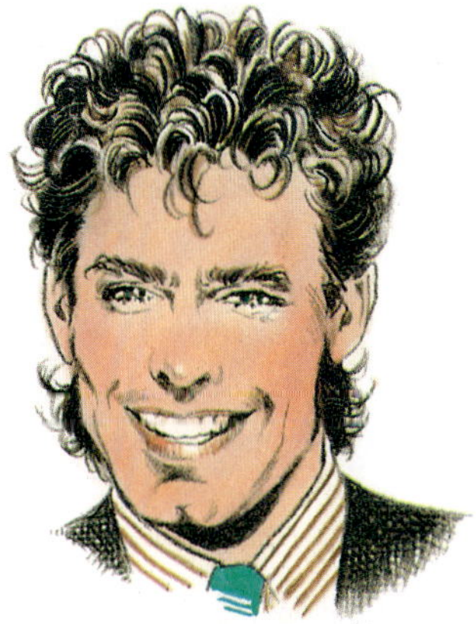

11.72—Man's medium length style.

PERMS FOR MEN

Many of your male clients need the added texture and fullness that only a perm can give. A perm can also help overcome common hair problems. A perm can redirect a cowlick, help limp or unmanageable hair more easily maintain a style, and make sparse hair look fuller.

Perming techniques are basically the same for both men and women. Most often, the partial perm technique gives you and your male clients the best results.

Keep in mind that men want waves for control. (Figs. 11.71–11.73)

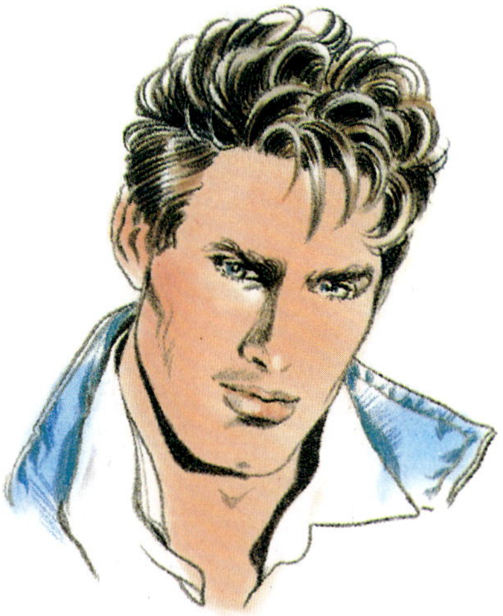

11.73—Man's short, wavy style.

HEATED CLAMP METHOD

This technique of perming involves the use of heated clamps applied directly over each wound rod. After the hair is wound on rods and thoroughly saturated with the waving lotion, a pre-heated clamp is placed on each curl. Processing begins as soon as the heat is applied. After the hair has been processed for a pre-determined period of time, the clamps are removed and the hair is rinsed and neutralized in the usual manner.

There are three special control features of the heated clamp method:

1. The temperature of the rods is strictly controlled.
2. The processing does not start until the heat is applied.
3. All curls are processed for exactly the same length of time.

SPECIAL SITUATIONS

There are certain hair types and conditions that require special attention. There also are hair types that should not be permed. If you have any doubt about perming the hair successfully, make a preliminary test curl.

1. Hair that shows signs of damage or breakage should not be permed. If the hair is excessively dry, brittle, or over-porous, it should be given reconditioning treatments until the condition improves and the damaged areas can be cut off. When you determine that the condition of the hair has improved, choose a mild perm formula and make a complete preliminary test curl before giving the perm.
2. Hair that has been previously treated with a sodium hydroxide or "no lye" relaxer (or any hair straightener that does not require a neutralizing step) should not be permed. Relaxers and perms break different bonds in the hair structure. Since the bonds are not all completely re-formed, the use of both products on the same hair can result in severe hair damage or breakage.
3. Tinted, bleached, highlighted/frosted, or previously permed hair in good condition can usually be permed successfully if the correct perm formula is chosen. Generally, these hair types vary in porosity so a product with a pre-wrap lotion to fill in porous areas is usually the best choice.

◆ NOTE: Tinted hair usually refers to hair that has been treated with a permanent hair color that is mixed with 20 volume peroxide. If the hair has been tinted with an ultralight shade or higher than 20 volume peroxide, it should be treated as bleached hair, which is usually more delicate and porous.

4. Hair treated with a semi-permanent hair color (color that is not mixed with peroxide/developer and therefore does not lighten the natural color) is frequently resistant to perming because semi-permanent color coats the surface of the hair and slows down penetration of the waving lotion. Hair treated

with a semi-permanent color should be considered more resistant than tinted or color-treated (tint mixed with peroxide) hair. Perming can also cause discoloration of semi-permanent color. If you perm hair that has been treated with a semi-permanent color, it might be necessary to apply a temporary rinse after perming in order to even out the color. One week after perming you may reapply the semi-permanent color to achieve more acceptable and long-lasting color results.

5. Hair color restorers or progressive hair color darkeners contain metallic salts. These metallic salts form a residue on the hair, which interferes with the action of the waving lotion and can result in very uneven curls, severe discoloration, or hair damage.

   To determine if hair has been treated with a hair color restorer or darkener, a 1-20 test is recommended. In a glass bowl, mix 1 oz (30 ml) of 20 volume peroxide and 20 drops of 28% ammonia. Into this mixture immerse at least 20 strands of hair for 30 minutes.

   - If there are no metallic salts present, the hair will lighten slightly. You can perm the hair.
   - If hair strands lighten very rapidly, the hair contains lead. Do not perm.
   - If there is no reaction after 30 minutes, the hair contains silver. Do not perm.
   - If the solution begins to boil within a few minutes and a very unpleasant odor is evident, plus the hair pulls apart easily, then the hair contains copper. Do not perm.

   Hair coated with metallic salts must not be permed. Do not perm until the product has been cut out of the hair. Rerun the 1-20 test to be sure that the hair is no longer coated with metallic salts before perming.

6. Unmanageable, naturally curly hair with an uneven curl pattern can be permed to form larger, more defined curls that are easier to manage. Generally, the procedure for a body wave (page 220) is the best approach. Keep in mind that naturally curly hair, even if it is coarse and dense, can be very porous, so choose the perm formula carefully.

7. Once the hair is permed, your client should return for another perm every 3 to 4 months depending on how quickly the hair grows, the type of curl given, and how frequently the hair is cut. Before re-perming, carefully analyze the hair again, and if necessary, use a pre-wrap lotion and/or a milder waving lotion formula. Note the product and procedure used and the results achieved on the client's record card. ✔

✔ Completed—Learning Objective No. 7

PERMING TECHNIQUES

REVIEW QUESTIONS

PERMANENT WAVING

1. Why is permanent waving beneficial to the client?
2. What is spiral wrapping?
3. What is croquignole wrapping?
4. What is a cold wave?
5. What is the purpose of a) waving lotion, b) neutralizer?
6. Define an acid-balanced perm.
7. What is "stop-action" processing?
8. What is an alkaline perm?
9. What is the main active ingredient or "reducing agent" in an a) alkaline perm, b) acid-balanced perm?
10. Name the acid-balanced perm that is heat activated by a chemical within the product.
11. What is the main ingredient in neutralizers?
12. What are the two main actions in permanent waving?
13. Define the three major components of hair.
14. Hair is composed almost entirely of a protein material called ____________________.
15. What bonds must be broken in order for the perming process to occur?
16. How do you decide which perming technique is right for your client?
17. Why is pre-perm analysis important?
18. What is hair porosity?
19. What is a pre-wrap lotion?
20. What is hair texture?
21. What two factors determine processing time?
22. What is hair elasticity?
23. Define hair density.
24. What factor determines the size of a curl?
25. Name two types of permanent wave rods.
26. Name two factors that must be considered in choosing rod size.
27. Why is sectioning and blocking important in permanent waving?
28. Name two rules to follow when wrapping a perm rod.
29. How must the hair be wrapped on a perm rod?
30. What is the purpose of end wraps?
31. What are the three methods of end wrap application?
32. What is a test curl and how is it taken?

HAIRCOLORING

12

LEARNING OBJECTIVES

AFTER COMPLETING THIS CHAPTER, YOU SHOULD BE ABLE TO:

1. Demonstrate the correct procedure for haircoloring, including consultation, analysis, and strand test procedures.
2. Explain the principles of color theory, and relate their importance to haircoloring.
3. List the classifications of haircolor, explain their activity on the hair, and give examples of their use.
4. Explain the activity of hydrogen peroxide in haircoloring.
5. Explain the uses of hair lighteners, and give examples of when each type of lightener would be preferred.
6. Demonstrate the single- and double-process tint application.
7. List preventative and corrective steps to avoid or solve haircoloring problems.
8. List the safety precautions to follow during haircolor procedures.

INTRODUCTION

Cosmetology is a career that offers you the opportunities to develop your creative talents in many different ways. One of the most exciting and challenging areas of creativity in your career as a professional cosmetologist will be haircoloring and lightening.

Haircoloring is both the science and the art of changing the color of hair. Haircoloring includes the processes of:

1. Adding artificial pigment to the natural hair color.
2. Adding artificial pigment to previously colored hair.
3. Adding artificial pigment to prelightened hair.
4. Diffusing natural pigment and adding artificial pigment in one step.

(The terms *tinting* and *coloring* are used interchangeably in this text.)

◆NOTE: Haircolor (one word) is an industry-coined term referring to artificial haircolor products and services. Hair color (two words) is the color of hair created by nature.

Hair lightening, or decolorizing, involves the diffusing of the natural or artificial color from the hair. Hair lightening involves the processes of:

1. Decolorizing the natural pigment to prepare the hair for the final color.
2. Decolorizing the natural or artificial pigment to the desired color.
3. Decolorizing the natural or artificial pigment for corrective coloring.
4. Decolorizing the natural or artificial pigment in selected areas (highlighting).

These are profitable sources of salon income because coloring represents repeat business. The client who has tinted or lightened hair usually returns for retouching at regular intervals. Satisfactory service and trust in their colorist encourages clients to remain loyal to the same salon.

Your success as a colorist depends only on the time and energy you are prepared to give to the continuous study and practice of your haircoloring skills. As you expand your skills and gain confidence, you may choose to specialize in haircoloring services, similar to medical professionals who practice in and develop one area of expertise.

Thanks to the styling revolution of the 1960s and 1970s, there are many stylists who have mastered hair cutting or perming, and concentrate their energies solely on these frequently requested services. Add *color* to that great haircut and perfect texture, and you've got a powerful attention-getting combination. Specialist hair colorists are less common than cutters, and their skills are in increasingly high demand due to renewed publicity and popularity.

Cosmetologists willing to develop their coloring skills and expertise can serve the needs of a huge and growing clientele.

REASONS CLIENTS COLOR THEIR HAIR

1. Graying

- To conceal premature graying.
- To keep and enhance their natural white or gray and eliminate yellow.

2. Self-Image Boost

- To alleviate boredom or depression.
- To promote a more professional appearance.

3. Experimental

- To subtly enhance their existing hair color.
- To create a fashion statement or trend that expresses their personality.

4. Artistic

- To accent their hairstyle design, making it look more finished.
- To enhance or minimize their features, using color to create illusions.

5. Corrective

- To eliminate the damaged look of sun-lightened hair ends.
- To remove the unsightly cast of chlorine or minerals caused by their water.
- To improve upon the results of previous color experimentation.

Almost everyone at one time or another has considered doing something a little different with their hair. Our potential clients may have already done some experimentation at home or in another salon by changing their haircut or style, their hair texture by perming, or their hair's natural color.

With the emergence and availability of nonprofessional products that your clients can buy, why should they come to you, a professional colorist, for advice and service? And who are the "typical" haircoloring clients today? (Fig. 12.1)

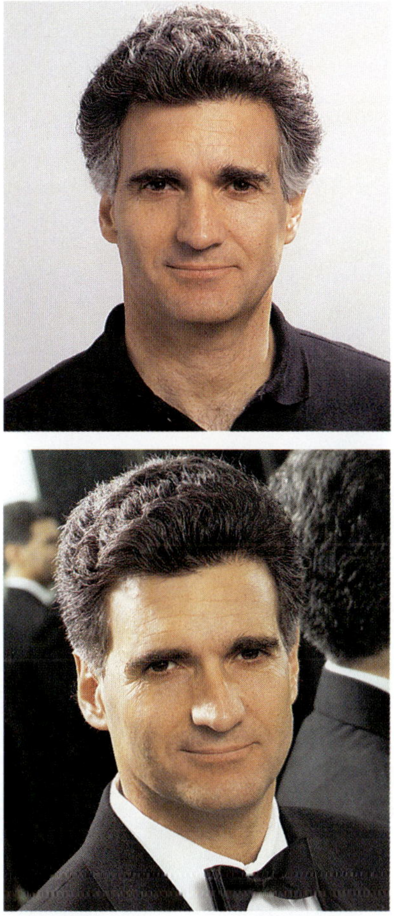

12.1—There are many reasons clients choose to color their hair. To cover gray hair is one. (Hair: Frederic Fekhai. Color: Mark Wofford. Both for Keralogie L'Oreal Technique Professionnelle. Photo: Keith Trumbo.)

TYPICAL CLIENTS

Haircoloring offers a wide variety of choices and therefore attracts the attention and interest of anyone who wants to look good and feel better. Gone are the stereotypes of the obviously tinted client—the damaged hair, the flat or unnatural appearance. Typical are those clients who want to cover or enhance their gray; teens, women, and men who enjoy frequent fashion changes; clients currently unhappy with their natural color or who want to improve the shine and texture of their hair; and current haircoloring clients who come in for their retouch applications and a little relaxation time to themselves. Even the male clientele for haircolor is growing rapidly and is expected to be the fastest growing category of haircoloring client this decade. (Fig. 12.2)

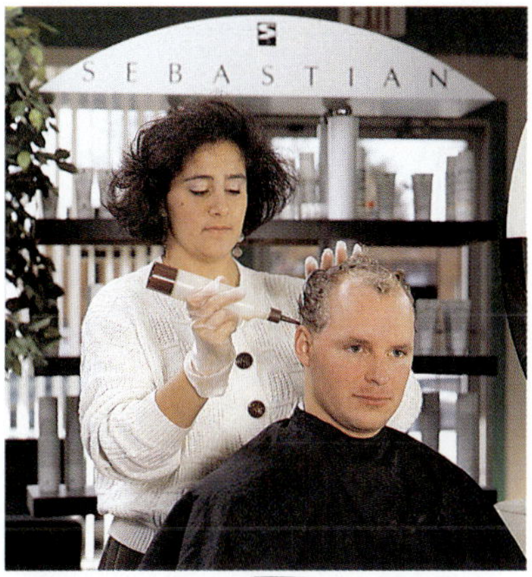

12.2—Haircoloring is a popular service for the male clientele today.

As a trained professional hair colorist, you will have access to licensed professional-only products that far surpass the ones your clients can purchase in selection, performance, and stability. You will have knowledge of which colors look best on your clients, which products and application techniques will best achieve the desired look, how to choose these products and customize them to fit hair conditions at different times of the year, and how haircoloring and lightening products will react on clients' hair. The key to your success in haircoloring is communication.

With continuously increasing technology and the latest advancements in haircolor education, haircoloring manufacturers are moving to standardize terminology to simplify learning and provide greater assistance to colorists.

◆ NOTE: This chapter contains many technical terms. You should refer to the Haircoloring Glossary on pages 311–318, which was prepared by the International Haircolor Exchange to provide a standard vocabulary of haircoloring for our industry.

THE COLORIST'S ROLE IN CLIENT COMMUNICATION

Observe

Simple observation gives you a chance to use your training and analyze clients' needs. Your eyes are your primary information-gathering tool. The following is a list of factors about hair that influence color choice. With time and practice, you will notice certain physical characteristics relevant to haircolor selection immediately upon seeing a client for the first time. These are items you will need to note when observing clients prior to a haircoloring service:

- Color Level
- Color Tone
- Eye Color
- Skin Tone
- Length
- Porosity
- Density
- Texture
- Form
- Percentage of Gray

Each of these will be described in detail as we go through a typical haircolor consultation.

The consultation is a time when your greeting and appearance are most impressive. The greeting establishes your credibility and trustworthiness. Your professional appearance, confident mannerisms, and use of professional industry terminology will establish you as an authority in a client's eyes.

You only have one chance to make a first impression on your clients so make it a good one. You, and you alone, are responsible for the image you project. Make sure your clients and potential clients see you as you want them to. Establish and maintain eye contact, make clients comfortable, and listen.

Listen

Listening allows you to find out how clients view their needs. The finest formulation combined with the most talented application will still result in color failure if clients are dissatisfied.

Despite all the activity in a busy salon, clients' thoughts are centered mainly on their own concerns. So naturally, all clients expect to be treated with courtesy and attention. The cosmetologist who recognizes this fact and gives clients respect, courtesy, and attention will win their confidence. And, when this cosmetologist sincerely recommends a haircolor service, clients are likely to listen carefully and seriously consider the recommendation.

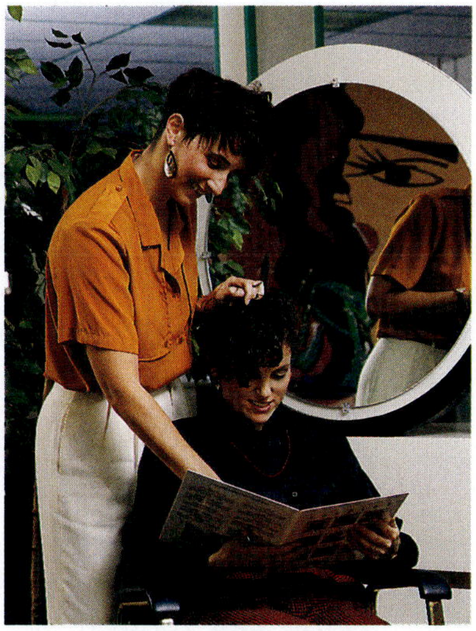

12.3—Good communication is essential when discussing a haircoloring service with a client.

Make Suggestions

To recommend a haircolor service with sincerity means to suggest a color only when you honestly believe that your clients would be happier and more attractive with the color service. You must be attentive to your clients' needs by listening closely, by being genuinely interested, and by treating every client as you would like to be treated yourself in the same situation. In doing so, you can be confident that your choice will reflect and meet your clients' needs, improve your clients' appearance, and enhance your reputation as a colorist. (Fig. 12.3)

Explain Time and Monetary Investment Involved

At the completion of your consultation, you should have an agreement with your clients as to what is needed, how long it will take, and how much it will cost.

Determine a Solution to Fulfill the Client's Needs

Haircolor is a wonderful service, and can make a tremendous difference for your client. Whether you choose a subtle change or something quite dramatic, the opportunity to create is greatly enhanced by being able to offer a haircolor service.

In the following pages, you will learn how to analyze your clients' needs and choose and perform a haircolor service. There are many choices and considerations. Haircoloring is an art, something to be learned over time, not simply by reading books. The people who walk into your salon to become your clients bring not only their hair, but their likes and dislikes, their hopes and dreams—a whole wealth of experiences in which you can share. Take your time, look carefully, listen well, and offer the gift of your art.

Career Path

COLOR SPECIALIST

Surveys of cosmetology students, stylists, managers, and salon owners have revealed that a lack of expertise in haircoloring is a major concern in the beauty industry. This fact can be financially devastating as haircoloring can easily become the number-one money maker in any salon. Because of this, salons are always looking for color specialists. If you have an eye for color and the willingness to work hard on becoming educated in this tricky area, you're almost guaranteed a job.

A color specialist may run the color department at a large salon, or may simply be the resident color stylist in a smaller salon. In either case, he or she will be expected to consult with clients and give advice on what color best suits them and which of the myriad of choices will best fit their needs—highlighting, permanent or semi-permanent color, nonperoxide color, and so on. Selling color and educating clients about the care and maintenance of colored hair are part of the job.

A color specialist can also teach private seminars, be a spokesperson for a large manufacturer, or even service celebrity clients and models.

The key to becoming a color specialist is to continue your education far beyond obtaining your license. Take advanced color courses whenever possible, attend seminars and workshops, attend shows, and buy all the haircolor videos and books you can. Most hairstylists know something about color; few know it in depth. Once you've learned all you can from others, it will be necessary to practice coloring again and again. Find a salon with a good color department and let the owner know you're interested in a career in color. Often other colorists will be willing to help you, since the field is open.

HAIRCOLOR CONSULTATION

The consultation is one of the most important steps in the haircoloring service. But first there are other important elements to consider that will allow you to "set the stage" for your consultation success.

SETTING THE STAGE: THE PROPER ENVIRONMENT

Adequate Lighting

Light, and how it plays with haircolor, is of prime importance to the hair colorist. Bright natural light makes haircolor appear different than does dim light. Electric lights of varying intensities and hues also alter the eye's perspective of color.

Perform the consultation in a well-lighted room, preferably with natural lighting. If this is not possible, arrange lighting so that there is incandescent in front of clients (around the mirror) and fluorescent behind the colorist (ceiling fixtures).

Incandescent lighting alone will make the hair and skin tones appear warmer than they truly are; fluorescent lighting alone has a cool cast and will give the skin and hair a pale and unnatural "gray" appearance. Always remember to consider the lighting in which your clients will most often see themselves; a beautifully subtle highlight in natural sunlight may disappear under office lighting. Conversely, a strong, attractive color in your salon lighting could become neon looking in the sunlight.

The best mix of lighting for haircolor is to use full-spectrum white fluorescent tubes, or consider adding track lighting spot lights (incandescent) to existing fluorescent lighting in most buildings.

Color of Consultation Area

Privacy and good lighting are important. Ideally, a separate room (or area) in the salon should be reserved specifically for consultations. If possible, the walls should be white or neutral, and neutral draping should be used to conceal the clients' street clothes, especially if they are strong colors that may influence your perception of the clients' hair and skin tonality. This would also be an excellent time for clients to put on chemical smocks to protect their clothes from stains.

Gathering and Utilizing Color Consultation Tools

In your consultation room or area, you will keep all of your professional haircoloring consultation tools—items that will make communication with your clients go smoothly. Keep a haircolor portfolio of your work or magazines and picture books with different haircolor levels, tones, intensities, and application techniques, so clients can show you the general hair color they have in mind. Ink colors on the page will not exactly match colored pigments in the hair, but if you tell your clients this you will both still be able to use these tools as a guide to understanding the desired color.

Manufacturers' paper color charts and haircolor swatches, although showing color on white paper or on white hair, will at least give you an idea of clients' wishes. After all, your idea of red and a client's idea of red may be different—as different as strawberry blonde and burgundy. Manufacturers also make available to colorists their natural level haircolor swatches, to help you judge the natural hair color depth or level based on their color product's system. (Fig. 12.4)

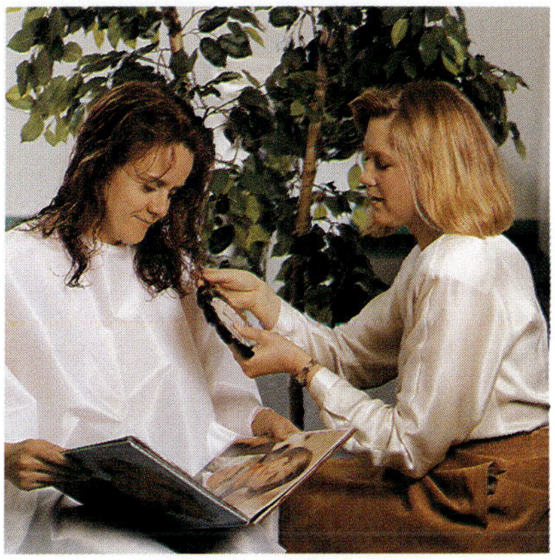

12.4—Use style books and color charts and swatches when consulting with a client on a haircolor service.

A client record card (see page 234) will be necessary to transfer your hair analysis, testing, and consultation information into a permanent file, along with your client's release statement. This is discussed more fully later. You will also want to gather together your materials for strand and predisposition tests, which will be performed prior to each service in this chapter.

STRAND TEST TO CONFIRM COLOR SELECTION

Before applying a tint, conduct a preliminary strand test to confirm your selection. You will learn the following information:

1. Whether the proper color selection was made.
2. Timing needed to achieve the desired results.
3. If further preconditioning treatments are needed.
4. If it is necessary to apply a filler.

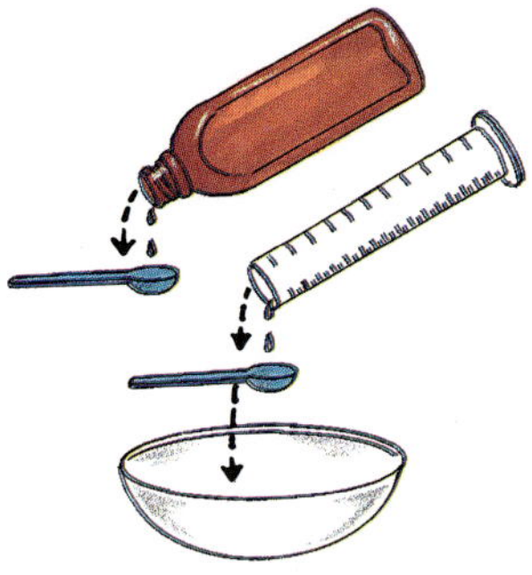

12.5—Mix color with peroxide.

Strand Test Procedure

1. Mix a small amount of color with peroxide according to the manufacturer's directions, using plastic measuring spoons to ensure accuracy of proportions. (Fig. 12.5)
2. Apply mixture to a ½" (.125 cm) section, usually in the crown area of the head. (Remember to test each area where the color varies. More than one formula may be necessary to achieve even results.)

◆ NOTE: It is important that the hair has received all pretreatments necessary according to your analysis before the strand test is given, so that the results will be accurate.

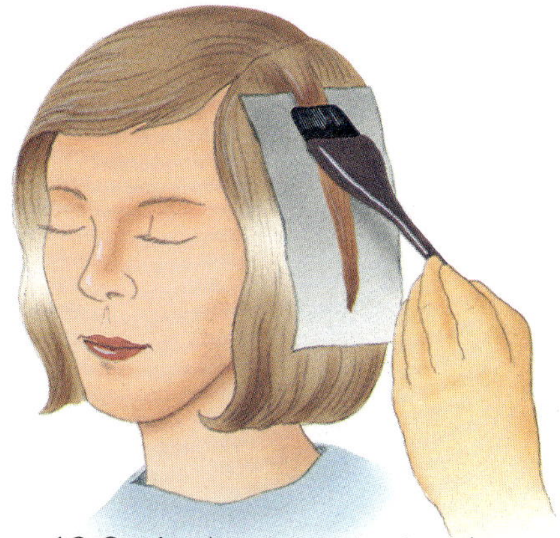

12.6—Apply mixture to strand.

3. Separate the strand from the rest of the hair using foil or plastic wrap. Process with or without heat according to the manufacturer's directions, keeping careful records of timing on the client's record card. (Fig. 12.6)
4. Rinse strand, shampoo, towel dry, and examine results. (Fig. 12.7) Adjust formula, timing, or precondition as necessary and proceed with tinting on the entire head.
5. If results are unsatisfactory, adjust the formula and repeat the process on a new test strand.

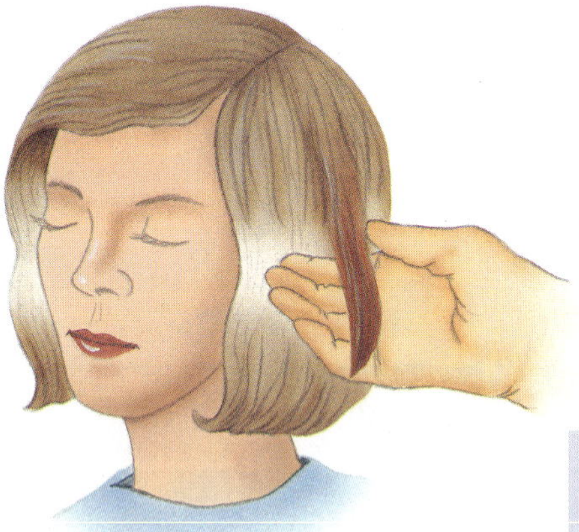

12.7—Examine results.

C A U T I O N

A predisposition test must be given before coloring the hair with an aniline derivative product. The client should be draped to protect clothing. Operator dermatitis, although rare, involves the same types of negative reactions to chemicals as the client can experience. Since a colorist's hands are in water and contact chemical solutions repeatedly throughout an average day, it is important to take proper precautions. You should protect yourself from allergic reactions by wearing gloves until the product is completely removed from the client's hair.

◆ NOTE: For further information regarding chemicals in the cosmetology field, refer to the Occupational Safety Hazards Act Guidelines. Safety data sheets are, by law, available from each manufacturer, detailing the materials of concern to cosmetologists in each of their products. Each workplace in every industry is now required to have these sheets on hand to explain the uses, possible health hazards, and safety procedures for products you may encounter in your profession.

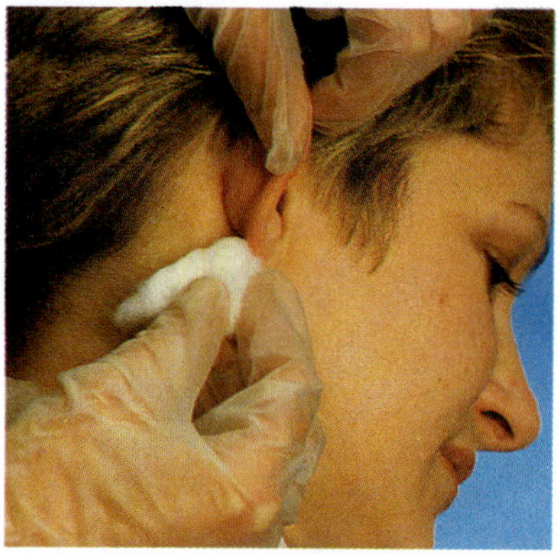

12.8—Clean patch test area.

PREDISPOSITION TEST

Allergy to aniline derivative tints is unpredictable. Some clients may be sensitive, and others may suddenly develop a sensitivity after years of use. To identify an allergic client, the U.S. Federal Food, Drug, and Cosmetic Act prescribes that a patch or predisposition test be given 24 to 48 hours prior to each application of an aniline tint or toner. The tint used for the skin test must be the same formula as that used for the haircoloring service.

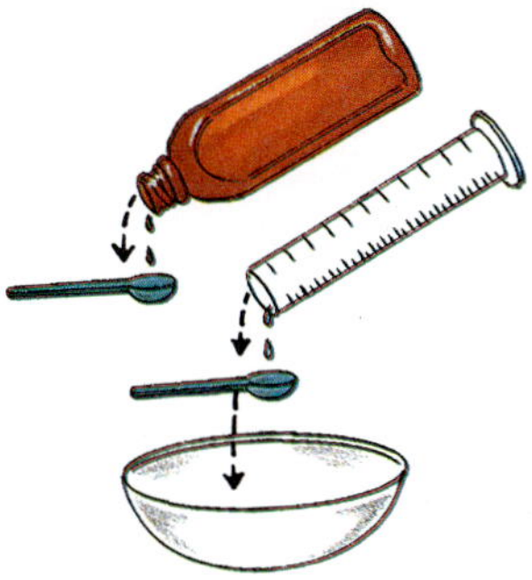

12.9—Mix tint and peroxide.

Procedure

1. Select a test area—behind one ear extending into the hairline or at the inside bend of the elbow.
2. Using a mild soap, cleanse an area about the size of a quarter. (Fig. 12.8)
3. Dry the area.
4. Prepare the test solution according to the manufacturer's directions. (Fig. 12.9)
5. Apply to test area with a sterile cotton swab. (Fig. 12.10)
6. Leave the area undisturbed for 24 to 48 hours.
7. Examine the test area.
8. Note results on the client's record card.

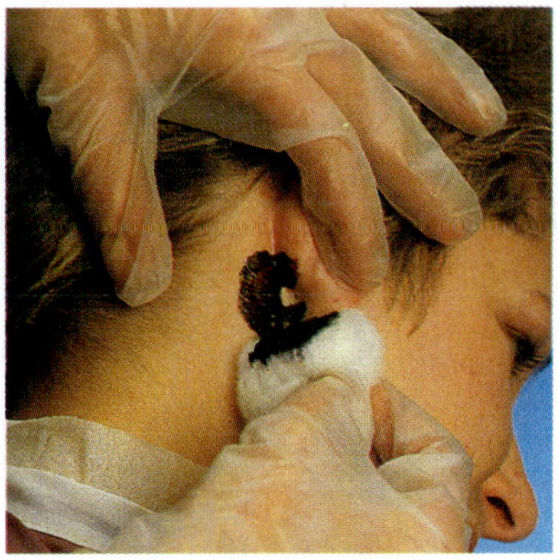

12.10—Apply tint mixture.

A negative skin test will show no sign of inflammation, and color may be safely applied. If the skin test is positive, you will see redness, swelling, burning, itching, or blisters. A client with these symptoms is allergic, and under no circumstances should receive the color service for which the test was performed. Application in this instance could result in a serious reaction for the client, and a malpractice suit for the hair colorist.

CAUTION

Aniline derivative tints must never be used on the eyelashes or eyebrows. To do so may cause blindness.

HAIRCOLOR RECORD

Name ______________________ Tel. ______________________

Address ______________________ City ______________________

Patch Test: ☐ Negative ☐ Positive Date ______________________

DESCRIPTION OF HAIR

Form	**Length**	**Texture**	**Density**	**Porosity**	
☐ straight	☐ short	☐ coarse	☐ sparse	☐ very porous	☐ resistant
☐ wavy	☐ medium	☐ medium	☐ moderate	☐ porous	☐ very resistant
☐ curly	☐ long	☐ fine	☐ thick	☐ normal	☐ perm. waved

Natural hair color ______________________

Level	Tone	Intensity
(1-10)	(Warm, Cool, etc.)	(Mild, Medium, Strong)

Condition

☐ normal ☐ dry ☐ oily ☐ faded ☐ streaked (uneven)

% of gray ________ Distribution of gray ______________________

Previously lightened with______________________for ____________(time)

Previously tinted with______________________for ____________(time)

☐ original hair sample enclosed ☐ original hair sample not enclosed

Desired hair color ______________________

Level	Tone	Intensity
(1-10)	(Warm, Cool, etc.)	(Mild, Medium, Strong)

CORRECTIVE TREATMENTS

Color filler used ______________ Conditioning treatments with ____________

HAIR TINTING PROCESS

whole head ____________retouch inches (cm) ________shade desired ____________

formula: (color/lightener) ____________ application technique ____________

Results: ☐ good ☐ poor ☐ too light ☐ too dark ☐ streaked

Comments: ______________________

____

____

____

____

Date	**Operator**	**Price**	**Date**	**Operator**	**Price**

CLIENT RECORD CARD

Always record the consultation on the client's record card. It is important to keep an accurate record so that successful services can be repeated and any difficulties encountered in one service may be avoided in the next. A complete record should be kept, containing all analysis notes, strand test and whole head results, timing, and suggestions for the next service.

RELEASE STATEMENT

A release statement is used for chemical services. It is designed to release the school or salon owner from responsibility for accidents or damages and is required for some malpractice insurance. A release statement is not a legally binding contract, however, and will not absolve the cosmetologist of responsibility for what has occurred to the client's hair. It is now used primarily to explain fully to clients whose hair is in questionable condition that their hair may not withstand the requested chemical treatment. It also encourages clients to be more truthful about any prior chemical experimentation that may affect your color selection and end result.

RELEASE FORM

I, the undersigned, ______________________________.
(name)

residing at ______________________________.
(street, address)

______________________________.
(city, state and zip)

about to receive services in the Clinical Department of

______________________________.

and having been advised that the services shall be performed by either students, graduate students, and/or instructors of the school, in consideration of the nominal charge for such services, hereby release the school, its students, graduate students, instructors, agents, representatives, and/or employees, from any and all claims arising out of and in any way connected with the performance of these services.

The Proprietor Is Not Responsible for Personal Property

Signed ______________________________.

Date ______________________________.

Witnessed ______________________________.

THIS RELEASE FORM MUST BE SIGNED BY THE PARENT OR GUARDIAN IF THE CLIENT BEING SERVED IS UNDER 21 YEARS OF AGE.

ANALYZING THE CLIENT'S HAIR PHYSIOLOGY

No two people are exactly alike. And no two heads of hair are exactly the same. Even an individual client's hair will vary from season to

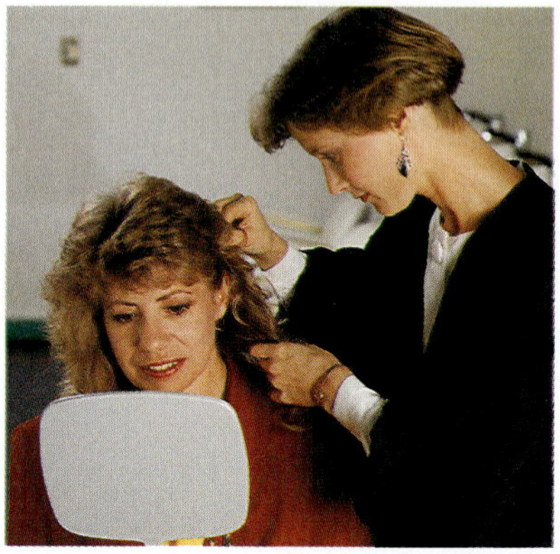

12.11—It is important to analyze a client's hair before performing a haircolor service.

season and from year to year. Every person has a natural hair color that is either a dark color, a medium color, or a light color, but no two people have exactly the same hair color. Inside the hair shaft, where you cannot see, the factors that create or affect hair color are always different from person to person. That is why the same hair-coloring formula and procedure will produce a different result for every client. (Fig. 12.11)

How Hair Structure Relates to Coloring

The hair is a remarkable and resilient fiber. Every haircolor service will affect or be affected by the structure of the hair. Some haircolor products cause a dramatic change in the hair's structure; others affect it very little. When a product significantly changes the hair structure, it usually creates a weaker strand of hair.

Knowing how products affect the structure will allow you to make choices. Your perceptions of what the hair can or cannot tolerate will allow you to be the best judge of what is most appropriate for each client. Briefly, we'll take a look at the structure of the hair and how nature creates color.

Generally every hair on a person's head is composed of three parts: the cuticle, the cortex, and the medulla. The ***medulla*** is at the innermost center of the hair shaft. The ***cuticle*** is the outermost layer of the hair. It is made up of overlapping bands of keratinized protein that is very similar to the protein that makes up our fingernails. It is translucent, allowing diffused light to pass through. The cuticle protects the interior cortex layer of the hair. The shiny appearance of the hair is dependent on this cuticle layer being smooth and intact. A healthy cuticle contributes 20% to the overall strength of the hair.

The ***cortex*** is the second layer of the hair. The natural color we see in the hair is in this layer. The cortex structure is made up of elongated, fibrous cells bundled together. Melanin pigment granules are scattered between the cortex cells. These granules are imbedded in the cortex layer like the chips in a chocolate chip cookie. The strength and elasticity of the hair are dependent on the cortex layer being intact. A healthy cortex contributes 80% to the overall strength of the hair.

Hair ***texture*** is described as the diameter of the individual hair strand. The terms *coarse, medium,* and *fine* are used to differentiate between large, medium, and small diameters. Texture has an effect on hair color because the hair's natural melanin pigment is distributed differently in the different textures. Each diameter also has a different resistance to the changes haircolor chemicals make on the hair shaft. (Fig. 12.12)

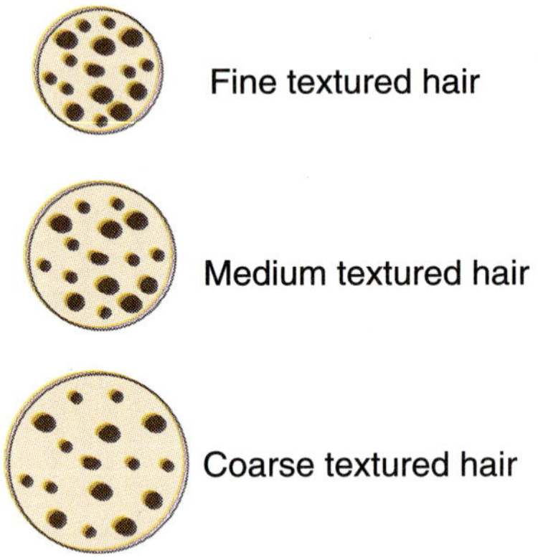

12.12—Diameters of various hair strands. The fine strand appears darker because the pigment is more closely grouped together.

Fine-textured hair's pigment is grouped more tightly together. Because of this tighter grouping, when you deposit color, you will have a darker result on fine hair. By the same token, fine hair is less resistant to lightening because there is less structure to resist the chemical. When lightening fine hair, a milder lightener can be used successfully.

Medium-textured hair will have average responses to haircolor products. Note any variations in texture throughout the hair. The face-line hair is usually finer in texture than the hair farther back on the head.

Coarse-textured hair has a more open grouping of hair pigment due to the larger diameter hair shaft in which the pigment is located. Because of this open grouping, you will have a slightly lighter result when depositing color. When lightening the hair, you will encounter greater resistance to the lightener, and a stronger lightening product may be needed.

Porosity is necessary for color to take properly. Each product we put on the hair requires a different degree of porosity.

Porosity, in simple terms, is the ability of the hair to absorb moisture. Porous hair will accept liquid (haircolor for example) more readily than nonporous hair. Uneven porosity can create problems if even color results are desired.

As hair grows longer, the ends are subject to frequent shampooing, drying, styling, and environmental influences. There will be visual and textural changes. The cuticle will be slightly abraded (worn away), and the rough hair fiber will lose some of its flexibility, body, and shine. There will also be some variation in color from strand to strand and even from the scalp area to the midshaft. Hair may be lighter and more faded out toward the ends.

This longer, older hair is described as overporous, a condition in which hair reaches an undesirable level of porosity. This hair will respond differently to haircolor products than the newer hair closer to the scalp. Those different responses can only be determined by performing a strand test. As a general rule, overporous hair will look more dull or flat and reflect more cool tones, while the healthier hair will reflect more warm tones.

Occasionally, a client's hair has a cuticle so smooth and compact that we need to create the proper porosity for the success of our haircoloring service. This hair is considered *resistant* to the swelling effects of alkalies that allow haircolor to penetrate, and, if necessary, cover gray hair. Presoftening of gray or resistant hair will be covered later. (Fig. 12.13)

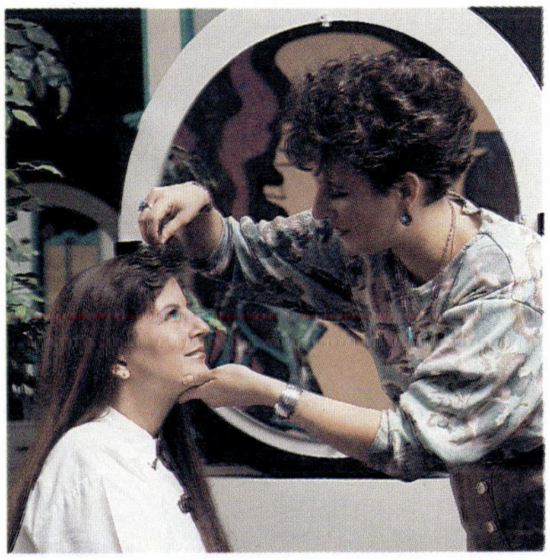

12.13—Checking the porosity of hair before a coloring service is important.

Hair ***density*** is the number of hairs per square inch on the scalp. Hair can be described as *sparsely, moderately,* or *thickly* distributed on the head. It is important to notice that hair density varies, even on the same head. For some, the hair around the face line is more sparsely distributed, and the hair over the crown is more densely distributed. For others, the opposite is true.

Note the variations in density. The dense areas of your clients' hair will require more product and a more careful application. Remember, for haircolor to work effectively, each hair shaft must be surrounded by product. (Fig. 12.14)

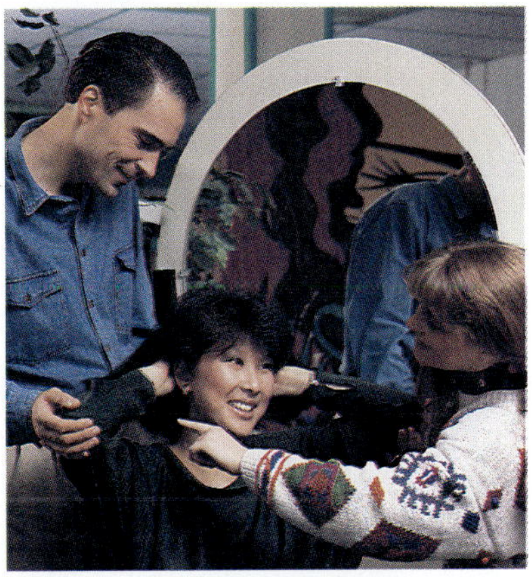

12.14—Note the variations in hair density prior to a haircoloring application.

Hair ***length*** will be a factor in your haircolor choice. The hair on our heads grows an average of ½" per month. This translates to 6" per year. If your client's hair is 12" long, the hair farthest away from the scalp is 2 years old.

Longer hair has been exposed to the elements for a longer period of time and is referred to as older hair. Older hair will vary in porosity throughout the length of the hair shaft.

Unequal reactions to liquid and chemicals along the length of the hair shaft are due to variations in porosity. To observe variations in porosity, hold several strands of hair away from the scalp by their ends. Note any variations in color or surface texture. Older, more porous hair will appear lighter in color and rougher in texture.

Since the hair is of a greater length, more haircoloring product may be needed for the application. Preconditioning treatments may be necessary prior to a color application to help equalize porosity and provide the foundation for even color results. Many colorists charge for long hair accordingly, and may also prefer to use the brush-and-bowl application technique (painting the color on with a tint brush instead of using a bottle) to ensure even distribution of the haircolor product along the hair shaft. (Fig. 12.15)

The ***formation*** of the hair as it grows from the follicle is a genetic trait and is described as being straight, wavy, or curly. The smoother the hair form, the more light reflection. The curlier forms will refract, or bounce back light, and hair colors may not reflect as strongly as on straighter hair forms. Careful color choice and application will create satisfactory color results on any hair texture. To compensate for excessively curly hair, a more intense or stronger tone may be used, as determined by your strand test. Polymer haircoloring products or those that fill in, or smooth, the cuticle layer may also increase the perception of color as well as shine.

As a colorist, you should work *with* the hair's natural attributes, and use texture, form, density, and porosity to your advantage. Follow the hair's natural pattern or style and insert highlights or lowlights to enhance a cut and give a more polished appearance. (Fig. 12.16)

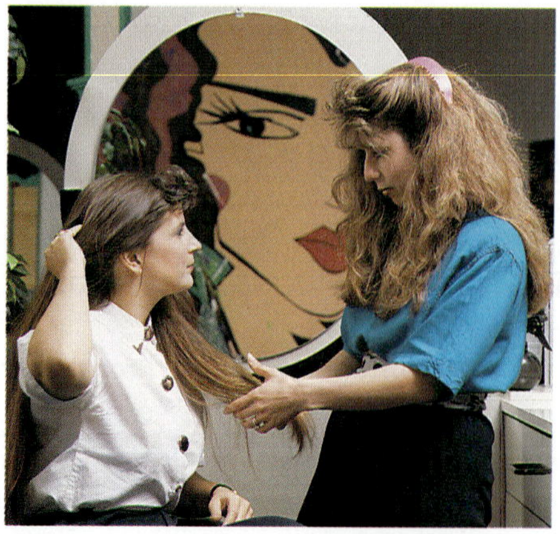

12.15—Hair length will be a factor in your haircolor choice.

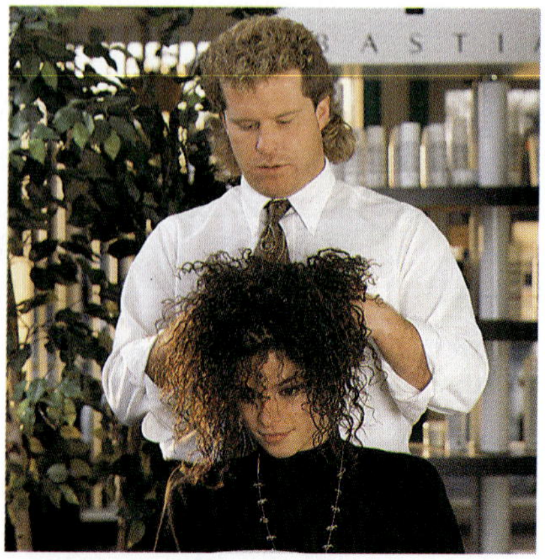

12.16—A curlier hair form may require a stronger tone.

Identifying the Natural Hair Color

Natural hair color is the base of the colorist's work. Understanding the science of natural color will help you develop informed haircoloring choices for each client. It is amazing to realize that nature creates an endless variety of hair colors, with no two alike, using a single substance called melanin.

Natural pigments are classified as melanins. Melanin is made of molecules capable of reflecting color. They are classified into two groups: black-brown or eumelanin (yu-**MEL**-ah-nin) and yellow-red or pheomelanin (**FE**-oh-mel-ah-nin). Special cells called ***melanocytes*** (**MEL**-uh-no-sights) receive the amino acid ***tyrosine*** (**TYE**-ro-seen) from the blood vessels at the bottom of each hair follicle. Within the melanocyte, a chemical reaction occurs. An enzyme known as ***tyrosinase*** (**TYE**-ro-sin-ace) gives oxygen to the tyrosine, and the result is a change in its molecular structure. This oxidation of tyrosine produces the melanin that creates all the natural hair color variations.

Once the melanin is developed, it is coated with ***melanoprotein*** (**MEL**-uh-no-pro-teen) to form a granule. While the hair is forming, these pigment granules called ***melanosomes*** are pushed up between the cells that are forming as cortex fibers and become a part of the hair structure. These melanin-filled granules are scattered through the cortex of the hair, in no set pattern or amount. This is how nature creates so many hair color variations from only one natural substance—melanin.

The natural hair color tone we see (black, brown, blonde, or red) will depend upon the type of melanin—eumelanin, pheomelanin, or a combination of both. The lightness or darkness of the hair will depend on the amount and distribution (whether closely packed or scattered) of melanin present in the hair.

The keratin protein of the hair is colorless. It is the melanin that gives hair its color. When hair turns gray, it is the same basic structure as it has always been, except without pigmented melanin. These melanocytes don't necessarily stop producing pigmented melanin all at once. Sometimes they produce less and less until gradually the hair appears lighter.

Often, clients will wish to color their hair long before the gray hair is noticeable, because their color lacks richness. When we lose all the pigment in a few of our hairs, we lose a little pigment in all our hair. This is a great motivation for coloring one's hair.

Understanding melanin is important to the professional colorist because melanin is a contributor to any new haircolor the colorist wants to create.

Whether it is natural or artificial pigment, when you are analyzing your client's color, you must first identify the color level. A ***level*** is the degree of lightness or darkness of a particular color, excluding tone.

In haircoloring, cosmetologists and haircolor manufacturers use a system to analyze the lightness or darkness of a color. It is called the ***Level System***. The materials you receive with your haircolor products will describe your particular manufacturer's system. Generally, in the majority of product labeling systems, a scale of 1 to 10 is used to describe the lightness or darkness. Level 1 colors are darkest; level 10 colors are lightest. Some manufacturers will elect to use a level system starting with zero; others extend their levels beyond 10 to 12. The scale works the same regardless of the starting and ending points—low numbers are darker; high numbers are lighter.

Haircolor manufacturers provide a chart depicting the colors in their product line. This color chart shows the level and tone of the various colors. Natural hair colors can also be analyzed with this tool. By comparing the manufacturer's color chart with your client's hair, you can determine the hair color level. You can then describe the lightness or darkness with a number from the level system.

To determine your client's natural hair color level, take a few strands of hair and hold them up and away from the head, allowing light to pass through. Holding the hair away from the scalp, take the manufacturer's level swatch and fan out the hair strands. Place it next to the hair closest to the scalp. Sometimes the hair will be a different level due to exposure to the elements or another chemical service. Be certain to identify the natural level at the base of the hair shaft, closer to the scalp. Also identify the level or levels of the midshaft and ends so you can adjust your formula accordingly.

Do not part the hair and hold it flattened against the scalp: this would produce an incorrect reading, as the hair will appear darker without light. Hair that is wet or heavily soiled will also give a darker appearance.

The natural hair color levels are: 1. black, 2. very dark brown, 3. dark brown, 4. medium brown, 5. light brown, 6. dark blonde, 7. medium blonde, 8. light blonde, 9. very light blonde, 10. lightest blonde. (Fig. 12.17)

◆ NOTE: The names for the natural hair color levels may vary from manufacturer to manufacturer. What is important for you to identify is the varying degrees of lightness to darkness that distinguish each level. Use the selected manufacturer's color chart as your guide in identifying your client's natural color level.

Levels 1, 2, and 3 are considered to be dark hair. People with dark hair comprise 75% of the population. Generally people with dark hair want their hair to stay dark. This is usually the best choice, because their skin and eye color are also strongly pigmented. The dark hair color in combination with richly toned skin and eye color creates an intense and exotic combination.

Levels 4, 5, and 6 are the medium levels. People with medium hair comprise 15% of the population. You will note the client's pigmentation in skin and eye color is also in the medium range. There are certainly more options for someone with a medium level hair color. Generally, you will select colors with richness or vibrancy for these clients.

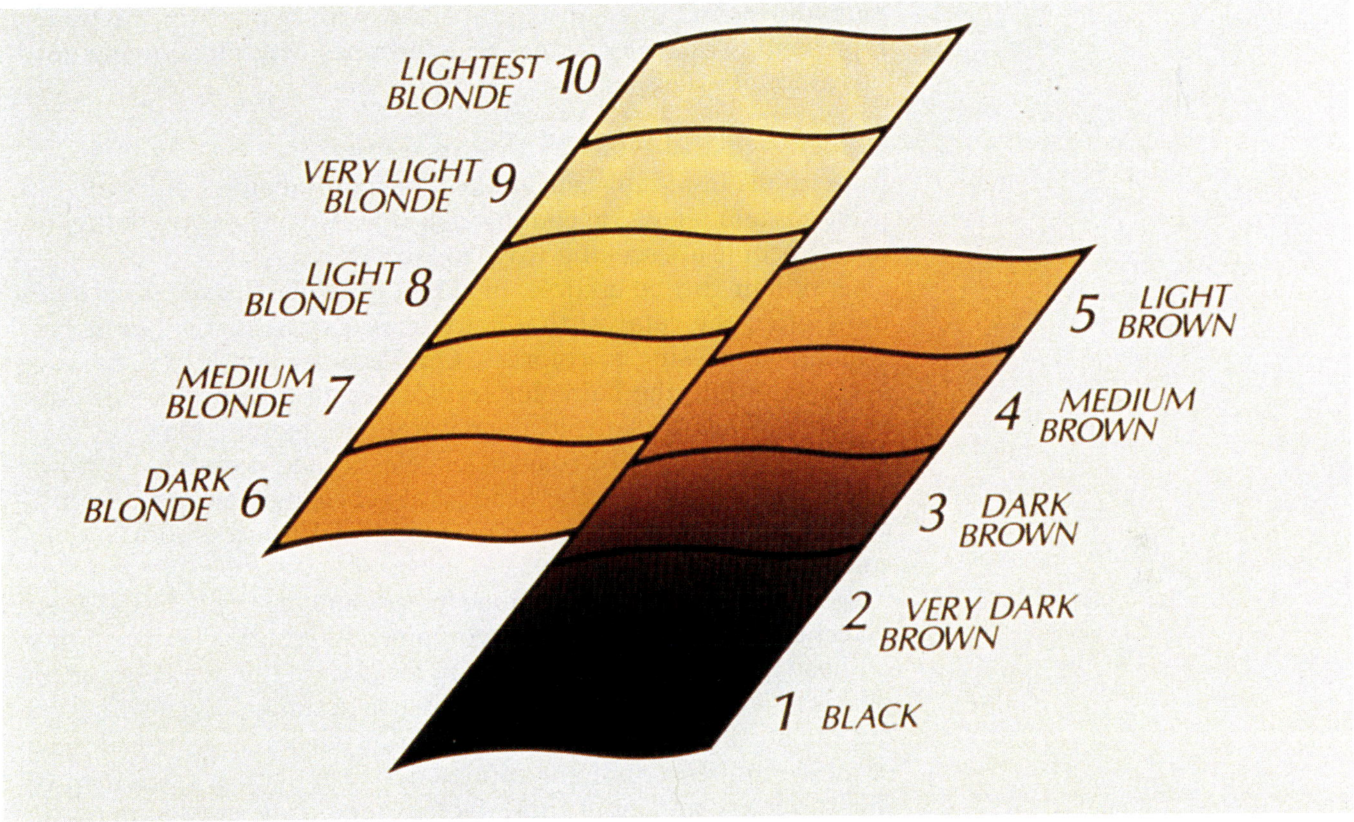

12.17—Natural hair color levels.

Levels 7 and 8 are the light levels. Again you will observe corresponding skin and eye pigmentation in this light range. People with a light color level comprise 9% of the population. Clients with light hair generally have the most options regarding their color choices. Darker or lighter hair works well.

Levels 9 and 10 are the very light levels. We don't see many of these people as clients. Their hair color is generally pleasing until it turns gray. We will discuss gray hair at a later point in the chapter.

The term ***tone*** is used to describe the warmth or coolness of a color. The manufacturer's color chart you used earlier to discover color level also describes hair colors by indicating their tone.

The warm tones are red, orange, and yellow, although some haircolor labels use different names like auburn, copper, gold, or bronze.

The cool tones are blue, green, and violet, often listed on labels as ash, drab, platinum, or smokey. Those words conjure up visual pictures of the properties or characteristics of the color tone.

Intensity refers to the strength of the tonality in a color. Intensity is described as being mild, medium, or strong. The difference in intensity can be as subtle as an auburn highlight or as strong as a traffic-stopping red. The strength of the warm or cool tone in a hair color is indicated in Figure 12.18, with neutral (in the center) representing an even balance of color tones without showing obvious amounts of either warm or cool colors.

Percentage and Distribution of Gray

Individuals in today's society are constantly being bombarded by print ads and television commercials that emphasize youth. Because of this people are seeking ways to look younger.

Gray hair can be a curse, or it can be a blessing. It is certainly most often the catalyst that convinces clients to color their hair, which is a blessing to colorists. On the other hand, gray hair can also complicate the haircolor service because it does not respond to haircoloring the same as the naturally pigmented hair.

Gray hair tends to be coarser, less elastic, and occasionally curlier than the other hair on the head. It also becomes more resistant to chemical services, and thus requires special consideration in haircoloring practice.

It is first necessary to determine the amount of gray hair (the actual percentage) on the head. Then you must determine the distribution of those gray hairs (where they are located on the head). A person who is 50% gray could have their gray hair sprinkled equally throughout the head or located only in the front portion of the head. Each of these requires a different approach to formulating. Therefore, we must identify and note these factors regarding gray hair on the client's record card.

DETERMINING THE PERCENTAGE OF GRAY

PERCENTAGE OF GRAY	CHARACTERISTICS
10%–30%	Mostly pigmented; difficult to see; generally most heavily located in temples and sides with some blending of colors throughout the head.
30%–50%	More pigmented than gray; easy to see in dark colors but may blend in with lighter natural hair.
50%–70%	More gray than pigmented; unnecessary to study hair to see gray.
70%–90%	Mostly nonpigmented hair; generally majority of remaining pigmented hair is located in back with rest blended over head.
90%–100%	Virtually no pigmented hair; tends to look white.

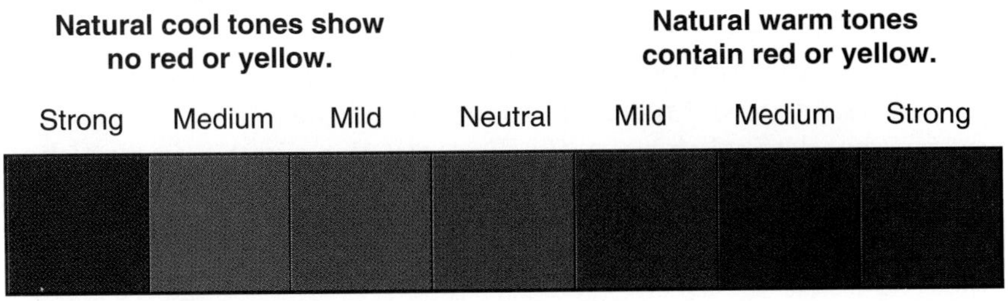

12.18—The strength of warm or cool tones is called intensity.

Another consideration when formulating for gray hair is recognizing the natural hair color that has not yet turned gray. Most people retain some dark hair as they turn gray. The situation in which hair appears gray occurs when there is a mixture of white and dark hair. This blending, known as salt and pepper, creates different shades of gray depending on the ratio of pigmented to nonpigmented hair. This hair must be analyzed for level and tone.

Be careful not to allow the reflection of the white or gray hair next to the pigmented hair to affect your judgment. In many instances, this will cause even the most experienced colorist to identify the naturally pigmented hair as lighter than it really is. By misjudging the depth of the natural level, you may not compensate adequately for the undertones present in the hair, which will create a warmer-than-expected end result when you begin to lift the natural hair color.

What occurs during the graying process? The melanin enters the hair shaft void of color. The melanin pigment granule is still nestled in the cortex of the hair shaft and will still be evident as it is affected by coloring processes. When you lighten hair that is gray or white (nonpigmented hair), the melanin pigment still diffuses the same as colored melanin. The strand would become weakened, the cuticle would become lifted, and the hair would become more porous. The only difference is that the hair would take on a yellow cast.

Another consideration when formulating for gray hair is what color the client's hair was prior to turning gray. The hair colorist must recognize that when the hair starts to turn gray, the remaining natural hair changes as well. Gray hair does a masterful job of concealing the undertones that still remain in the hair. The undertones are there and are no less intensified than they were before the hair turned gray.

Each person is born with a particular combination of natural pigment. There is harmony between the hair, eye, and skin tones. At the point graying clients come to you for color service, their hair has changed dramatically from that original birth color. By knowing what color their hair was when they were children, you will be able to anticipate the changes that hair will undergo during treatment with an oxidative haircolor product. The answer to this question will indicate the intensity of pigmentation with which you will be dealing.

Not all colors are appropriate for all people. Clients often have unrealistic desires and wish to be lighter or more neutral toned than is possible. They do not realize how much their hair color has changed since it started turning gray. Finding out the client's original hair color will provide some additional information to assist you in your decision-making process.

This method of organizing hair colors is called Natural Hair Color Categories. Let us explore what each natural hair color category goes through when the hair starts to turn gray.

The B Category, dark brown and black: People born with black or dark brown hair. Levels 1, 2, and sometimes 3 are in the black/dark brown category. They may have some reddish highlights. Their hair darkens with age until it turns gray.

The hair is generally on the cool side so there is no major change in the natural hair color when the hair grays. The hair colorist must determine when you no longer color the gray hair dark to match the natural hair color. At some point in clients' lives they can no longer continue to wear the dark haircolors that they could when they were younger. It is at this point that the hair colorist must lighten the hair and at the same time minimize the red/orange tones that are generally unflattering to clients in this category. The red tones that this category can wear most successfully are the darker red or blue/red tones.

The hair of someone in the B category will decolorize through as many as 10 different stages. During decolorization, all changes in color are warm in tone. If warm tones are desired, they exist in the hair and can be enhanced. If warm tones are not desired, caution must be exercised to avoid their appearance. An oxidative haircolor will almost always produce a warm result or will fade to a warm tone. If warm tones are not desired, a deposit-only or semi-permanent product would be a better choice. A light, cool result would require double-process lightening followed by a cool-toned tint or toner.

The W Category, warm brown: People born with blonde hair that gradually darkens before adolescence.

Even before the hair begins to gray the natural hair color loses its warmth and starts to flatten. What the hair colorist must always be aware of is that the undertones that were present prior to the hair turning gray are still there. These clients can generally wear red tones very well and often will request them. These clients also wear highlights very well.

An oxidative haircolor would lighten the hair nicely, but it would always retain some warm tones. To achieve a cool color result, you would have to use a double-process lightening product.

The L Category, light brown: People born with blonde hair that remained blonde through adolescence. Their hair gradually darkens in their teens to a soft brown color.

The soft brown category is usually level 5 or 6. The natural hair is light and does not make for an attractive contrast when the hair color begins to gray. The color usually takes on a drab, dreary look. This category does not have the red/orange undertones that the B and W categories do. Remember these clients were blonde when in high school so they would generally not be averse to once again being blonde.

Clients in the L category generally can achieve attractive blonde colors with the light blonde shades of oxidative tints. Pale cool colors would probably require prelightening.

The R Category, red: People born with red hair that remains red throughout adolescence. Their hair gradually darkens or loses warmth with age. The red category usually falls in the levels 5, 6, and 7.

The red category does not gray gracefully. The once-vibrant red hair becomes a muddy red color. Many times the changes in hair color happen so gradually that clients may not realize that their hair is losing its glow.

Blonde has not been noted as a category. People with blonde hair, levels 8, 9, and 10, do not color their hair until it darkens. At this point they are in the L category.

Knowing the Natural Color Category, in addition to identifying the level, will assist you in recommending the proper haircolor service to accomplish the desired end result, and the haircolor formula that is best suited for your client. (Fig. 12.19)

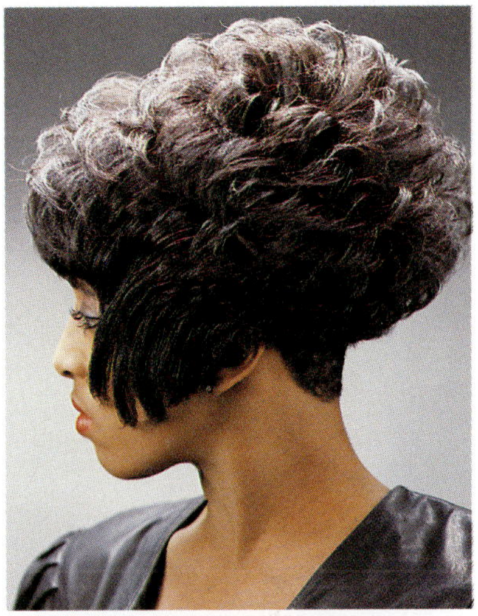

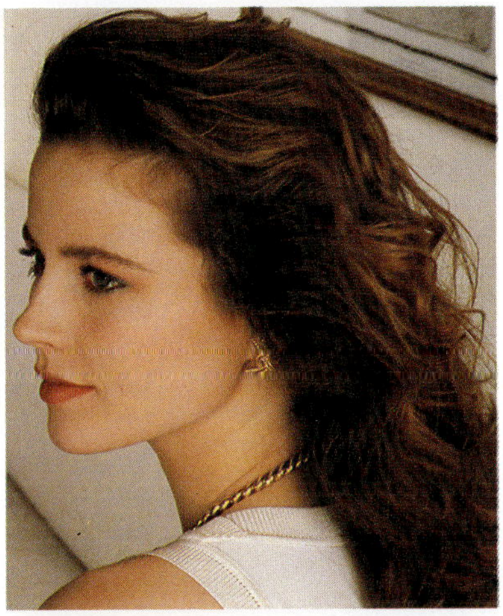

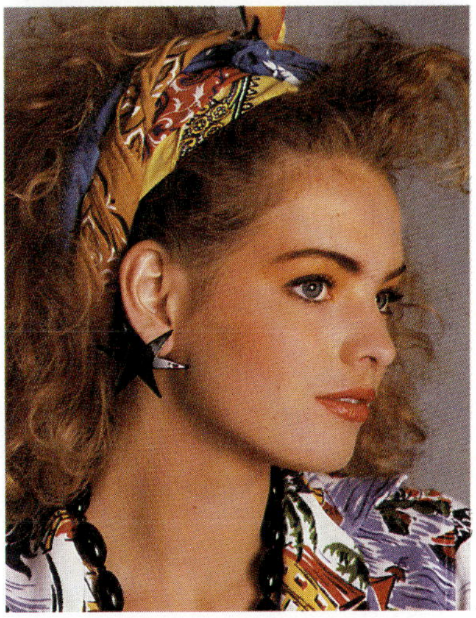

12.19—Achieving natural haircolors with the Level System.

Selecting Color for Desired Result

Every haircoloring service must begin with a professional assessment of the client's current hair color and what changes need to be made. Only then can the best procedure and formula be selected.

Basic Rules for Color Selection

1. Make sure the client's hair is clean and dry.
2. Look through the hair. To see level as well as tone, raise the hair by pushing it up with the hands against the scalp.
3. Analyze the level present in the hair. Does the client want to go lighter or darker?
4. Analyze the level of the desired color. Add or subtract from the natural color to determine the level of color necessary.
5. What are the natural tones? What highlights does the client want? Select the color within the level that will supply those tones, or determine what primary additive should be used.
6. Know the properties of the product you are using. Consult the manufacturer's information on each color and how it reacts on different hair color levels (light, medium, or dark hair).
7. Analyze the condition of the hair, especially its porosity. Does the hair need to be conditioned prior to the service to help the color be true and prevent excessive fading?

Each manufacturer's color product's directions will indicate their formulation for adequate lift and/or deposit, and what haircolor classification and volume of developer (if any) is required to achieve the desired results, based on your thorough analysis of your client's hair and needs.

Examining the Scalp

Carefully examine the scalp to determine the presence of any factors that would make it inadvisable to use a haircoloring product. An oxidative tint solution should not be used if the following conditions exist:

1. Positive skin test (predisposition or patch test)
2. Scalp abrasions, irritations, or eruptions
3. Contagious scalp disorders

Examining the Hair

Examine the hair to determine what, if any, pretreatment may be necessary prior to your haircolor service. Elements to consider are:

1. Evidence of prior chemical treatments (either color, permanent wave, or relaxer)
2. Different degrees of porosity over the length of the hair shaft due to sun, harsh chemicals, or hair length
3. Variations in texture at the facial hairline, crown, or nape.

In some cases it may be advisable to postpone the haircolor service due to excessive damage or the presence of noncompatible chemicals in the hair.

The results of such an examination may indicate the need for any of the following:

1. Reconditioning treatments
2. Color removal
3. Removal of metallic coloring
4. Postponement of service due to breakage or some other problem

All information about the condition of the client's hair should be recorded on the client's record card.

Discuss Client's Expectations and Hair Limitations

The difference between your client's current hair color and what is desired will indicate the haircolor category and formula to use. Does your client want a temporary change or a more permanent one? Does your client want something close to the current color or a dramatic color change? Based on your thorough analysis, you can choose the proper product and technique that will fulfill the client's expectations, but also respect the hair's limitations.

Be realistic in discussing color selection with your client. It is best to select a general range of color lightness and tone, rather than to promise an exact shade. Some clients will be able to change their color in one process, creating the right level and tone at the same time. Other clients will need two separate products and processes to create the same effect. Be sure to consider carefully all the factors that will influence your client's decisions.

Consider the Client's Lifestyle

A coloring procedure that requires a great deal of care may be impractical for a very active person. Pale blonde may be the wrong choice for someone who swims regularly (pool chemicals can turn blonde hair green). An iridescent eggplant color would be inadvisable for someone who works in a conservative law firm. All of these factors must be considered.

An office job would dictate a more conservative color choice than a freelance fashion photographer. A full-time mom might need a lower maintenance color service. A businessman would wish for an undetectable line of demarcation between the haircolor and his new growth.

Sun lovers will have different color results than people who avoid sun exposure. Tennis, boating, and convertible cars all mean more sun. Pool swimmers have constant exposure to chlorine, which changes the texture and color outcome. People who engage in heavy daily exercise need to shampoo their hair more often; this could cause their color to fade.

Medicines can affect haircolor results. Sulfur-based drugs can add warmth to light blonde colors. High doses of vitamins and minerals can darken the natural haircolor level. Always ask your clients and note any medications they are taking on the record card.

Home care products are of great importance for haircolor clients. A shampoo for controlling dandruff or psoriasis will change your color result. Rapid fading can occur because of highly alkaline, nonprofessional products. Some mousses, conditioners, and hair sprays can build up and coat the hair shaft. This will alter the porosity of hair, causing uneven color results.

Educating your clients on how to care for their color-treated hair will improve your results. Healthy, well-cared-for hair will be a positive reflection on your workmanship. Teaching your clients proper maintenance is the most professional approach to beautiful hair color. (Fig. 12.20)

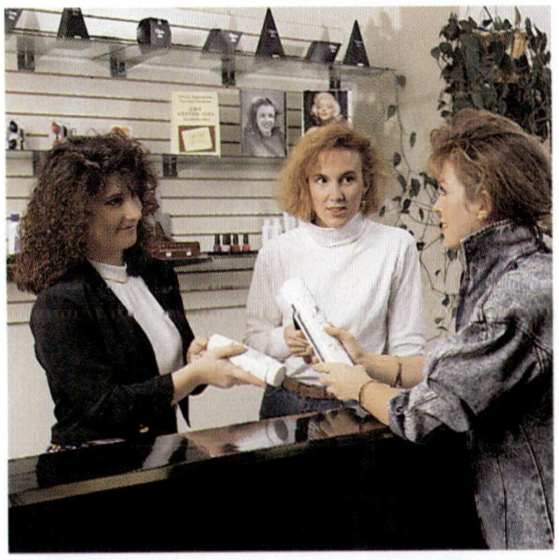

12.20—Discuss products and proper maintenance for color-treated hair with clients.

Time spent in the salon for services is a point of discussion. For some, primping is a form of self-indulgence; for others, it's pure torture. Frequency of maintenance must be presented during your consultation.

The time and money involved in committing to a color service should be spelled out in advance. Your conversation should be something like: "This color (show a picture or swatch) can be achieved by (indicate the type of color service i.e., weaving, single-process color, etc.). The cost of your service today will be ($00.00). To maintain this color, it is important that you have this service every (number of weeks) and the cost each time will be ($00.00). Does that work for you?"

This is a time to make direct eye contact with your client and wait for the answer. If the time or cost is objectionable, alter your suggestion. Continue this conversation until you and your client agree to the maintenance schedule you have presented. At this point, you will have an agreement with your client and can begin your service.

Choosing Level, Tone, and Intensity

If necessary you will adjust the haircolor formula for each individual texture or condition. Remember the findings of your analysis, listed on your client's record card. Include the client's current color in formulating for level, tone, and intensity. Generally speaking, a change of 1 to 2 levels will produce the most natural results. Any tone can be enhanced or subdued to the client's wishes by using the law of color in selecting your formula. Adjust for gray, porosity, and length. Natural-looking haircolors are a balance between all three primary colors, including the client's contributing pigment and the artificial color selected.

Selecting the Appropriate Application Technique

After a thorough discussion with your client, you must then choose the method that will achieve the desired effect. Sometimes a combination of application techniques is necessary to first cover gray, then add carefully placed highlights, to make the transition from the lightness of gray to the contrasting darkness of a solid color. Another example would be the use of a double-process blonding technique for clients with dark natural coloring who choose to be a pastel color with a cool tone. Whatever you select, make sure the client understands each step of the procedure and the technique necessary to achieve your objective. This will avoid startled looks from clients when they see unexplained things happening to their hair during a procedure.

USING COLOR KEYS TO FIND THE MOST FLATTERING COLOR FOR THE CLIENT

Analyzing Skin and Eye Coloring

The color of clients' eyes can be a clue as to what their haircolor could be. Eyes are rarely one color. Usually they are combinations of two or even three colors. Basically there are brown, blue, and green eyes. Look more closely. Brown eyes with olive green, reddish brown, or gold flecks are quite common. Blue eyes may also have flecks of white, gold, or gray. Green eyes can range from gray-green to hazel (with brownish overtones) to yellow-green.

We can categorize eye color as warm or cool. Warm eye colors contain red, orange, yellow, or gold flecks through the iris of brown, blue, or green.

Warm eye colors are:

- Brown with red, orange, yellow, or gold
- Blue with yellow or gold
- Green with reddish brown, orange, yellow, or gold

People who have warm eye colors can wear warm haircolors.

Cool eye colors contain black, gray-brown, gray-green, blue, violet, gray, or white flecks through the iris of brown, blue, or green.

Cool eye colors are:

- Brown with black, gray-brown, gray-green, or gray
- Blue with white, blue, gray, or violet
- Green with blue or gray

People with cool eye colors look most attractive in cool or neutral haircolors.

The depth of eye color is another factor in your color choice. Lighter eyes reflect a lighter pigmentation throughout the client's coloring. A lighter intensity color choice would be indicated. Medium eyes reflect stronger pigmentation, and more intense color options are available. Dark eyes reflect the strongest pigmentation. A deeper color choice is advisable. To choose a color that will harmonize with the client's natural pigmentation, include the depth of eye color (light, medium, or dark) in your color equation.

◆NOTE: Many clients choose colored contact lenses to enhance their appearance. This can affect your color choice. If you are not certain of the client's natural eye color, always ask.

Skin tone can be broken down into four simple categories: olive, red, golden, and neutral. It is easiest to observe the natural skin tone by looking at the skin on the neck, close to the clavicle. Facial and arm skin is often affected by sun exposure, which masks the skin tone, making it difficult to determine.

Olive skin tones have an underlying tone of gray, green, or yellow. Olive-toned clients look best in cool or neutral colors. If a warm shade is desired, it should be in a darker level.

Red skin tones have an underlying tone of red-brown, red, or blue-red. Red-toned clients look best in cool or neutral colors. Warm colors are not recommended for these clients.

Golden skin tones have an underlying tone of golden brown, gold, or peach. Golden skin tones look best in warm colors. The level chosen would be affected by the client's natural level.

Neutral skin tones are a balance of warm and cool. Neutral skin can have an underlying tone of pink and yellow in combination. You will not observe one predominant underlying skin tone. Generally these skin tones are described as ivory, beige, or brown skin. Neutral skin tones look well in either warm or cool colors.

How does this information indicate a color choice? The chart on page 252 will help you in your selection. Remember that each person is unique, however, and consult with your instructor. Gradually, as your skill develops, you will see these items automatically. (See also Fig. 12.21)

Color Key 1

YOUR NATURAL EYE COLORS

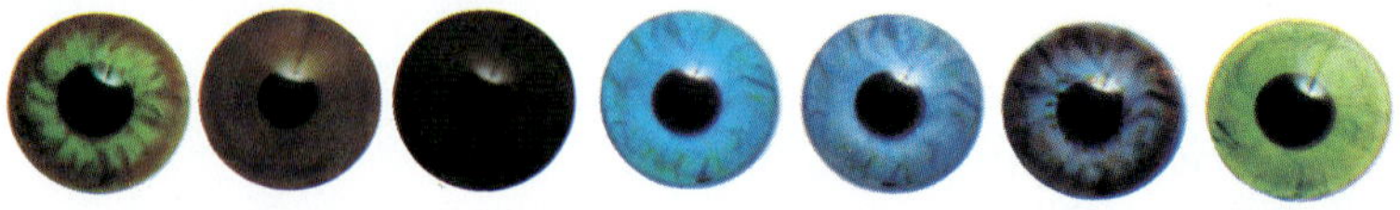

YOUR NATURAL HAIR COLORS AND MOST FLATTERING TINTS

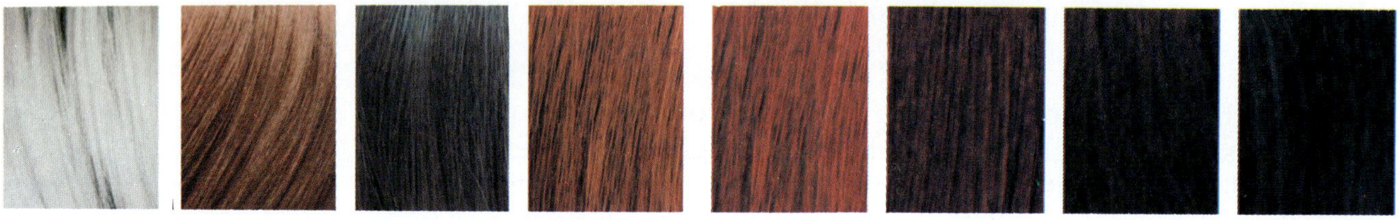

YOUR NATURAL SKIN COLORS

MAKEUP AND WARDROBE COLORS FOR PERSONS IN COLOR KEY 1

The purpose of this chart is to help you select your client's best colors for makeup, haircolor, and wardrobe; colors that will harmonize with their complexion tones. In Color Key 1, blue pigmentation predominates the undertones of the skin. When selecting a person's Color Key, the natural eye colors in the chart will be helpful in determining their correct Color Key. Light-skinned people who have a blue-pink undertone to their complexions, therefore, fall into Color Key 1. Some people in Color Key 1 have an olive undertone. Dark-skinned people in Color Key 1 may have a charcoal or occasionally an ashen gray hue to their dark complexions. If you determine that a client's personal coloring is in Color Key 1, always choose colors from the Color Key 1 selection.

12.21—The Color Key System.

Color Key 2

YOUR NATURAL EYE COLORS

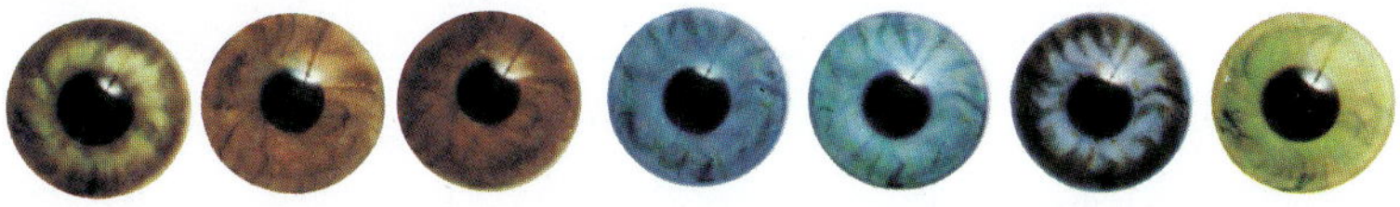

YOUR NATURAL HAIR COLORS AND MOST FLATTERING TINTS

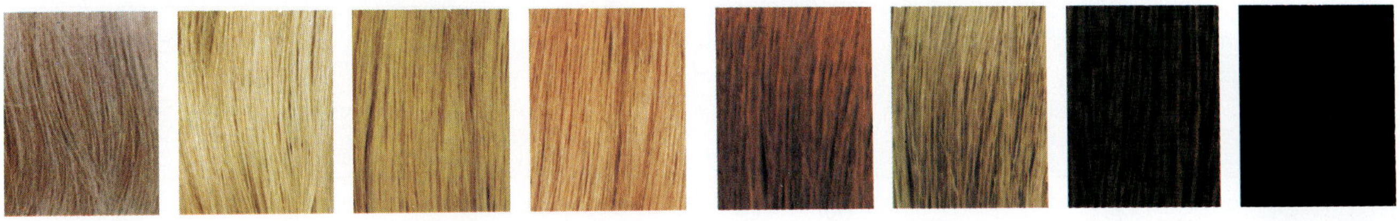

YOUR NATURAL SKIN COLORS

MAKEUP AND WARDROBE COLORS FOR PERSONS IN COLOR KEY 2

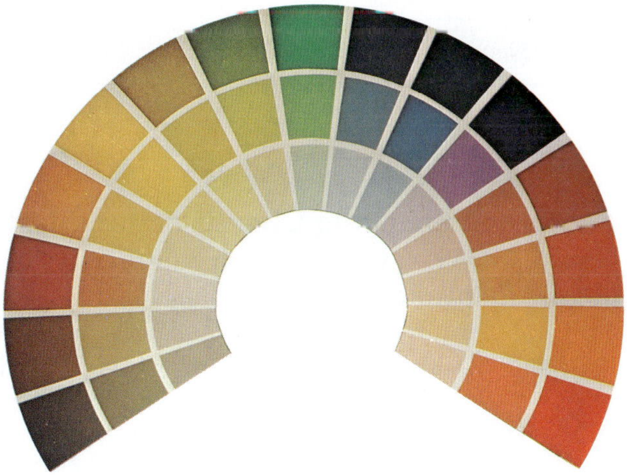

The purpose of this chart is to help you select your client's best colors for makeup, haircolor, and wardrobe; colors that will harmonize with their complexion tones. In Color Key 2, yellow pigmentation predominates. Light-skinned people with a peach-pink undertone to their complexion will, therefore, fall into Color Key 2. Dark-skinned people in Color Key 2 have a golden undertone. If you determine that a client's personal coloring is in Color Key 2, always choose colors from the Color Key 2 selection.

HAIRCOLOR SELECTION CHART

Natural Level	1 2 3	4 5 6	7 8	9 10
Category	"B" Dark Brown and Black	"W" Warm Brown "R" Red	"L" Light Brown	
Suggested Levels	Dark Hair	Medium Hair	Light Hair	Very Light Hair
	Recommendation: Stay close to natural level.	Recommendation: With rich or vibrant colors.	Recommendation: A wide range of possibilities. Lighter or darker options.	Generally, you will not see as clients.
Eye Color	Cool		Warm	
	Brown with black-gray, brown-gray, green-gray. Blue with blue-gray, violet. Green with blue-gray.		Brown with red, orange, yellow-gold. Blue with yellow-gold. Green with reddish brown, orange, yellow-gold.	
Haircolor Option	Neutral Color Choice		Warm or Neutral Color Choice	

Skin Tone	Red Red-brown, red-blue, red underlying tone.	Olive Gray, green, yellow underlying tone.	Golden Golden brown, gold, peach underlying tone.	Neutral Brown, beige, ivory, pink, and yellow combined. The underlying tone is a balance of warm/cool.
Haircolor Option	Cool or Neutral	Warm or Neutral	Warm	Cool or Warm

Enhancing Client's Natural Coloring

When working with hair that has not been colored, you will notice a natural harmony in the hair tone, skin tone, and eye color tone. Maintaining that natural harmony will give you a pleasing, natural effect. A more avant-garde effect will be achieved by using complementary color tones. The key to maintaining harmony in color tone is understanding the Law of Color.

Consider how tones change with maturity. Many clients initially want to return to the color of their youth. They do not realize that the pigment of their skin is aging in a process similar to that of the hair. To tint the hair back to the natural color of their youth creates a severe contrast that can be harsh. Generally, a color of a similar tone but lighter level will be more flattering.

There will always be clients who break these rules. Many do so with great success. Attractiveness is a quality that incorporates esthetics, the laws of art and balance, along with the client's personality and self-expression. ✔

✔ **Completed—Learning Objective No. 1**

CONSULTATION AND ANALYSIS

COLOR THEORY

It is important that you understand the theory of color pigment before you begin applying haircoloring products to clients' hair. It is only through knowledge of color theory that you can think your way through color problems to the correct color formulation for each situation.

THE LAW OF COLOR

The Law of Color is a system for understanding the relationships of color. When combining colors, you will always get the same result from the same combination. Equal amounts of red and blue mixed together will always make violet. Equal amounts of yellow and blue will always make green. Equal amounts of red and yellow will always make orange. This system is called the Law of Color because these relationships have been tested over and over and have proven to be true.

Primary Colors

Primary colors are pure or fundamental pigments (colors that cannot be created by mixing colors together). The primary colors are, in order of their dominance, blue, red, and yellow. (Fig. 12.22, page 254) Understanding the order and size is essential to understanding haircolor theory. All other colors are created from these three primaries. Colors with a predominance of blue are cool toned colors. Colors with a predominance of red or yellow are warm-toned colors.

Blue is the darkest of the primary colors. When you add blue to your mixture, you will make a color darker and cooler in appearance. Blue is the only cool primary, and when it is added to any primary, secondary, or tertiary color, it is dominant. The resulting new color will also be cool. (Fig. 12.23, page 254)

In addition to a cool tone, blue also adds depth or darkness to any color in which it is added. Its molecular size, or pigment weight, is very important; it is the primary color with the largest size and the heaviest pigment concentration. Because of this, blue is closest to the outer cortex, positioned just below the cuticle layers. During an oxidative service (such as perming or coloring), the blue primary color dissipates, leaving the hair shaft first because of its location on it. When the hair is oxidized by ammonia in a perm or haircoloring solution, the hair shaft expands sufficiently to allow the blue molecule to oxidize and escape. The result is a loss of depth and coolness in the hair shaft, revealing the undertones created by the two remaining (warm) primaries—red and yellow.

The next primary by weight is red, and again, its molecular size and placement within the cortex is important. It explains why red is difficult to remove during lightening. Red pigment contains a high percentage of the hair's sulfur content (from the sulfur bonds),

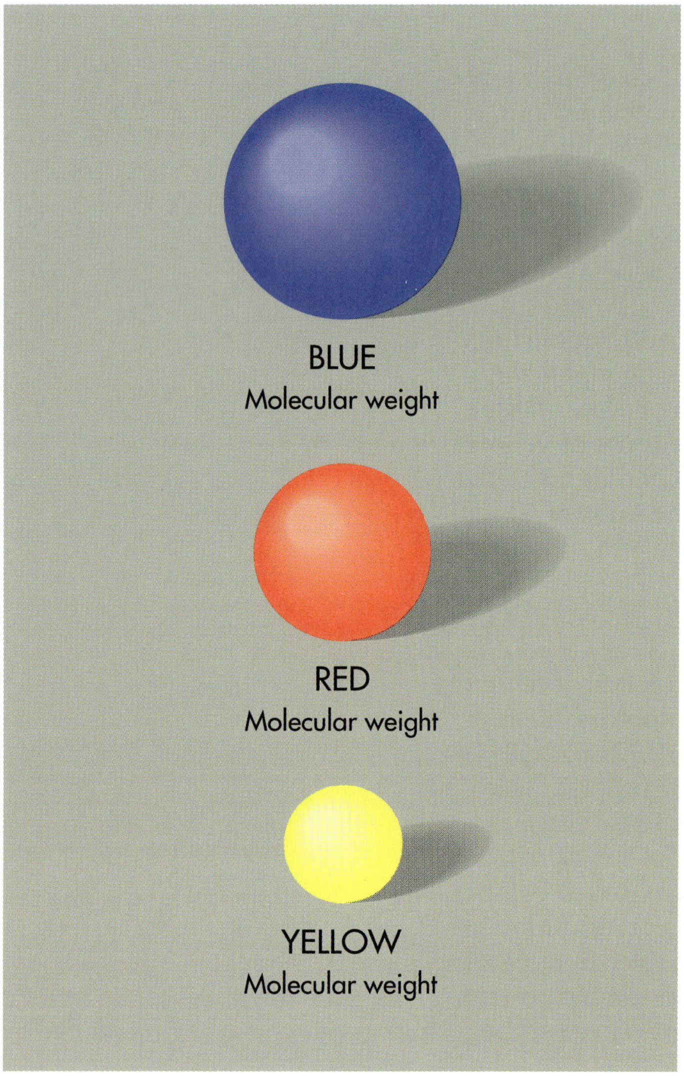

12.22—Primary colors arranged by molecular size or pigment weight.

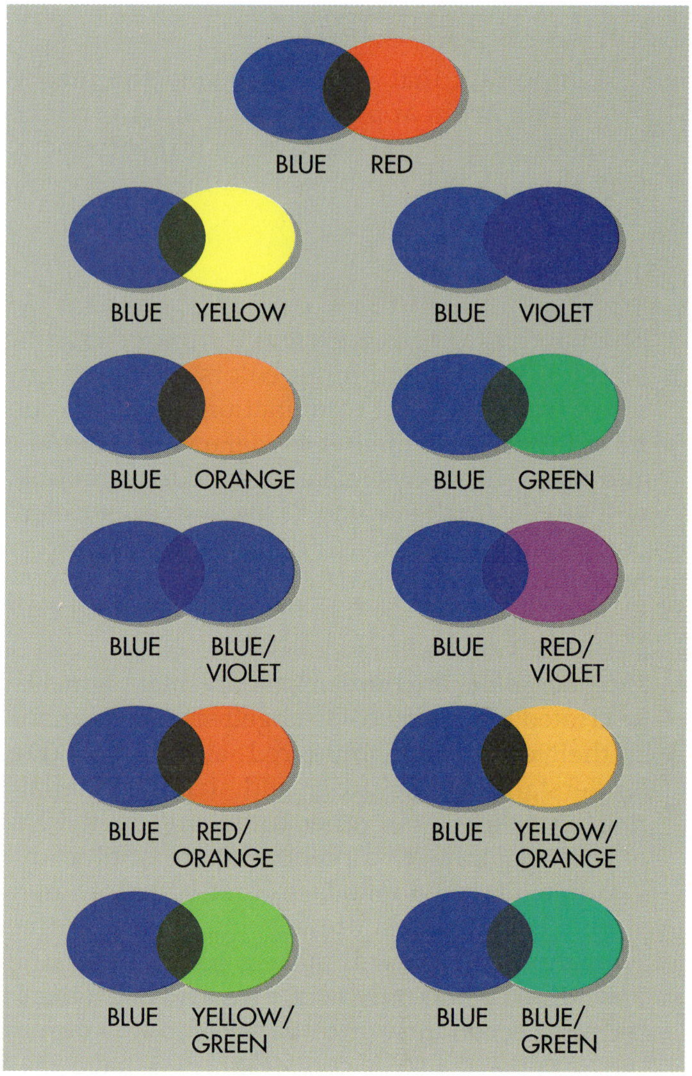

12.23—Blue shown in combination with any secondary or tertiary color creates a cool result.

helping to give the hair strength and invaluable to many chemical processes' success. Red is positioned deeper in the hair shaft than blue, so in order to remove it, you must swell or expand the hair shaft large enough and for a long enough time to allow oxidation to affect the red molecule, so it will sufficiently dissipate. When you add red to your mixture, you will make a color richer and warmer in appearance. So along with a loss of warmth, the departure of red from the hair shaft also leaves the hair appearing lighter, due to the remaining and third primary, yellow.

Last of the primaries is yellow, which is found deepest within the hair shaft. The yellow molecule is very hard to remove completely for the same reasons that red is. As the last color pigment to leave the hair during oxidation, it also takes with it a great deal of the hair's remaining integrity, or internal strength. Bleach is the surest—and in most cases the easiest—way to completely remove yellow.

Yellow is the lightest of the primary colors. When you add yellow to your mixture, you will make a color lighter and brighter in appearance.

When all three primary colors are present in equal proportions, the resulting color is black in its highest concentration, with shades of gray to white in its lightest level and intensity. Unequal proportions of the three primaries will produce a neutral brown or blonde, depending on the amount of pigment present. For example, unequal proportions of red, yellow, and blue with a majority of red will produce a reddish brown. A predominance of yellow would create a golden brown, and more blue than red or yellow becomes a dark or drab brown.

Secondary Colors

Secondary colors are green, orange, and violet. They are created by combining two, and only two, primary colors in equal proportion. Green is a combination of blue and yellow. Orange is a combination of red and yellow. Violet is a combination of blue and red. Green and violet both have blue in them, so they are cool tones. Orange has red and yellow, so it is a warm tone. (Fig. 12.24)

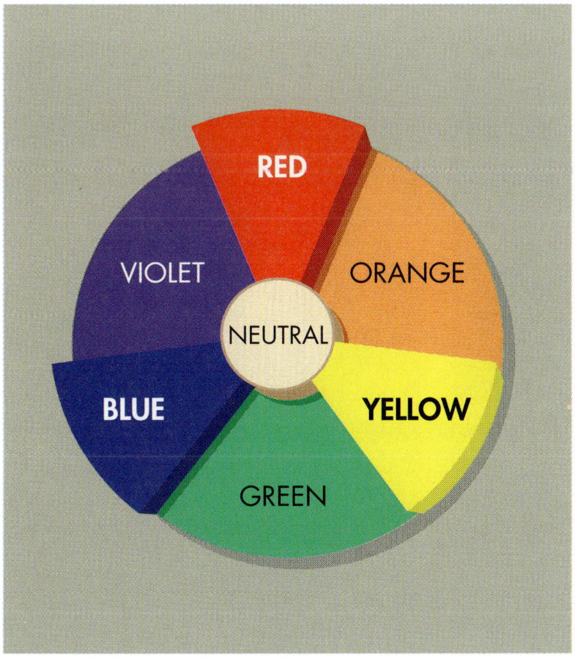

12.24—Secondary colors are created from equal parts of two primaries.

Tertiary Colors

Tertiary colors are blue-green, blue-violet, red-violet, red-orange, yellow-orange, and yellow-green. When relating this basic information to haircolor, we notice that haircolor is never one primary color. Natural-looking haircolor is made up of a combination of primary and secondary colors.

Tertiary colors are created by mixing a primary color with the adjacent secondary color on the color wheel. Blue-green and blue-violet are cool tones. Red-violet is also cool but not as cool as the other two because of the predominance of red. Red-orange and yellow-orange are warm tones. Yellow-green is a warm tone but not as warm as the other two because of the presence of blue. (Fig. 12.25)

Complementary Colors

The term *complementary* comes from the word complement, which means to make complete or to mutually make up what is lacking. Complementary colors are a primary and secondary color positioned opposite each other on the color wheel. Combinations are blue and orange, red and green, and yellow and violet.

When mixed together these colors neutralize each other. When formulating, you are often attempting to neutralize or refine unwanted warmth in your end result. Knowing the complementary relationships can direct you in choosing the appropriate tone to haircolor. For example, when mixed in equal amounts, red and green neutralize each other, creating brown. Orange and blue neutralize each other, and yellow and violet neutralize each other. (Fig. 12.26)

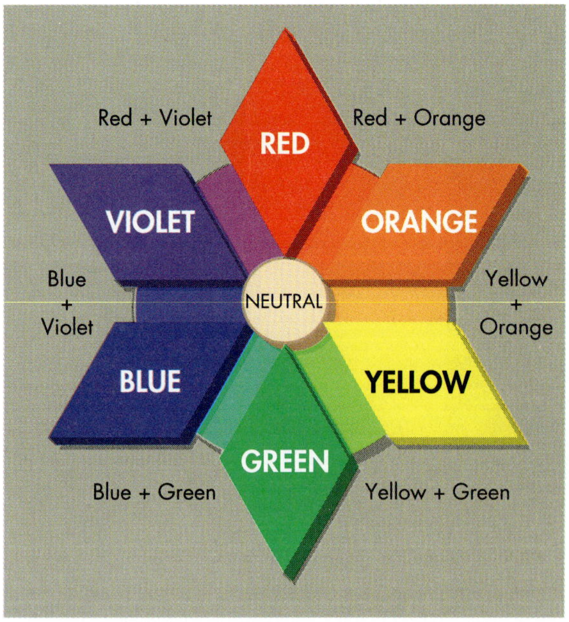

12.25—Wheel showing how the combination of primary and secondary colors creates tertiary colors.

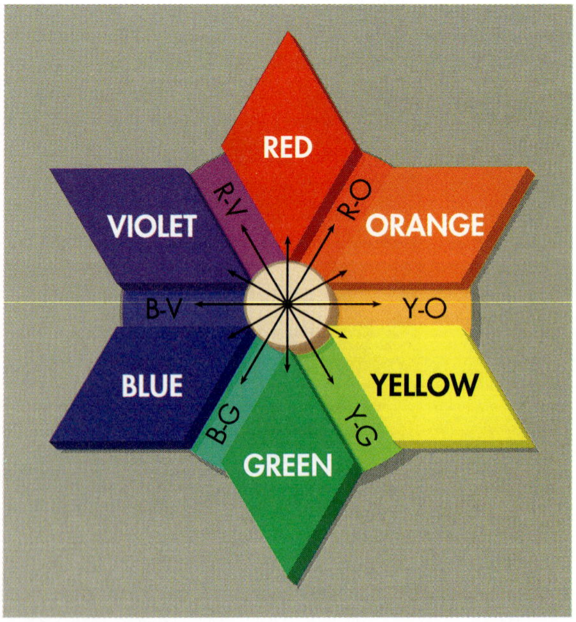

12.26—Complete color wheel with arrows to indicate which colors neutralize others.

There are different ways of using this complementary relationship. By placing complementary colors side-by-side, you create maximum contrast. This means the two colors' appearances intensify when placed next to each other. For example, red hair (which is actually orange) and bright blue eyes create a vibrant color combination.

Another way colorists use the complementary relationship is by mixing two complementary colors together. Knowing the complementary relationships gives you the key to knowing how to create a neutral color. Complementary pairs always consist of all three primary colors. For example, if you look at the color wheel, you see that the complement of red (a primary color) is green (a secondary color). Green is made up of blue and yellow (both primary colors), so all three primaries are represented in this complementary pair.

When formulating haircolor, we always work with a combination of colors. That combination may be your client's natural pigment and one haircolor product. Or, it may be several colors blended together. Your client's own natural pigment contributes warm tones to the end result. Knowing how much warmth will be contributed takes practice and experimentation with each color level.

We have learned that the warm tones are red, orange, and yellow. When these warm tones are unwanted, you can refine your result by using the complementary tone, opposite on the color wheel.

Red pigment is only a factor in the very darkest hair (other levels will have more orange than a true red). Level 1 or 2 may need a haircolor product with a green tone to refine or neutralize the unwanted red tone.

The unwanted tone we hear our clients comment on most often is orange. Our clients may call this unwanted tone "brassy" or "red." It will be up to your educated eye to determine whether the actual tone is orange. The complementary color to orange is blue. A blue-based haircolor product will help to neutralize orange highlights in the hair.

One word of caution: The level of your correction must be the same or slightly darker than the problem. For example, if you have a client whose hair is level 6 orange and she wants it to be more neutral looking, you would need to use a level 5 or 6 blue-toned haircolor to correct the warmth. A level 7 in a blue-toned haircolor will not have enough pigment to overcome the level 6 orange.

Another unwanted tone we may need to correct is yellow. In this case, the complementary color is violet. A violet-toned haircolor product will refine yellow.

Sometimes, we see green in the hair. This is usually caused by a chemical. It may occur from swimming in a chlorinated pool or because of an improper color choice. Because this hair is also likely to be over-porous, strand test to ensure the proper tonal value and intensity necessary to correct the greenish cast without overpowering.

CREATING NATURAL-LOOKING HAIRCOLOR USING ARTIFICIAL PIGMENTS

Most hair colors represent a balance of colors, which means that they generally contain a balance of each of the primary colors. However, colors will have a predominant base and a level of lightness or darkness that must be identified before formulating a tint for the hair.

Oxidation tints are identified by the predominant base and the level of color formulated by the manufacturer. Most manufacturers provide literature that identifies the level and base color for you. You may identify the level and base color of the client's hair by comparing it to the manufacturer's color identification chart (as a guide, not an absolute).

All colors—warm, cool, or neutral—can be formulated in tones that range from the lightest blonde to the darkest black, using the basic theory related to the Law of Color.

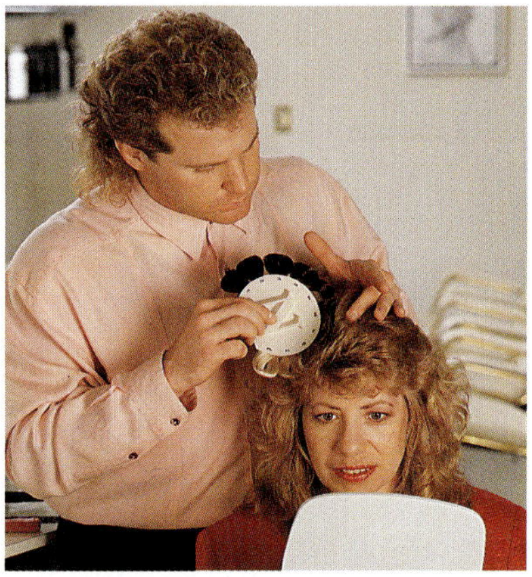

12.27—A manufacturer's color guide along with the color wheel are tools that can be used for creating natural-looking haircolor.

Referring to the Color Wheel to Predict Results

The color wheel is a professional tool colorists use to create custom formulas. It is based upon the universal method of creating different colors by combining the primary, secondary, and tertiary colors. This tool, together with the colorist's knowledge of artificial coloring products, will enable the colorist to enhance or subdue tones present in the hair during the coloring process. Manufacturers' materials may provide other visual tools to clarify this information, along with recommendations for color formulation. (Fig. 12.27)

Using Level, Tone, and Intensity in Selecting a Color

When you have decided on the haircoloring products to use, you must next find the correct level, tone, and intensity to achieve your desired result. In many manufacturer's product lines, you may find more than one color choice at each level. However, each of these shades will create a different tonality. Choose the one closest to what you need to achieve the desired result. To give the new haircolor the exact tonality and intensity desired, the basic shade can be adjusted or modified by adding a small quantity (¼ to ½ ounce) of a cooler or warmer shade on the same level, or by using an accent additive (usually added drop by drop) to enrich or drab the final formula.

The Four Rules for Natural-looking Haircolor

In order to more easily mimic the characteristics of virgin hair color, consider the following in determining your choice of color and application technique:

1. The hair should be lighter on the ends than at the base of the hairshaft.
2. The hair should be lighter on the surface than underneath.

3. Face-line hair should be lighter than the hair behind it (crown and nape).
4. The darker hair should always be the dominant color, i.e., in reverse highlighting, always have more dark hair than light on the head. ✔

✔ Completed—Learning Objective No. 2

COLOR THEORY

CLASSIFICATIONS OF HAIRCOLOR

Haircoloring falls into four main categories: temporary, semi-permanent, deposit-only, and permanent. These classifications refer primarily to staying power (lasting ability), but also reflect their actions on the hair. These characteristics are determined by chemical composition and molecular weight, or size, of the pigments within the products found in each classification.

TEMPORARY HAIRCOLORING

Temporary colors utilize the largest pigments of all four classifications of haircolor. The large size of this color molecule prevents penetration of the cuticle layer of the hair shaft and allows only a coating action on the outside of the strand. The chemical composition of a temporary color is acidic and makes only a physical change rather than a chemical change in the hair shaft. (Fig. 12.28)

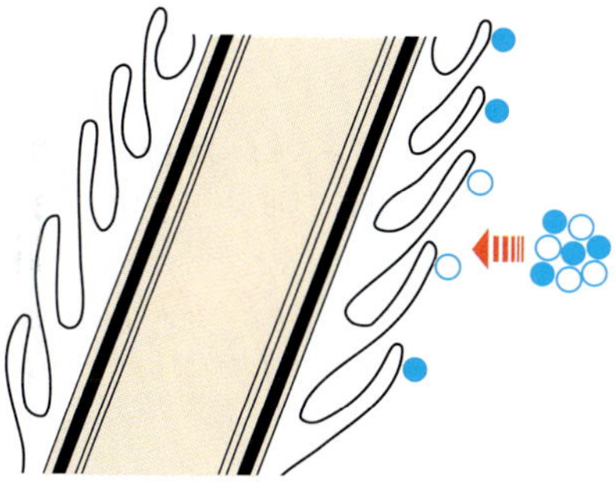

12.28—Action of temporary haircolors.

Action of Temporary Colors on the Hair

Since the color remains on the cuticle and does not penetrate into the cortex, it lasts only from shampoo to shampoo. However, excessive porosity can allow temporary color to penetrate, making it last much longer. Temporary colors usually contain certified colors—colors that have been approved by the Food and Drug Administration (FDA) for use in cosmetics.

Temporary colors can be used for the following:

1. To temporarily restore faded hair to its natural color.
2. To neutralize the yellowish tinge in white or gray hair.
3. To tone down overlightened hair without creating further chemical damage.
4. To temporarily add color to the hair without changing its condition.

Temporary haircolors have several disadvantages:

1. Color is short of duration; it must be applied after every shampoo.
2. Coating is thin and may not cover hair evenly.
3. Color may rub off on pillows or collars and may run with perspiration or other moisture.
4. They can only add color; they cannot lift.
5. Staining may result if the hair is porous or if a dark color is used on very light hair.

Temporary colors come in a wide array of shades from light to dark, warm to cool. They are easy to apply and are valuable as an introduction to haircoloring, or as a "quick fix" in corrective coloring situations when the hair may not tolerate a stronger chemical.

A patch test is usually not necessary for this type of haircolor, although the recent introduction of noncertified direct dyes does not always make this claim a certainty. Consult the manufacturer's directions for recommendations.

Types of Temporary Haircoloring

A wide variety of products are available within this classification: color rinses; color shampoos; color sprays; color gels, mousses, and creams; color crayons; mascara; and color powders.

Coloring crayons and **mascara** are temporary colors used to add color to eyebrows and lashes.

The primary purpose of haircolor crayons is to blend regrowth between retouches. They are manufactured in stick form and in a small variety of colors, and have a wax base. The wax base of color crayons retards the absorption of liquids and thereby makes it necessary to completely remove the coloring from the hair before the next chemical service.

Mascara crosses the line between a haircoloring and makeup product. It is considered a temporary haircoloring because it temporarily colors the hair of the eyelashes with a variety of neutral shades—brown and black—as well as the colors of an artist's palette—blue, violet, and teal, just to name a few. Mascara also gives the illusion of density and length to the lashes.

Coloring mousses and **gels** are now available.

Color mousses are one of the most contemporary ways to temporarily color the hair. They offer a wide array of colors that are fast and easy to apply. Color mousses serve many of the same purposes as temporary color rinses. They can brighten, tone gray, disguise regrowth lines, and blend uneven color as well as create dramatic effects.

Color mousses stay put on the hair shaft. They do not drip, run, or blow off the hair when blow-drying. This characteristic, and the fact that they do not appear to be a traditional haircolor, makes them popular with men. They also give the hair body and volume. Some mousses also have detangling and conditioning abilities.

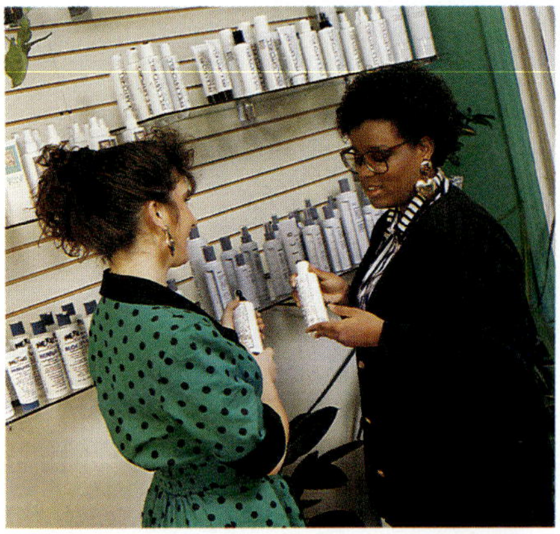

12.29—A variety of color mousses and gels are available.

The color gels and creams are available in a variety of shades, some natural, others wild and vibrant. These colors are designed to shampoo completely out, but because they tend to be tones of great intensity, they may stain porous, bleached, or very dry hair. (Fig. 12.29)

Spray-on haircoloring is applied to dry hair from aerosol containers. These are generally used for special or party effects.

Temporary color sprays can be sprayed over the entire head of hair to create an even tone, such as brown or auburn, but they are more popular for creating special and exotic effects.

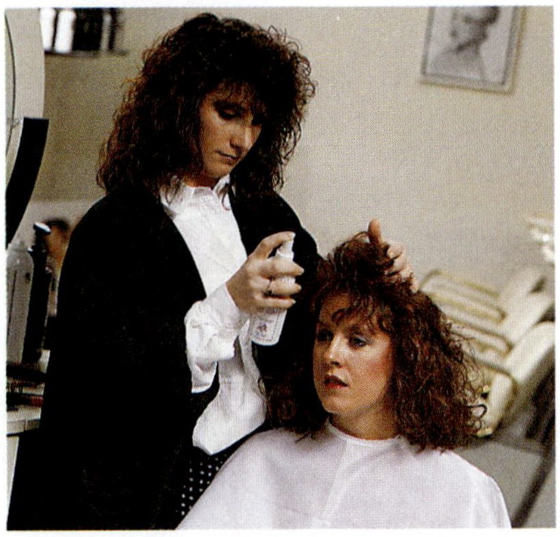

12.30—Spray-on haircoloring products are popular for creating special effects.

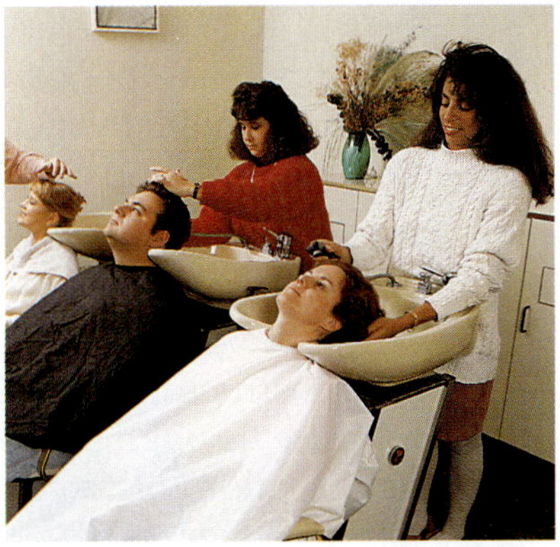

12.31—Color-enhancing shampoos combine the action of a color rinse with that of a shampoo.

The metallic salts in color sprays can build up after repeated use and cause an adverse reaction with future chemical services. These products are also extremely flammable, so they cannot be used around clients who are smoking. (Fig. 12.30)

Color-enhancing shampoos combine the action of a color rinse with that of a shampoo. These shampoos add color tones to the hair.

Color shampoos are also known as highlighting shampoos. They are a combination of rinse and shampoo, which act similarly to temporary color rinses in that they give only slight color changes that are removed with plain shampooing. Color shampoos are used to brighten, impart slight color, and eliminate unwanted tones. (Fig. 12.31)

Temporary color rinses are prepared rinses used to add color to the hair. These rinses contain certified colors and remain on the hair until the next shampoo. Temporary rinses are also known as water rinses, since they are a simple aqueous-alcoholic solution combined with various dyes.

The pigment molecules are designed to attach to hard keratin. Skin and hair are composed of similar types of keratin, with the soft keratin of the skin and scalp even more reactive than the hard keratin of the hair. This allows rinses to stain the scalp as well as the skin. Therefore, it is advisable to wear gloves to protect your hands even though the solution itself is relatively harmless.

Application of Temporary Rinses

There are many methods of application, depending upon the product used. Your instructor will help you interpret the manufacturer's directions.

Implements and Materials

Neck strip	Towels	Protective gloves
Shampoo cape	Comb	Applicator bottle (optional)
Temporary color	Shampoo	Record card

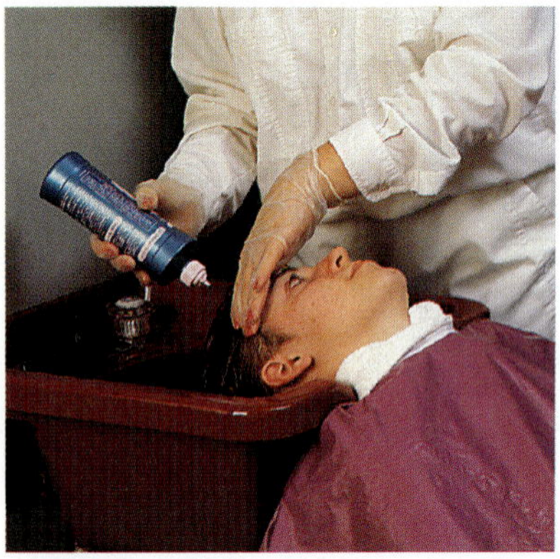

12.32—Apply temporary rinse.

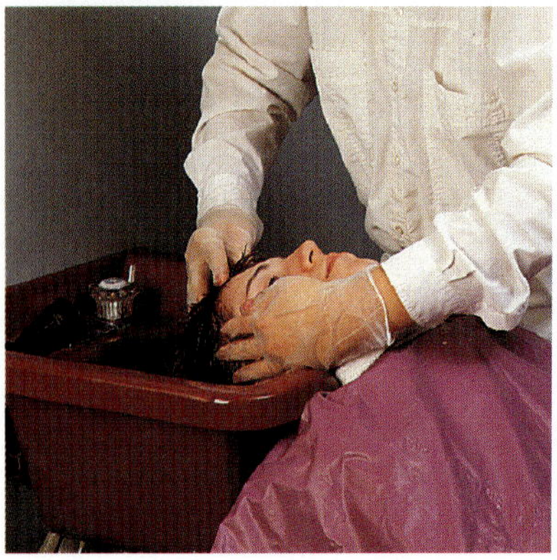

12.33—Blend rinse through hair.

Procedure

The hair is first shampooed and towel dried. Make sure that the client is protected with the neck strip and cape as temporary coloring can easily stain skin and clothing.

1. Client should be comfortably reclined at the shampoo bowl.
2. Shake product thoroughly to blend any pigments that may have settled. Apply color. Use an applicator bottle as directed by your instructor. (Fig. 12.32)
3. Blend rinse through entire hair shaft. (Fig. 12.33)
4. Blend the color with a comb, applying more color as necessary.
5. *Do not* rinse hair.
6. Proceed with styling as desired.

Cleanup

1. Discard all disposable supplies and materials.
2. Close containers, wipe them off, and store in proper place.
3. Clean and sanitize implements.
4. Organize and sanitize work area.
5. Wash and sanitize hands.
6. Record results and file record card.

Alternate Application Methods

Temporary color is also available in the form of gels, mousses, foams, and sprays. To apply, return the client to your work area and apply color as directed by the manufacturer.

TRADITIONAL SEMI-PERMANENT HAIRCOLORING

Semi-permanent color offers a form of haircoloring suitable for the client who is reluctant to have a permanent color change. The semi-permanent color is formulated to be more lasting than temporary but milder than permanent color techniques.

Semi-permanent color may be excellent for clients who feel that their hair is dull, drab, or showing gray, but are not ready to begin permanent haircoloring. Semi-permanent color can blend gray and deepen color tones without altering the natural color, since there is no lightening action on the hair.

Semi-permanent color is available in a wide range of shades. It can be purchased as a gel, cream, liquid, or mousse. Semi-permanent color is often chosen by younger clients as fashion trends change. Semi-permanent color can deposit a dramatic color, or even be used for special effect streaks in bright colors. Providing the hair's porosity is normal, the color will naturally fade without a regrowth, so the client can change the color at any time or discontinue the effect.

Semi-permanent haircolor is formulated to last approximately 4 to 6 shampoos. No developer is required. The color molecules penetrate the cuticle somewhat so that the color gradually fades with each shampoo. Due to this gradual fading of color tone from the hair, regrowth may be less noticeable (depending upon the color applied) and retouching may not be required as frequently. If the hair is extremely porous, or if heat is used with some types of semi-permanent color, the results can be more permanent. Results depend on the hair's original color and porosity, processing time, and technique.

Semi-permanent coloring can have the following advantages:

1. The color is self-penetrating.
2. The color is applied the same way each time.
3. Retouching is not necessary.
4. Color does not rub off on a pillow or clothing.
5. Hair returns to its natural color after approximately 4 to 6 shampoos.

◆ NOTE: Semi-permanent tints containing aniline derivatives require a patch test. Follow the manufacturer's directions carefully.

Types of Semi-Permanent Haircolors

1. Semi-permanent tints that blend or cover gray completely, but do not affect the remaining pigmented hair.
2. Semi-permanent tints that enhance gray hair without changing the natural pigment.
3. Semi-permanent tints that add color and shine to hair that is not gray.
4. Translucent tints that add gloss, tone, and sometimes special effects to the hair. These colors vary in their effect according to porosity, heat application, and timing. Consult your instructor and manufacturer's information for assistance with these products.

Semi-Permanent Haircolor Uses

1. **To enhance hair's natural color.** Semi-permanent colors can be used to add golden or red highlights, and to deepen the color of the hair. This type of color is especially effective on ethnic clients and clients whose natural hair color is too light or too drab to set off their complexions.
2. **To tone prelightened hair.** Semi-permanent colors can serve as a nonperoxide toner for prelightened hair. Prelightened hair is porous and the toner will penetrate.
3. **To refresh faded tints.** Excellent for between permanent color services and for corrective work, when a nonperoxide alternative is desired.
4. **To add color to gray/white hair.** Most semi-permanent colors are designed to cover hair that is 25% or less gray or create a blending effect on higher percentages. They are also recommended for clients who want to keep and enhance their gray or white hair.

Figure 12.34 indicates how this type of haircoloring works on the hair shaft.

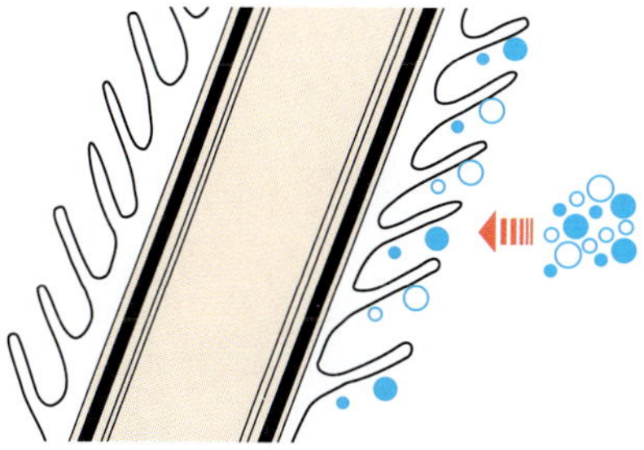

12.34—Action of semi-permanent haircolor.

Action on Hair

Traditional semi-permanent colors are formulated with pigment molecules that are smaller than those of the temporary colors but larger than those of the permanent tints. They have a mild penetrating action that results in a gentle addition of color in the cortex as well as some coating of the cuticle.

The chemical composition of semi-permanent colors falls within the approximate pH range of 8.0–9.0, thus causing an alkaline reaction on the hair. The alkali swells the cuticle, opening imbrications and allowing the molecules to enter the cortex. However, this solution is mildly alkaline, which causes limited swelling and opening. Only a small number of these medium-sized molecules enter and remain in the cortex.

The pigment molecules are trapped within the cortical layer of the shaft as the hair shrinks back toward normal during the rinsing step of the service. A neutral or slightly acid after-rinse helps to close the imbrications and hold the pigment molecules within the cortex. However, even the mild swelling that occurs with shampooing allows some of the color to fade.

Traditional semi-permanent colors have several distinct differences from temporary and permanent colors. They last longer than temporary colors and do not rub off. They are also easy to use, requiring no retouch application. Because semi-permanent colors make no significant permanent changes in the structure of the hair, they are less damaging. Some brands even give a conditioning effect. They are excellent for toning bleached hair that is too weak or porous to accept another peroxide treatment and for use on hair that is exceptionally fine or damaged from permanent wave or relaxer services.

Semi-Permanent Color Selection

The following steps, used in conjunction with the manufacturer's color chart, offer a guide to selecting the correct color with which to perform a strand test:

1. On solid hair (no gray) select a level of semi-permanent color that is two levels lighter than the desired shade. (For gray coverage, see chart on page 309.)
2. Due to the absorption of light, the use of an ash or cool shade will create a color that the eye interprets as darker than if a warm shade is applied.
3. Due to the reflection of light, the warm colors will appear shinier.

The addition of artificial color molecules to the natural pigment of the hair shaft will create a color that is darker than the sample on the color chart. Most color charts show the approximate color that will be achieved on white hair. This color is to be used as a guide to estimate the color results when it is applied to natural hair.

The natural hair color must be considered as half the formula. Think of it as "½ artificial color and ½ natural color." Semi-permanent colors lack the strong oxidizers necessary to lift; therefore they deposit color and do no substantial lifting. Think back to laws of intensity and remember that color applied on top of color makes a darker color.

Since these products "take" based on the hair's porosity, be cautious to avoid creating ends that are darker than the base of the hair. Semi-permanent colors, due to their depositing nature, may also build up on the hair's ends with subsequent applications. A strand test will determine your formula and timing before each service.

Many semi-permanent colors are used just as they pour from the bottle. However, others require the mixing of an activator prior to application. This activator is an oxidant that helps to swell the cortex and open the cuticle for color penetration. This mild oxidizer also develops the color pigments within the formula.

Some semi-permanent colors include a color balancer in the packaging. This crystal need be added only if the semi-permanent color is to be applied immediately following the removal of a lightening or bleaching product. It stops the residual oxidation that occurs on the hair shaft until the normal pH is completely restored.

Some semi-permanent colors come packaged with an "after-rinse." This rinse is acid balanced to close the cuticle and trap the color molecules within it. This helps prevent fading to a lighter color as well as fading off-tone. The chemical composition of the after-rinse is designed to leave the hair soft, pliable, and easy to comb. Whether or not the product you select is packaged in this way, it is always a good idea to finish your service with a mild conditioning rinse.

Application of Semi-Permanent Haircolors

Implements and Materials

Neck strip	Applicator bottle or brush	Finishing rinse
Towels	Plastic cap (optional)	Plastic clips
Tint cape	Cotton	Protective cream
Protective gloves	Mild shampoo	Record card
Comb	Selected color	Color chart
Timer		

Preliminary Steps

1. Give preliminary patch test if required. Proceed only if test is negative.
2. Thoroughly analyze hair and scalp. Record results on client's record card.
3. Assemble all necessary supplies.
4. Prepare client. Protect clothing with a towel and tint cape. Ask client to remove jewelry and put safely away.
5. Apply protective cream around hairline and over ears.

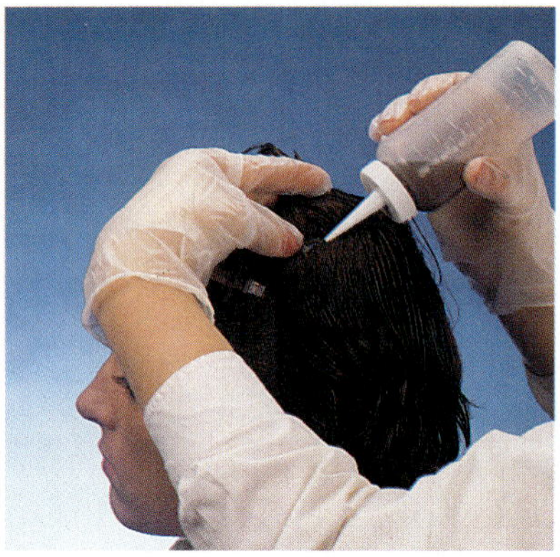

12.35—Apply semi-permanent color.

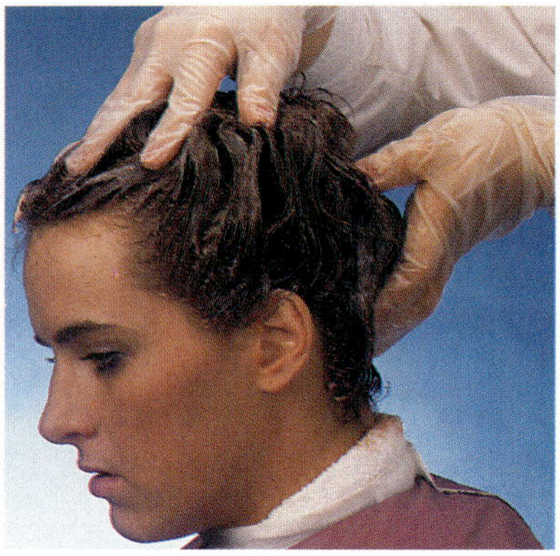

12.36—Gently work color through hair.

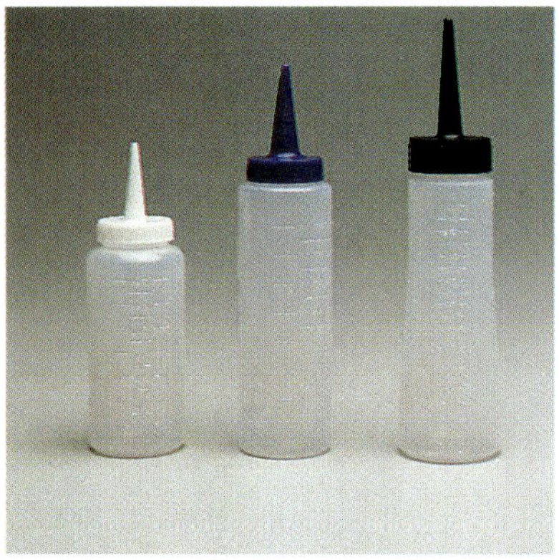

12.37—Tint applicator bottles.

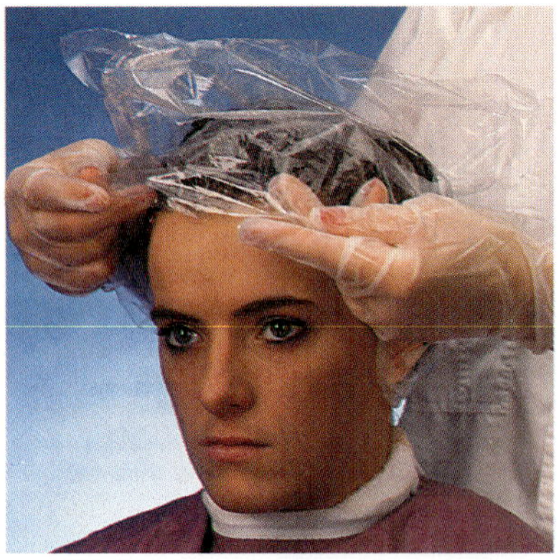

12.38—Use plastic cover if required.

6. Put on protective gloves.
7. Perform a strand test.
8. Record results on client's card.

Procedure

1. Give a mild shampoo, if required.
2. Towel dry hair.
3. Put on protective gloves.
4. Apply semi-permanent tint to entire hair shaft, (Fig. 12.35) starting near the scalp and gently working color through ends. (Fig. 12.36) Apply with bottle or brush according to the consistency of the color selected and your instructor's directions. (Fig. 12.37)
5. Pile hair loosely on top of head.
6. Follow the manufacturer's directions about using a plastic cap or heat. (Fig. 12.38)
7. Process according to strand test results.
8. According to the timing instructions provided by the manufacturer, when color has developed, wet hair with warm water and lather.
9. Rinse then shampoo, if the manufacturer recommends it, then rinse again with warm water until water is clear. (Fig. 12.39)
10. Use a finishing rinse to close the cuticle and set color. (Fig. 12.40)
11. Rinse and towel blot hair. Style as desired.
12. Complete record card and file.

Cleanup

1. Discard all disposable supplies and materials.
2. Close containers, wipe them off, and store safely.
3. Clean and sanitize implements, tint cape, work area, and hands.

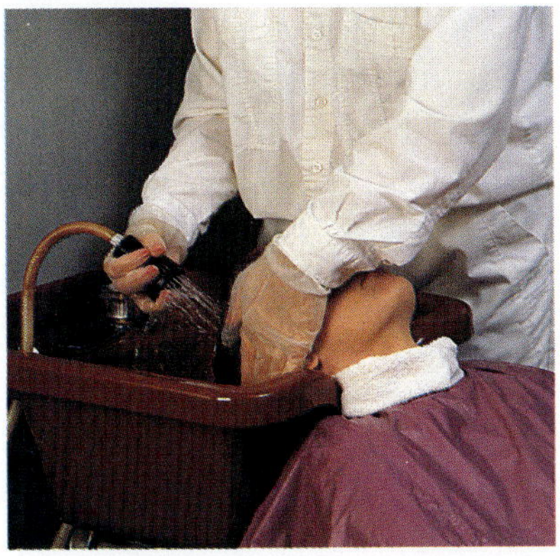

12.39—Rinse hair with warm water until water is clear.

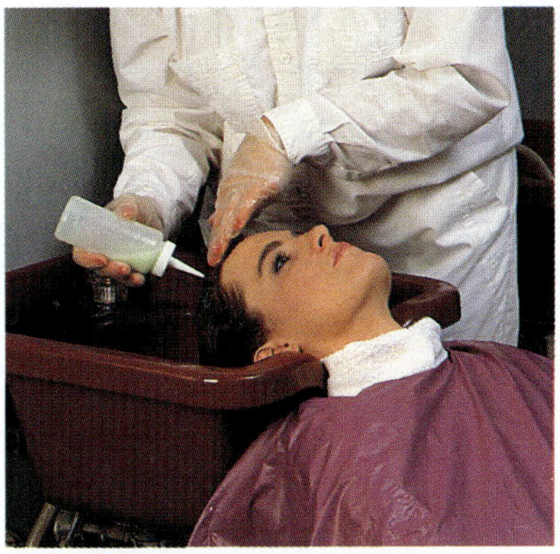

12.40—Give a finishing rinse.

Polymer Semi-Permanent Haircolors

The polymer colors are classified as semi-permanent colors because they use direct, disperse application and include certified dyes that require no oxidation process or the addition of an oxidizer for color development. However, they are distinctly different from traditional semi-permanent colors in color results, color fastness (holding ability), and chemical composition.

A **polymer** is a substance or product containing long chain-like structures. This structure actually inhibits its penetration of the cuticle and its ability to adhere to the keratin of the hair shaft. However, the dyes in polymer colors are extremely concentrated so that regardless of the long-chain structure, the color becomes well fixed to the hair. The polymers are designed to coat and penetrate the hair shaft, creating translucent shine and accent hues rather than complete coverage of the natural color.

The color fastness or staying power of the polymer colors differs from traditional semi-permanent colors. The polymer colors are advertised as colors that are removed gradually by shampooing. However, in many cases colorists have found this *not* to be true. The higher the heat and the longer the processing time, the deeper the color penetration and the greater the color fastness. Polymer colors have been known to become so well attached to the structure of the hair that even bleaches or dye solvents prepared with hydrogen peroxide will not remove them. Regardless of the experience of the colorist, performing a strand test is the most professional method of color selection.

The natural melanin within the hair shaft will not be changed by this type of coloring. The color achieved will be the direct result of the addition of the polymer pigment to the natural pigment of the shaft. After perming or relaxing services, the softened state of the shaft allows for more deposition than can be achieved on non-chemically treated hair.

The polymer semi-permanent colors were originally available in only highly intense primary and secondary colors that added a high-fashion accent to natural hair color. They are currently also available in more natural shades, including a neutral or clear color designed to fill in the cuticle and give hair a shinier, healthier appearance.

DEPOSIT-ONLY HAIRCOLOR

When semi-permanent colors were first introduced years ago, clients shampooed their hair weekly, making the lasting ability of the semi-permanent of the time a satisfactory 4 to 6 weeks. Today, however, with more clients shampooing daily, a color that lasts 4 to 6 shampoos may be unsatisfactory. For a color that will act similarly in nature to the semi-permanent colors but will produce a longer-lasting effect, manufacturer's have introduced a new category of haircolors called "Deposit-only colors."

Composition and Action

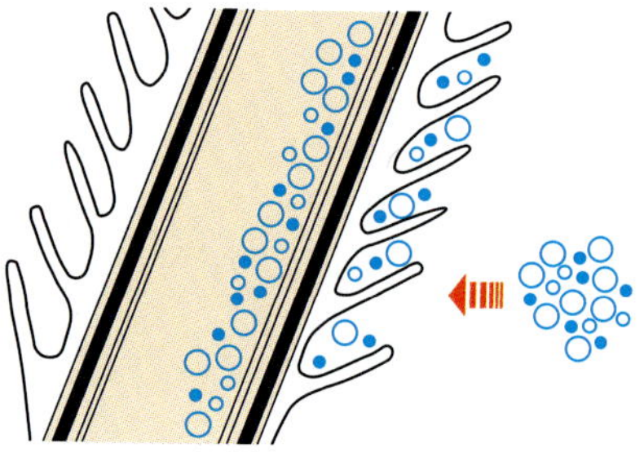

12.41—Action of deposit-only haircolor.

The effect of a deposit-only haircolor lies between those of the semi-permanent and permanent color classifications. Deposit-only colors use a form of a catalyst, such as low volume developers, to gently swell and open the cuticle layer and drive the color into the cortex. Deposit-only haircolors have small- and medium-sized dye molecules. The small-sized molecules slightly penetrate into the cortex, and the medium-sized dye molecules penetrate the cuticle layers, resulting in a color that has the gentleness of a semi-permanent color with the longevity of a permanent haircolor. Deposit-only colors last 4 to 6 weeks, gradually fading from the hair and producing a diffused line of demarcation. (Fig. 12.41)

Selecting and Formulating a Deposit-Only Color

Deposit-only haircolors are ideal for gray coverage, to refresh faded permanent tints, for corrective coloring and reverse highlighting, and for depositing tonal changes without lift.

By its very nature, a deposit-only haircolor will darken the natural hair color when applied. Remember when formulating that half of your formula will be the client's natural hair color and half will be the depositing color you have selected. Since color on top of color always appears darker, select a deposit-only color lighter than the client's natural level if your intent is to keep the same amount of depth but add tone.

Since gray hair is absent of pigment and appears lighter, it is important to consider the gray hair in your formulation of a deposit-only haircolor. As there is no lift, the resulting depth of color when covering gray may appear too extreme unless you allow for some brightness in your formulation. It is often inadvisable to make gray hair one even shade when coloring with any product, since natural hair color has different depths and tonalities that give the hair the added life that gray hair is lacking. (Since there is no lifting ability with deposit-only haircolors, use the chart for semi-permanent colors on page 309 when selecting color.)

It is always better when taking a client from lighter to darker to err on the side of lightness, because a darker tone can easily be used to deepen the color if necessary. A too-dark result, on the other hand, will involve corrective procedures to lighten or remove the artificial pigment before reapplying to achieve the desired color.

Hair previously treated with another color service will have a greater degree of porosity, which must be considered carefully when formulating and applying a deposit-only haircolor.

Application Procedure for Deposit-Only Colors

The application procedure for a deposit-only haircolor is similar to that of a semi-permanent color, since both colors do not alter the hair's natural melanin or produce lift. Follow the manufacturer's application and timing guidelines for the product that you have selected.

For successful haircoloring services, the technician must follow a definite procedure. A system makes for the greatest efficiency, and the most satisfactory results. Without such a plan, the work will take longer, results will be uneven, and mistakes will be made.

PERMANENT HAIRCOLOR

Permanent haircolors are prepared from a variety of materials: vegetables, flowers, herbs, salts of heavy metals, organic and synthetic chemicals. All of these permanent colors fall into one of four classifications: vegetable tints, metallic dyes, compound dyestuffs, or oxidative tints.

PERMANENT HAIRCOLOR TYPES

Vegetable Tints

In the past, before technology brought us the beauty industry as we now know it, many vegetable materials such as chamomile and henna were used as haircoloring ingredients.

Chamomile flowers can be ground into a powder and used as a paste that is applied in a manner similar to a henna pack, with a processing time that ranges from 15 to 60 minutes. It gives a lighter, brighter effect to the hair. Shampoos and rinses containing powdered flowers are intended to add a bright yellow color in the hair. However, chamomile's effectiveness is limited to a minimal color change.

Henna is the most noteworthy and popular of the vegetable colors and comes from plants grown in moist climates throughout Africa, Arabia, Iran, and the East Indies. The henna leaves are removed before the flowering cycle, dried, and ground into a fine powder. Hot water is added to create a paste.

Henna is a natural product that esthetically appeals to the young client and the type of consumer that prefers organic products and avoids synthetics. Its "natural" qualities appeal to many.

Current technology has brought to the market hennas in black, chestnut, and auburn, plus a lightener. These hennas are made of concentrated herbal extracts that have both a cumulative and a semipermanent effect. The dye coats the hair and is partially removed by shampooing.

The coating action of henna creates a hair strand that becomes thicker, and thus helps to give body to fine, limp hair. Because it makes no structural changes in the hair, it can be used on weak hair without damaging it. Henna fills in a roughened cuticle and holds together a split end to provide a slick, light-reflective surface. This, coupled with the additional warmth, creates hair that shines.

However, it is important to remember that excessive application will build up on the outside of the shaft and can create an unnatural brassiness. If overused, the build-up can become so heavy that conditioners cannot penetrate to the hair shaft and the hair becomes dry and coarse.

Henna has a coating that, if overused, can build up on the hair and prevent penetration of other chemicals. Henna also penetrates the cortex and attaches to the salt bonds. Both of these actions may leave the hair unfit for other professional treatments. Always perform a strand test prior to application.

It is sometimes possible to remove henna when it becomes excessively built up on the shaft or when it is incompatible with a future chemical service. The following procedure outlines the steps to removal of henna build-up.

Application Procedure

1. Apply 70% alcohol to the hair shaft, avoiding direct contact with the scalp. Allow to set 5–7 minutes.
2. Apply mineral oil directly over the alcohol, completely saturating each strand from the scalp to the ends.
3. Preheat hood dryer.
4. Tightly cover the head with a plastic bag.
5. Place under the dryer for 30 minutes.
6. Without rinsing, apply concentrated shampoo for oily hair and work into the oil.
7. Allow to set in for 3 minutes.
8. Massage the hair again.
9. Add comfortably hot water and rinse thoroughly.
10. Shampoo again. (Three shampoos may be necessary.)

Technically the alcohol should loosen the henna coating the hair shaft. However, more than one treatment may be necessary to loosen it enough to slide off. Always perform a strand test to determine if removal was successful before applying the next chemical treatment.

Metallic Hair Dyes

Metallic haircolors can be recognized by the descriptive terms used by manufacturers in their packaging even before reading the ingredients list. Metallic dyes are known as "progressive haircolors" and "color restorers." They are referred to as progressive because the hair progressively turns darker and darker upon each subsequent application. The term color restorer is used because the natural hair color *appears* to be gradually restored. When the desired color is reached, the consumer is to reduce the frequency of application to maintain the color.

Metallic hair dyes comprise a minor portion of the home haircoloring market and currently are never used professionally. Nevertheless, it is crucial for the professional colorist to be informed of the chemical composition, characteristics, and methods of removal because metals react adversely with oxidation results.

Clients occasionally request chemical services without knowing the incompatibility of metallic color with professional products. Consumers generally do not even realize that they used a product containing metal. The colorist must be able to analyze and prescribe safe, professional treatments to avoid hair damage and discoloration.

The metallic salts react with the sulfur of the hair keratin, eventually turning the protein brown. In this reaction, the quality of the keratin is lowered from the use of this chemical.

The physical result is a colored film coating the hair shaft, which gives the hair a characteristic dull metallic appearance. The metallic coating also builds up on the surface of the hair shaft. Repeated treatments leave the hair brittle and conflict with future chemical services that include in their formulation hydrogen peroxide, thioglycolate, ammonia, and/or most other oxidizers.

Resulting damage has been discoloration, breakage, poor permanent waving results, and even destruction to the point of a melted hair shaft due to the heat created in this adverse chemical reaction.

Compound Dyes

Compound dyes are a combination of metallic or mineral dyes with a vegetable tint. The metallic salts are added to give the product more staying power and to create different colors. Like metallic dyes, compound dyes are not used professionally.

Many clients use haircoloring products at home. Therefore, you must be able to recognize and understand their effects. Such coloring agents must be removed and the hair reconditioned prior to any other chemical service.

Hair treated with a metallic or any other coating dye looks dry and dull. It is generally harsh and brittle to the touch. These colorings usually fade to unnatural tones. Silver dyes have a greenish cast, lead dyes leave a purple color, and those containing copper turn red.

Test For Metallic Salts:

1. In a glass container, mix 1 ounce (30 ml) of 20 volume (6%) peroxide and 20 drops of 28% ammonia water.
2. Cut a strand of the client's hair, bind it with tape, and immerse in the solution for 30 minutes.
3. Remove, towel dry, and observe the strand.

Hair dyed with lead will lighten immediately. Hair treated with silver will show no reaction at all. This indicates that other chemicals will not be successful because they will not be able to penetrate the coating.

Hair treated with copper will start to boil and will pull apart easily. This hair would be severely damaged or destroyed if other chemicals such as those found in permanent colors or perm solutions were applied to it.

Hair treated with a coating dye either will not change color or will lighten in spots. This hair will not receive chemical services easily, and the length of time necessary for penetration may very well damage the hair.

Preparations designed to remove metallics and nonperoxide dye solvents may assist in the removal of metallic and coating dyes from the hair. Performing a strand test will indicate whether the metallic deposits have been removed. The most effective guarantee of future successful chemical services is to cut the tinted hair off.

Procedure

1. Apply 70% alcohol to hair, and allow to stand for 5 minutes.
2. Without rinsing the alcohol, apply a heavy oil (mineral, castor, vegetable, or commercially prepared color removing oil) thoroughly to the hair.
3. Cover hair with a plastic bag, and place under hot dryer for 30 minutes.
4. Remove mixture from hair using a concentrated shampoo for oily hair.
5. Work shampoo into oil for 3 minutes, then rinse with warm water.
6. Repeat shampoo steps until oil is completely removed.

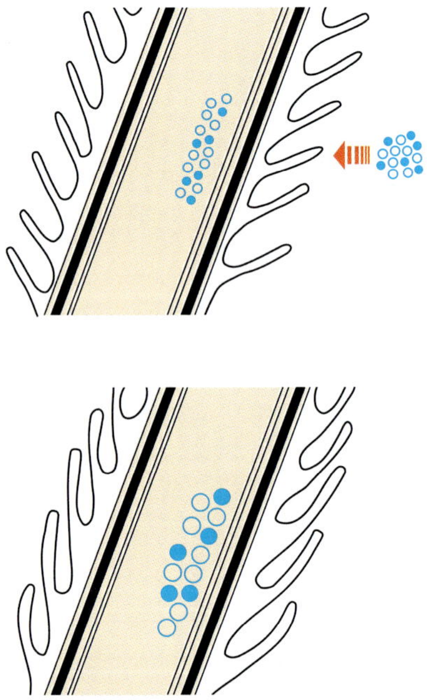

12.42—Action of permanent haircolor.

Oxidative Haircolor

Permanent oxidative haircolors can lighten and deposit color in one application, a feat performed by no other color classification. This ability to create an infinite array of levels, tones, and intensities has made permanent colors irreplaceable in the industry. These tints penetrate the cuticle of the hair and enter the cortical layer. Here, they are oxidized by the peroxide added into color pigments. These pigments are distributed throughout the hair shaft much like natural pigment. (Fig. 12.42)

Toners also fall into the category of permanent color. Toners are aniline derivative products of pale, delicate shades designed for use on prelightened hair, and will be covered more thoroughly later.

Application Classifications

Permanent haircolor applications are classified as either single-process coloring or double-process coloring.

Single-process coloring achieves the desired color with one application. Although the application itself may have several different steps, the desired color is achieved with a single application. Lightening of the hair's natural pigment and deposit of the artificial pigment in the cortex is done simultaneously as the haircoloring product processes. Some examples of single-process coloring are virgin tint applications and tint retouch applications.

Double-process coloring achieves the desired color upon completion of two separate product applications. It is also known as double-application tinting and two-step coloring. Two examples are bleaching followed by a toner application and presoftening followed by a tint application. Because the lightening action and the color deposit are independently controlled, a wider range of haircolor possibilities is opened up for each client.

To more fully understand the effects of permanent coloring products on the hair, it is first important to explain what the hair goes through when both single- and double-process haircoloring products are applied to it. ✔

✔ Completed—Learning Objective No. 3

CLASSIFICATIONS OF HAIRCOLOR

HYDROGEN PEROXIDE DEVELOPERS

Although other oxidizers are available, hydrogen peroxide serves as the oxidizing agent most commonly used in haircoloring. An **oxidizer** is a substance that causes oxygen to combine with another substance, such as melanin. As the oxygen and melanin combine, the peroxide solution begins to diffuse (break apart and spread out) and lighten the melanin within the hair shaft. This new smaller structure and spread-out distribution of the diffused melanin gives hair its light appearance.

Forms of Hydrogen Peroxide

Hydrogen peroxide (H_2O_2) is distributed for cosmetology use under a variety of names such as *oxidizer, generator, developer,* or *catalyst.* (Some manufacturers also use the word "catalyst" to mean protinator, an additive to lightening or bleach mixtures used to increase product strength.) Regardless of which name is used, hydrogen peroxide comes in three forms: dry, cream, and liquid.

Dry peroxide, in either tablet or powder form, is dissolved in liquid hydrogen peroxide to boost the volume. The availability of liquid peroxides in a variety of volumes has made this product somewhat obsolete.

Cream peroxide contains additives such as thickeners, drabbers, conditioners, and an acid for stabilization. The thickeners help to create a product that is easy to control. This extra control helps to prevent dripping during the use of brush-and-bowl method of application. This thicker formula is also advantageous when used in foil-weave wrapping, hair painting, or highlighting because the bleach mixture is less likely to "bleed" onto places where it is not wanted. The creamy formula also tends to stay moist on the hair longer than liquid peroxide, which prevents the hair lightening or coloring mixture from drying out and stopping the product action before full development is complete. However, the thickening additives in cream peroxides may dilute the strength of the formula, and make it undesirable to use when full product strength is needed, such as in tinting to cover gray.

Liquid peroxide contains no additives, only a stabilizing acid that brings the pH to 3.5–4.0. Liquid peroxide is convenient because it can be used in almost every bleach and tint formula on the market today. Another plus is that the formula for liquid peroxide is basically the same from one manufacturer to another rather than varied as with the cream peroxide. This offers the colorist consistent results regardless of the brand used. The lack of additives in liquid hydrogen peroxide creates a color formula that generally covers gray effectively.

The minuses to be considered in choosing liquid peroxide over cream are that the haircoloring and lightening products tend to dry out faster, and the conditioning agents are not present. However, one peroxide is not superior to the other. They are just different. It is the responsibility of the colorist to read the manufacturer's recommended directions and select the best product for the job.

Strengths of Hydrogen Peroxide

A variety of strengths of both liquid and cream peroxide are available. Consult your manufacturer's directions for the recommended strength. Although scientists identify the different strengths of hydrogen peroxide by percentages, cosmetologists identify the various strengths by volume, because it is the "freeing" of a certain volume of gases that creates the desired chemical reaction in hair coloring. Thus, 20 volume and 6% hydrogen peroxide are the same strength.

Uses of Hydrogen Peroxide in Haircoloring

The majority of permanent coloring products use 20 volume hydrogen peroxide for proper color development. Those that recommend the use of 40 volume are designed to achieve a greater breakdown of melanin, resulting in a lighter color than may be achieved with a standard lightening tint formula.

Formulas recommending the use of less than 20 volume are designed to allow more deposit than lift. Such formulas may be used when there is no need for breakdown of melanin to achieve the desired color.

CAUTION

Increasing the strength or volume used in a formula beyond the manufacturer's recommended directions may cause excessive damage to the hair and chemical burns to the skin and scalp.

It is especially risky to mix the higher levels of hydrogen peroxide with bleach formulated for use with 20 volume because the ingredients in the product itself, such as boosters, activators, or protinators, also work to increase the strength of the formula. However, a volume lower than 20 will not release enough oxygen to lighten the hair properly.

As the volumes of oxygen gas in any strength of hydrogen peroxide are set free, it reverts to water (H_2O). This is considered an advantage, because no dangerous residue is formed and left behind to damage the hair.

Most hydrogen peroxide solutions are packaged in opaque bottles because light causes them to break down. Heat has the same effect. Therefore, the manufacturers recommend storage in a cool, dry place. If stored safely, a stabilized, uncontaminated bottle, either partially or completely full, is expected to retain its quality for up to 3 years (always check your manufacturer's recommendations).

A hydrometer can be used to measure the volume of liquid peroxide for the purpose of adjusting its strength or simply confirming that the product is still potent. Occasionally a cap is left off or a product gets pushed to the back of a shelf, and it is best not to assume it is still potent. The hydrometer can also be a money-saving device. It is more economical to purchase the higher volume and dilute it in the salon than to buy an equivalent of prepackaged lower volumes. The hydrometer looks much like a thermometer, and must be handled delicately and stored carefully to prevent breakage.

When diluting high volumes of hydrogen peroxide, use the following charts:

130 Volume Hydrogen Peroxide Chart

For 16 oz. Total Quantity

12½ oz. of H_2O_2 + 3½ oz. of H_2O (water) = 16 oz. of 100 volume H_2O_2

7½ oz. of H_2O_2 + 8½ oz. of H_2O (water) = 16 oz. of 60 volume H_2O_2

6½ oz. of H_2O_2 + 9½ oz. of H_2O (water) = 16 oz. of 50 volume H_2O_2

5 oz. of H_2O_2 + 11 oz. of H_2O (water) = 16 oz. of 40 volume H_2O_2

3½ oz. of H_2O_2 + 12½ oz. of H_2O (water) = 16 oz. of 30 volume H_2O_2

2½ oz. of H_2O_2 + 13½ oz. of H_2O (water) = 16 oz. of 20 volume H_2O_2

1¼ oz. of H_2O_2 + 14¾ oz. of H_2O (water) = 16 oz. of 10 volume H_2O_2

100 Volume Hydrogen Peroxide Dilution Chart

For 10 oz. Total Quantity

6 oz. of H_2O_2 + 4 oz. of H_2O (water) = 10 oz. of 60 volume H_2O_2

5 oz. of H_2O_2 + 5 oz. of H_2O (water) = 10 oz. of 50 volume H_2O_2

4 oz. of H_2O_2 + 6 oz. of H_2O (water) = 10 oz. of 40 volume H_2O_2

3 oz. of H_2O_2 + 7 oz. of H_2O (water) = 10 oz. of 30 volume H_2O_2

2 oz. of H_2O_2 + 8 oz. of H_2O (water) = 10 oz. of 20 volume H_2O_2

1 oz. of H_2O_2 + 9 oz. of H_2O (water) = 10 oz. of 10 volume H_2O_2

It is important to use clean implements in measuring, using, and storing hydrogen peroxide. Even a small amount of dirt or impurity can cause peroxide to deteriorate, and can cause inconsistent color results. Once hydrogen peroxide is poured from its original container, it should not be returned to that or another stock bottle.

Never measure the needed amount of hydrogen peroxide by pouring it into the lid of another product. The residue will cause the container to oxidize as it sits on the shelf, thus making it unusable. Product frothing, a popping or hissing sound when opening the bottle, or a bulging or rounded bottle signals peroxide that has begun to break down or deteriorate.

✔ Completed—Learning Objective No. 4

HYDROGEN PEROXIDE

Contact with any metal (whether from metallic haircoloring products, a metal clip, or mixing bowl) has an adverse reaction on hydrogen peroxide and should be avoided. Metal speeds up the release of the oxygen molecules, and can cause hydrogen peroxide to oxidize the product and lose strength before it can penetrate the cuticle and cortical layers, reach the melanin, and allow for proper color development. ✔

HAIR LIGHTENING

Hair lightening, removing pigment from the hair, is always a popular salon service. Changing styles determine if the entire head is lightened, or just one area, or if a special effect is created. Lighter strands draw attention to the individual. (Fig. 12.43)

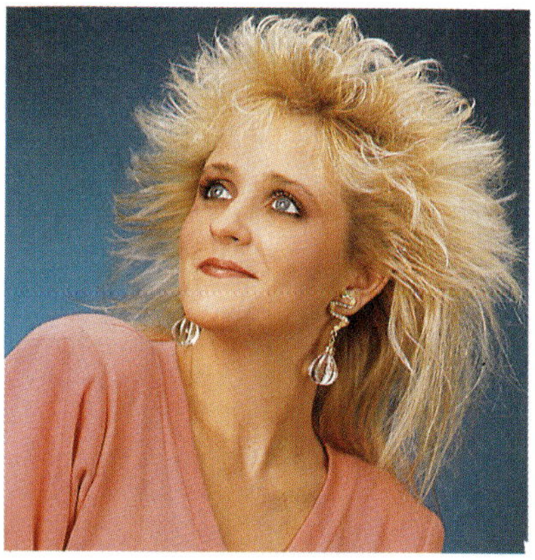

12.43—Special effects hair lightening.

Lighteners may be used for two purposes:

1. As a color treatment, to lighten the hair to the final shade.
2. As a preliminary treatment, to prepare the hair for the application of a toner or tint (double-process application).
   a) **Toner**—A lightener is always necessary before applying delicate toner shades.
   b) **Tint**—If the client desires a shade much lighter than the natural shade, a lightener can be used to remove some color before the tint is applied.

Lightening creates a desired color foundation. This new color foundation may be the finished result, or it may be the first step of a double-process application. Before beginning the lightening process, it is important to understand that achieving the desired shade requires that you consider not only the virgin hair color, how long the product should be left on to achieve the desired stage of lightening, and the resulting porosity of the hair shaft, but also selection of the appropriate product to achieve the desired color foundation.

The hair becomes more porous during the lightening treatment, a condition necessary to permit penetration of a toner. Even naturally light hair or gray hair may need a prelightening process in order to achieve the necessary degree of porosity for the acceptance of a toner or tint.

CAUTION

Clients with dark hair may not be able to be lightened to a very pale blonde color without extreme damage to their hair.

Hair lighteners, used according to the manufacturer's directions, can:

1. Lighten the entire head of hair for toner application.
2. Lighten hair to a particular shade.
3. Brighten and lighten existing shade.
4. Lighten only certain parts of the hair.
5. Lighten hair that has already been tinted.
6. Remove undesirable casts and off-shades.
7. Correct dark streaks or spots in lightened or tinted hair.

Types of Lighteners

Today's colorists have at their disposal three basic types of lighteners: oil, cream, and powder. Each classification has unique abilities, chemical characteristics, and formulation procedures.

Oil bleaches are the mildest of the three types of lighteners and have the least amount of lightening action. This product is appropriate when only one or two levels of color lift are desired. Oil bleaches are generally milder than some high-lifting oxidative dyes when mixed with higher volumes of hydrogen peroxide. Oil bleach can be used as a single-application color to achieve moderate color change of the entire head, or in a weaving to achieve a very subtle color change. It is also a popular product for presoftening resistant gray hair prior to a tinting service. Because oil bleach is so mild, it is used professionally to lighten excessively dark facial and body hair.

The benefits of ***cream lighteners*** are:

1. Conditioning agents give some protection to the hair and scalp.
2. Bluing agents help to drab gold tones.
3. Thickeners give more control during application.
4. Cream does not run or drip, which helps prevent overlapping during retouch.

Cream lighteners are the most popular type because they are easy to apply and do not run, drip, or dry out easily. The weak hydrogen peroxide and ammonia solution of cream bleaches is strong enough to do pastel blonding, but gentle enough to be used on the scalp.

Many manufacturers add a drabber to reduce brassy tones. Green, blue, and violet are effective because these tones on the color wheel are complementary to and may help neutralize some of the red, orange, gold, and yellow tones that naturally occur as the melanin goes through decolorization. Other manufacturers prefer to leave their lighteners a pure white in color so that the colorist can monitor the lightening process without wiping the product off.

Liquid and cream lighteners are generally mixed with accelerators, sometimes called boosters, protinators, or activators, in the form of dry crystals to increase the lifting power. The greater the number of protinators, the greater the strength of the formula:

- 0 activator—formula comparable to oil bleach in mildness.
- 1 activator—will lighten light brown hair.
- 2 activators—will lighten medium to dark brown hair.
- 3 activators—will lighten resistant dark brown hair.
- 4 activators—equivalent of powder bleach. Not used on scalp.

The manufacturer's recommended amount of booster has the effect of doubling the strength of the hydrogen peroxide solution. It is for this reason that no higher than 20 volume is recommended for on-the-scalp application, and also in order to protect the integrity of the hair fiber.

Powder bleaches, like cream bleaches, are strong enough to do pastel blonding. However, powder bleach cannot be applied to the scalp because it does not contain the oil and conditioners that make a cream lightener safe for on-the-scalp application. Application to the scalp would result in severe skin irritation and possible chemical burns. Powder bleach lighteners are used exclusively for off-the-scalp applications and special effects, such as foil-wrapped weaving, highlighting with plastic caps, and hair painting.

Like oil and cream lighteners, powder bleaches contain ammonia. In this instance, however, it is in a dry form. The ammonia begins the oxidation process when it mixes with liquid or cream hydrogen peroxide.

Powder lighteners, also called quick lighteners, contain oxygen-releasing boosters for quicker and stronger action. They may dry out more quickly, but they do not run or drip. Most powder lighteners expand and spread out as processing continues and should not be used for retouch services. Powder lighteners are recommended for off-the-scalp applications on resistant hair.

Action of a Lightener

One of the most frequent questions a colorist asks when lightening hair is, "Where does the color go?" It cannot be seen washing down the drain when the bleach is removed, nor does it appear to be absorbed into the bleach. In the early 60s many cosmetologists were told that the bleaching agent "ate" the natural pigment. This theory was demonstrated and "proved" by the addition of a bottle of tint to a bleach formula. The color tint would disappear before your very eyes!

The addition of hydrogen peroxide to a bleach formula (a process known as oxidation) occurs within the cortical layer of the hair shaft. The gases crash into the melanin or pigment with enough force to diffuse the molecules of color.

The oxidation process that is occurring within the bleach formula causes heat, and this chemical heat is enhanced by the body heat. Therefore, the stronger the chemical formula and the closer it is placed to the scalp, the greater the diffusion of melanin (decolorizing) within the shaft.

As soon as hydrogen peroxide is mixed into the bleach formula, it begins to release oxygen and the volume decreases. This process continues until the product either dries out or releases all available oxygen molecules.

Manufacturers of lighteners produce bleach mixtures in different degrees or strengths in a variety of formulas, but all diffuse, rather than remove, color. The eye interprets this diffusion of color, whether within the hair shaft or in a bowl of bleach to which tint has been added, as a lighter shade.

Lighteners cause the shaft to swell and lift the cuticle layer to allow penetration to the cortex. When the lightener is removed and the pH of the shaft is restored to normal, the shaft shrinks back down toward its prior size, but never quite reaches it. Some of the cuticle layer remains raised and thus each strand of hair becomes "fatter" or coarser.

Another structural change occurs with the breaking and restructuring of cortical bonds within the shaft. The weakening of these bonds makes the hair more pliable and less resistant. This additional pliability is considered an asset especially in conjunction with competition hair styling, fingerwaving, sculpture curling, roller setting, and backcombing.

The elasticity of the hair is also altered by lightening, and especially by bleaching. It is the most crucial factor to monitor during the lightening process. Healthy hair will stretch approximately ⅕ of its length and then bounce back to normal.

If the hair is over-lightened, moist strands will stretch more than ⅕ of their length and not bounce back. They can even be stretched to the point where the hair snaps and breaks. In its dry form, the natural elasticity of over-lightened hair will appear to be decreased. In fact, in this condition, the hair becomes dry, brittle, and can snap just from normal combing and brushing.

With each level of color lift, the hair will exhibit signs of increased dryness, porosity, and pliability. The dryness is easily treated with moisturizers, and the porosity is treated with protein treatments so that the hair retains the benefits of increased pliability without becoming excessively dry, elastic, or porous.

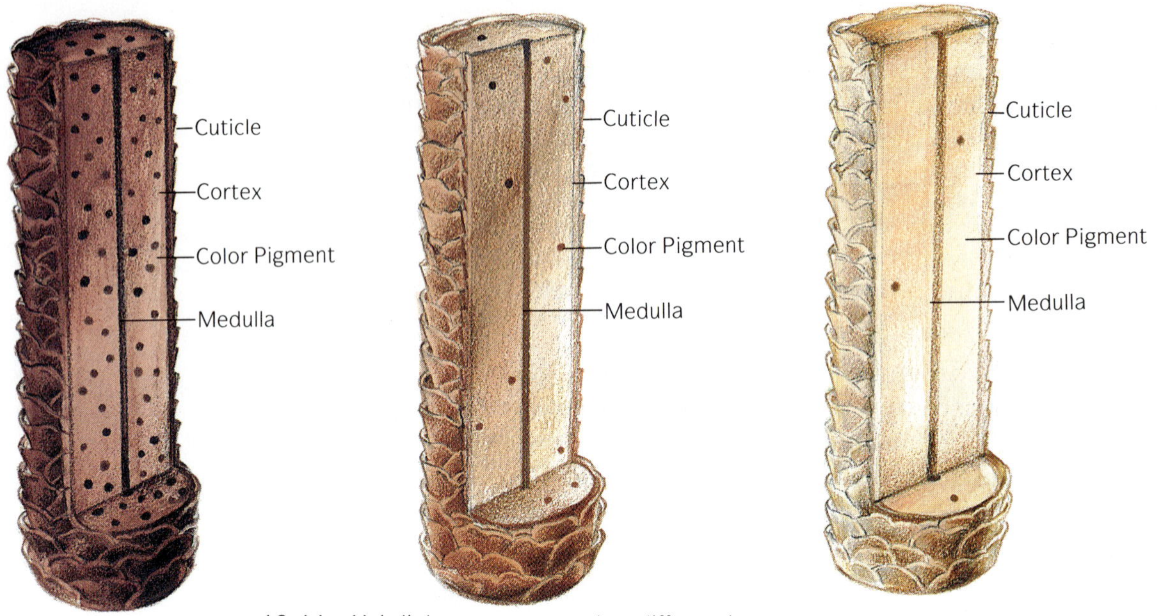

12.44—Hair lighteners are used to diffuse pigment.

The Decolorizing Process

A lightening product is used to diffuse pigment. (Fig. 12.44) The hair pigment goes through different stages of color as it lightens. The amount of change depends on how much pigment the hair has and the length of time the lightening product is processed.

The Degrees (or Stages) of Decolorizing

During the degrees of decolorizing, hair can go through as many as 10 stages. (Fig. 12.45)

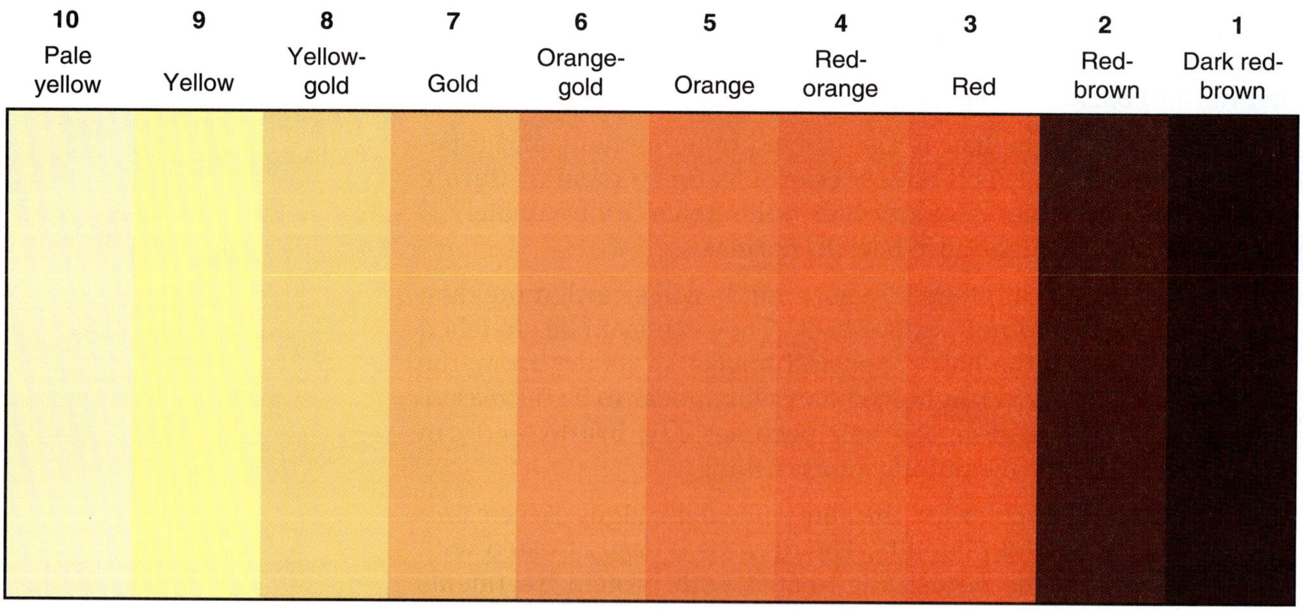

12.45—Ten degrees of decolorization.

10. Pale Yellow
9. Yellow
8. Yellow-Gold
7. Gold
6. Orange-Gold
5. Orange
4. Red-Orange
3. Red
2. Red-Brown
1. Dark Red-Brown

Contribution of Underlying Pigment

Decolorizing the hair's natural melanin pigment allows the colorist to create the exact degree of contributing pigment needed for the final result. First, the hair is decolorized to the appropriate level. Then, the new color is applied to deposit the desired tonality and intensity. Lightening the hair to the correct degree is absolutely essential to a beautiful, controlled, final haircoloring result because the natural pigment that remains in the hair contributes to the artificial color that is added by the colorist, giving you the final result.

Generally, on-the-scalp lighteners are made to work for up to 2 hours. Since the strongest lightening action takes place within the first 60 minutes, it is sometimes helpful when decolorizing very resistant hair to remove the first lightening mixture after 1 hour and apply a fresh one.

It is extremely important to be patient. Red-orange (degree 4) and gold (degree 7) require the most decolorization time to get through. Often, a colorist is tempted to remove the lightener too early. When color is then added to warm contributing pigment, the results will not be as desired.

Most heads of healthy hair can be safely lifted to the pale yellow stage. It is the job of the professional colorist to analyze the hair prior to lightening, and to closely observe the stages of lightening to determine how light the color can be taken. Performing a preliminary strand test takes the guesswork out of this procedure.

The hair is never safely lifted past the pale yellow stage to a white with bleach. The extreme diffusion of color necessary to give a white appearance to the eye causes excessive damage to the cuticle and cortex, and sometimes even the medulla. The result is that wet hair feels "mushy" and will stretch without returning to its original length. When dry, the hair will be harsh and brittle. Such hair often suffers breakage and will not accept a toner properly. However, this does not mean that only those born with blonde hair can be a white blonde. The baby-blonde look can be achieved by lightening to pale yellow and neutralizing the unwanted undertone with a toner.

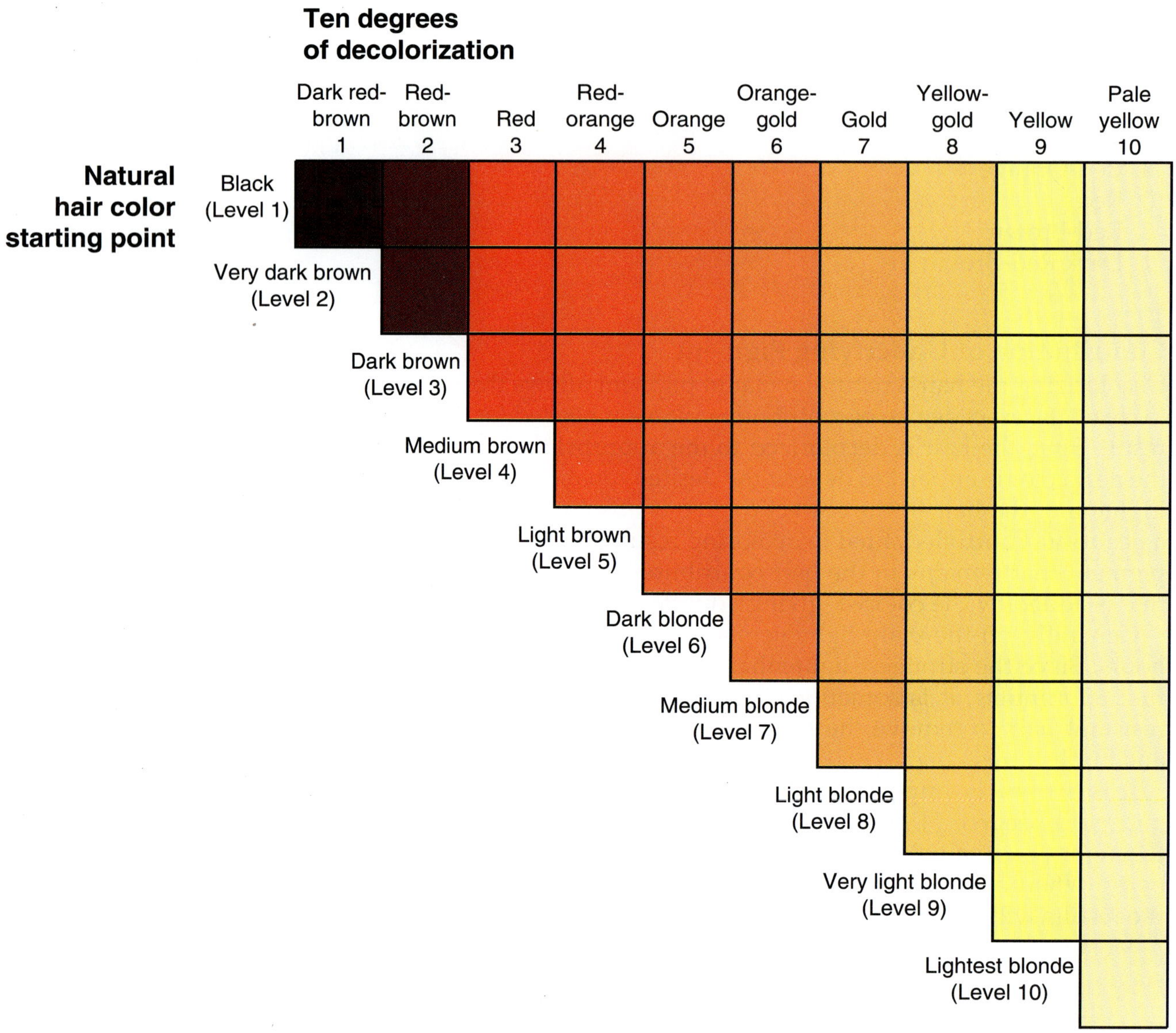

12.46—Contribution of underlying pigment.

Not all hair will go through all 10 degrees of decolorization. Each natural hair color starts the decolorization process at a different stage. Only black hair will pass through all 10 degrees of lightening to reach pale yellow. Remember, the goal is to create the correct degree of contributing pigment as the foundation for the final haircolor result. (Fig. 12.46)

Time Factors

The darker the natural hair color, the more melanin it has. The more melanin it has, the longer it takes to diffuse the color to give a lighter appearance to the hair. The amount of time needed to lighten the natural color is also influenced by the porosity. Porous hair of the same color level will lighten faster than hair that is nonporous because the bleaching agent can enter the cortex more rapidly.

Tone also influences the length of time necessary to lighten the natural hair color. The greater the percentage of red reflected in the natural color, the more difficult it is to achieve the pale, delicate shades of blonde. The ash blondes are especially difficult to achieve because the melanin must be diffused sufficiently to alter both the level and tone of the hair.

The strength of the product also affects the speed and amount of lightening. The stronger bleaches achieve the pale shades in the least amount of time.

Because heat, used in conjunction with lightening chemicals, softens the hair, creating a fragile state, caution must be exercised when using heat. Excessive heat can cause the motion of the molecules to become so great that extreme damage can occur as cuticle layers are removed and cortical bonds are destroyed.

Heat leads to quicker lightening, thus shortening the time needed for decolorization. The stages of lightening must be carefully observed to avoid excessive lift that could lead to the diffusion of so much natural pigment that the desired toner shade may not develop properly in the hair shaft. When this occurs, the toner shade may "grab" the base color, giving the hair an ashy, gray tone. However, beautiful blondes can safely be achieved by anyone with proper analysis, products, and techniques.

Lightening Virgin Hair

A preliminary strand test is necessary before lightening in order to determine the processing time, the condition of the hair after lightening, and the end results. Carefully record all data on client record card.

Preliminary Test Results

1. If test shows the hair is not light enough:
   a) Increase strength of mixture and/or
   b) Increase processing time.
2. If hair strand is too light:
   a) Decrease strength of mixture and/or
   b) Decrease processing time.
3. Watch strand carefully for reaction to lightening mixture and for discoloration or breakage. Reconditioning may be required prior to toning.
4. If color and condition are good, proceed with lightening.

◆ NOTE: A patch test must be taken 24 to 48 hours prior to the application of a toner containing aniline derivatives. To save the client's time, the strand test for lightening should be made the same day as the patch test.

Implements and Materials

Towels	Comb	Protective gloves
Plastic clips	Tint cape	Plastic or glass bowl
Shampoo	Peroxide	Acid or finishing rinse
Cotton	Record card	Applicator bottle or brush
Lightener	Timer	Protective cream

Procedure

The following general instructions may be changed by your instructor for particular lightening effects or products.

1. Prepare client. Protect client's clothing with towel and tint cape.
2. Analyze scalp and hair, and record on client's card. Do not perform the service if the client has abrasions or inflammation of the scalp.
3. Do not brush hair.
4. Check patch test area if toner is to be used. Proceed only if test results are negative.
5. Section hair into four quarters.
6. Apply protective cream around hairline and over ears.
7. Put on gloves to protect your hands.
8. Prepare lightening formula. Use immediately to prevent deterioration.
9. Apply lightener. Begin application where hair seems resistant or especially dark, usually the back of the head. Use ⅛″ (.3125 cm) partings to apply lightener. Start ½″ (1.25 cm) from the scalp and extend lightener up to, **but not through**, the porous ends. Apply lightener to top and underside of subsection in quick, rhythmic movements. (Fig. 12.47)

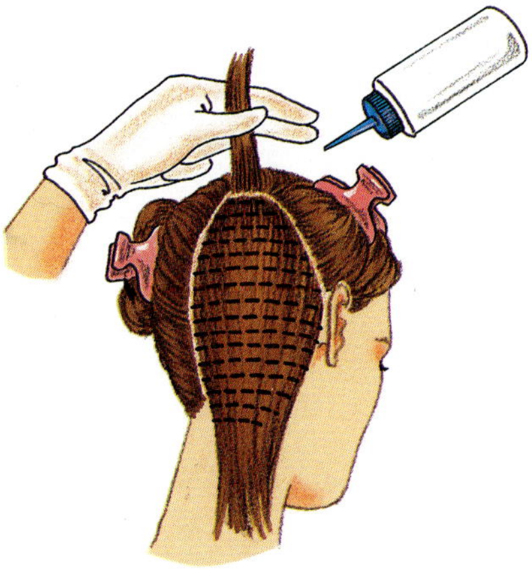

12.47—Apply lightener to underside of strand.

10. Continue to apply lightener. Double check application, adding more lightener if necessary. Do not comb lightener through hair. Keep lightener moist during development by misting the hair lightly with a spray bottle or reapplying lightener as the mixture dries.
11. Test for lightening action. Make first check about 15 minutes before time indicated by preliminary strand test. Remove mixture from strand with damp towel. Towel dry and examine. If strand is not light enough, reapply mixture and continue testing frequently until desired level is reached.
12. Apply lightener to hair near scalp with ⅛″ (.3125 cm) parting. (Fig. 12.48) If necessary, prepare fresh lightener. Process and strand test until entire shaft has reached desired stage.

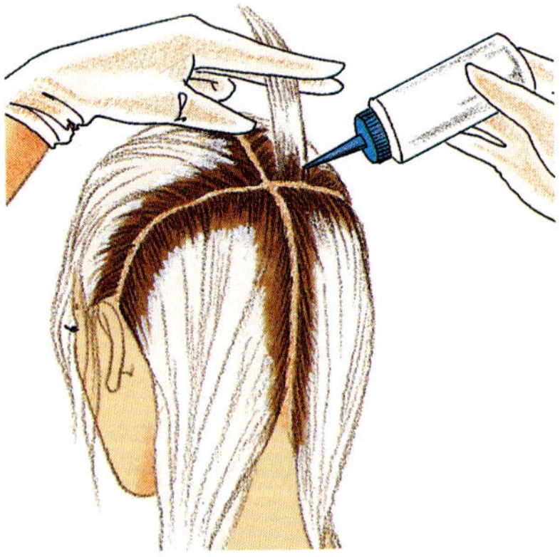

12.48—Apply lightener at scalp.

13. Remove lightener. Rinse thoroughly with cool water. Shampoo gently with acid-balanced shampoo, with hands under hair to avoid tangling.
14. Neutralize the alkalinity of the hair with an acid or a normalizing rinse. Recondition if necessary.
15. Towel dry hair, or dry completely under cool dryer if manufacturer requires it.
16. Examine scalp for abrasions. Analyze condition of hair.
17. Proceed with toner application.
18. Complete record card and file.
19. Clean up in usual manner.

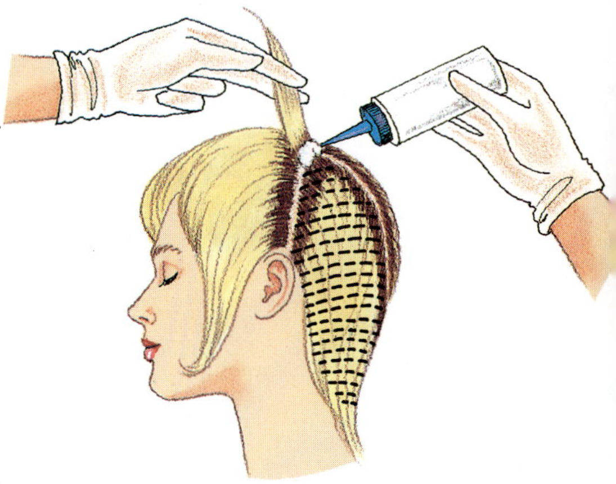

12.49—Apply lightener to new growth.

Lightener Retouch

As the hair grows, dark regrowth will be very obvious. A lightener retouch corrects this problem and matches the regrowth to the rest of the lightened hair. During retouch, the lightener is applied to the new growth only, with the following exceptions:

1. If another color is desired.
2. If a lighter shade is desired.
3. If color has become dull from repeated applications.

In each case, lighten the regrowth first. Then bring remaining lightener mixture gently through the hair shaft. Process for 1 to 5 minutes until problem is corrected.

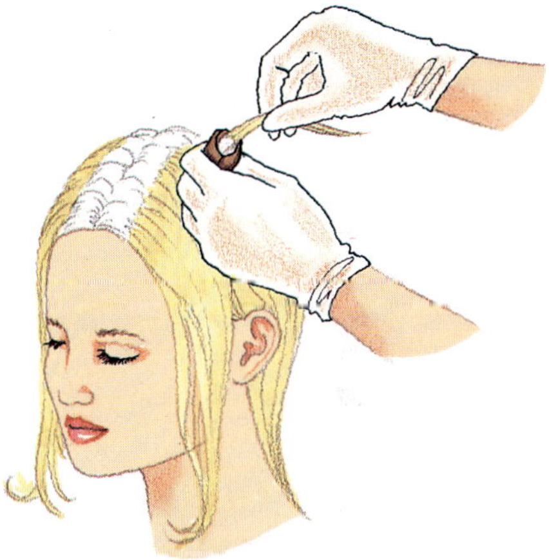

12.50—Strand testing.

Procedure

Always consult the client's record card to tell you about lightener formula, timing, and other pertinent information. The procedure for a lightener retouch is the same as that for lightening a virgin head of hair, except that the mixture is applied only to the new growth of hair. (Figs. 12.49–12.51)

A cream lightener is generally used for a lightener retouch because its consistency helps prevent overlapping of previously lightened hair, and it is gentler on the scalp. Overlapping can cause severe breakage and lines of demarcation.

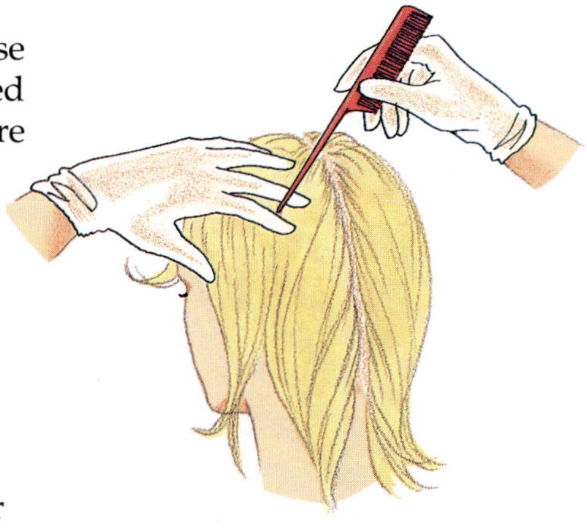

12.51—Check for complete coverage.

Safety precautions

1. Give a patch test 24 to 48 hours before toner application.
2. Read manufacturer's directions before preparing lightener.
3. Always wash your hands before and after servicing a client.
4. Drape client properly to protect clothing.
5. Examine scalp carefully. Do not apply lightener if irritation or abrasions are present.

6. Do not brush hair. If shampoo is required, avoid irritating the scalp.
7. Analyze condition of hair and give any necessary reconditioning treatments.
8. Wear protective gloves.
9. Use only sanitized applicators and towels.
10. Conduct strand test prior to lightener retouch.
11. Cream lightener should be the thickness of whipped cream to avoid dripping, running, or overlapping.
12. Always use lightener immediately after mixing. Discard left-over lightener.
13. Apply lightener to resistant areas first. Use ⅛" (.3125 cm) partings to ensure accurate coverage.
14. Apply rapidly and neatly for even lightening.
15. Give frequent strand tests until desired stage is reached.
16. Check skin and scalp after application and gently remove any lightener with cool, damp towel.
17. Lightener can be safely left on the scalp area a maximum of 1 hour.
18. If towel around client's neck becomes saturated, remove and replace to avoid skin irritation.
19. Cool water and mild shampoo should be used to remove lightener. Avoid tangling fragile hair.
20. Cap all bottles to avoid contamination. Store carefully.
21. Complete record card and file.

Spot Lightening

Uneven lightening, streaking, or dark spots are usually due to careless lightener application. It is necessary to correct these areas to ensure even color.

To correct streaked hair:

1. Prepare lightening formula.
2. Apply mixture only to darker areas.
3. Allow mixture to remain on hair until all streaks are removed.
4. Shampoo lightener from hair.

Toners

Toners are aniline derivative tints and require a 24 to 48 hour patch test. They consist of pale and delicate colors, and are applied to the lightest degrees of contributing pigment from the decolorizing process.

Toners require a double-process application:

1. The first process is the lightener.
2. The second process is the toner.

Pre-Lightening to Create a Foundation for Toners

After the hair goes through decolorizing, the color left in the hair is known as its foundation. Achieving the correct foundation is necessary to create the degree of porosity required for proper toner development.

Manufacturers of toners provide literature that recommends the proper foundation to achieve your desired color. As a general rule, the paler the desired color, the lighter the foundation must be. It is important to follow the guide closely because:

1. Over-lightened hair will "grab" the base color of the toner.
2. Under-lightened hair will appear to have more red, yellow, or orange than the intended color.

It is not advisable to prelighten past the pale yellow stage. This will create over-porous hair with inadequate amounts of natural pigment left in the cortex for your toner to bond to. Refer to the laws of color to select a toner that will neutralize or tone the prelightened hair to the desired shade.

In addition to achieving the correct foundation stage for toning, you must also achieve a sufficient porosity for toner development. Occasionally, virgin blonde, gray, or white hair reaches the correct color foundation without achieving sufficient porosity. You must make adjustments in your color mixture to achieve the desired color.

Preliminary Toner Application

1. Give 24- to 48-hour patch test prior to toner application.
2. Strand test may be given on same day as patch test to save time.
3. Proceed with application only if test results are negative and hair is in good condition.

Implements and Materials

Towels	Comb	Protective gloves
Plastic clips	Tint cape	Plastic or glass bowl
Shampoo	Peroxide	Acid or finishing rinse
Cotton	Protective cream	Record card
Toner	Applicator bottle or brush	Timer

Preparation

1. Arrange all supplies.
2. Prepare client.
3. Wear protective gloves.
4. Prelighten hair to desired stage of decolorization.
5. Shampoo hair lightly, rinse, and towel dry.
6. Acidify and recondition as necessary.
7. Select desired toner shade (indicated by the degree of prelightening previously required to achieve desired tonal result).
8. Apply protective cream around hairline and over ears.
9. Strand test and record results on client's record card.
10. Mix toner and developer if using an oxidative toner in a nonmetallic bowl or bottle according to manufacturer's directions.

Procedure

Wear gloves for protection throughout the application. Speed and accuracy of application are crucial for good color results.

Application of low or nonperoxide toners may vary. Your instructor will direct you.

1. Divide hair into four equal sections. Use the end of tail comb or tint brush. Avoid scratching the scalp.
2. At crown of a back quarter, part off ¼″ (.625 cm) partings and apply toner from scalp up to but not including the porous ends.
3. When the strand test confirms proper color development, gently work toner through ends using brush or fingers.

◆ NOTE: Do not bring toner mixture through porous ends until the last, and then only if changing tonal value or significant fading has occurred. To do so will only make the hair even more porous and more susceptible to continued fading. If ends tend to absorb too much color, dilute remaining mixture with mild shampoo, conditioner, or distilled water before applying to ends.

4. Apply additional mixture to hair, if needed, and blend. Leave hair loose to permit air circulation or cover hair with cap if required.
5. Time according to strand test results. Test frequently until desired shade is reached evenly throughout shaft and ends.
6. Remove toner by wetting hair and massaging toner to lather.
7. Rinse, shampoo gently, and rinse well.
8. Apply finishing rinse to close cuticle, lower the pH, and help prevent fading.
9. Remove any toner stains from the skin, hairline, and neck.
10. Style as desired. Use caution to avoid stretching the hair.
11. Complete record card and file.
12. Clean up in usual manner.

Toner Retouch

A toner retouch requires careful analysis of the hair. The new growth must be prelightened to the same stage as the hair was for the first toner application. Based on your analysis and strand test, you will either apply the toner to the entire shaft as in the original application, or you will apply toner to the new growth only. When that area is nearly processed, you can work diluted toner mixture through the remaining hair if necessary.

SPECIAL EFFECTS HIGHLIGHTING

Special effects highlighting involves any technique of partial lightening or coloring. Lightening for special effects is a fashion technique. As styles change, you only need to adapt placement of lightened strands and colors for the trend.

You may create special effects by strategically placing the light and dark colors in the hair. Some colors appear to advance, others appear to recede. Light colors will cause the area to advance toward the eye, appear larger, and make detail more visible. The contrasting dark areas will cause the area to recede, appear smaller, and make detail less visible.

Many do their own haircolor at home with a fair degree of success, but home haircoloring is limited. Special effects and advanced techniques cannot be achieved by an untrained person. It is for that reason that at-home haircolor will never replace professional haircoloring.

As you begin to expand your knowledge and expertise in haircoloring and lightening, you will find greater degrees of creativity in application techniques. Tone on tone, reverse highlighting, dimensional coloring, and scrunching are but a few ways to create special effects. Your instructor will assist you in mastering the basic techniques, and the rest is up to you. The possibilities are limited only by your imagination.

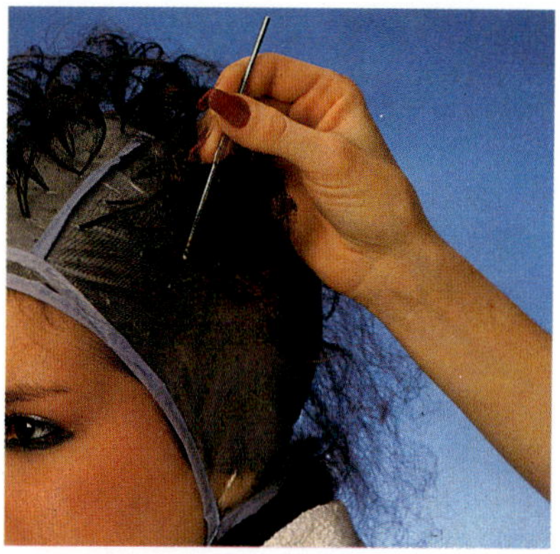

12.52—Draw strands through holes in cap with hook.

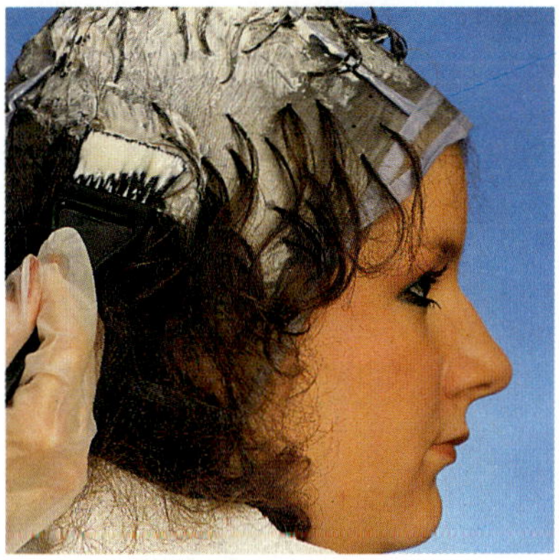

12.53—Apply lightener to selected strands.

Methods for Highlighting

There are several methods to achieve highlights. The most frequently used are:

1. Cap technique
2. Foil technique
3. Freehand technique

The **cap technique** involves pulling clean strands of hair through a perforated cap with a hook. (Fig. 12.52) The amount of strands pulled through depends upon the amount of lightness desired. Pull small strands and leave holes empty for a subtle look. The lightening will be greater if all holes are used, and more dramatic if larger strands are pulled through the holes.

The hair is then lightened, usually with a powder or "quick" lightener, or with a tint that can lift a great deal. (Fig. 12.53) The lightener is removed by first rinsing with lukewarm water, then gently cleansing with an acid-balanced shampoo. After towel-blotting and conditioning if necessary, the lightened hair is toned, if desired. (Figs. 12.54, 12.55)

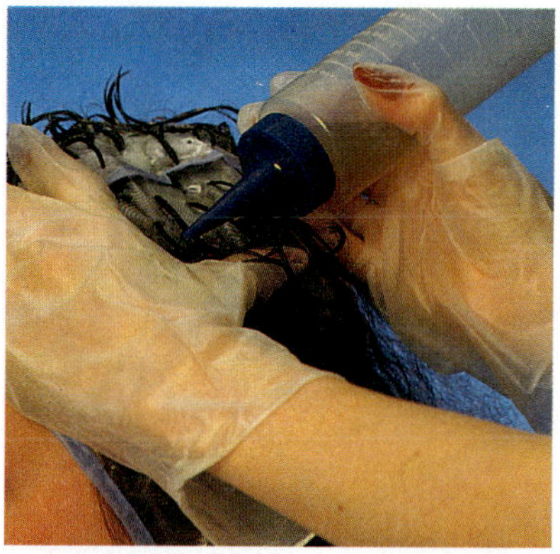

12.54—Apply toner to prelightened strands.

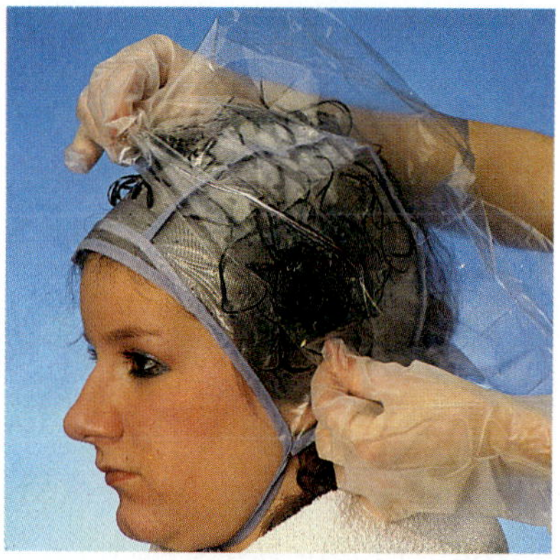

12.55—Cover loosely with a plastic cap.

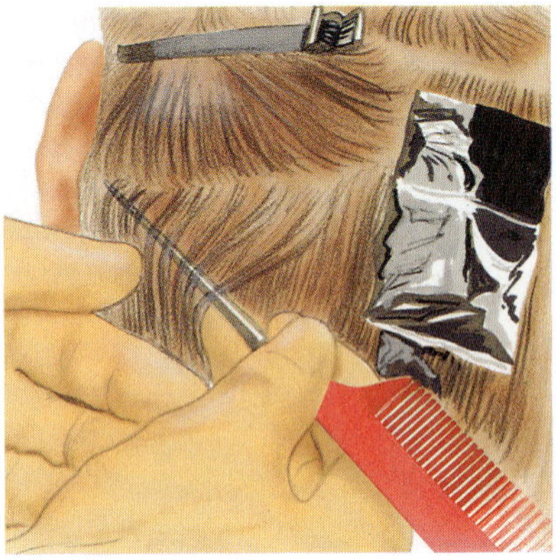

12.56—Weave subsection with a tail comb.

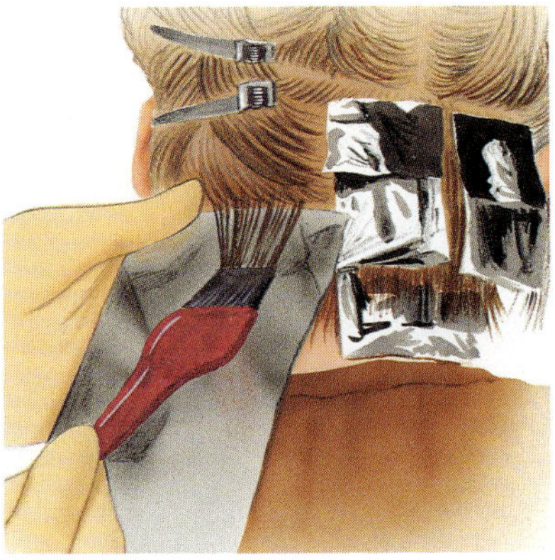

12.57—Place hair in foil packet as shown.

✔ Completed—Learning Objective No. 5

HAIR LIGHTENING

The **foil technique** involves weaving out (selecting) alternating strands from a subsection. (Fig. 12.56) The selected strands are then placed over foil or plastic wrap, and the appropriate lightener or high-lift tint is applied. The foil is folded to prevent lifting any unwoven hair. (Fig. 12.57) With this technique, the colorist can strategically place highlights.

Freehand techniques involve the placement of a lightening compound directly onto clean, styled hair. The lightener can be applied with a tint brush, an applicator bottle, or even with gloved fingers. Effects are extremely subtle, and can be used effectively to draw attention to a waveline or an upsweep movement.

Toning Over Highlighted and Dimensionally Colored Hair

When the hair is decolorized to the desired level and tonality during a highlighting service, the use of a toner is often eliminated. However, if a cool tonality is desired, then the use of a toner will cancel out the unwanted yellow contributing pigment.

When using a toner on highlighted hair, it is important to consider not only the varying degrees of porosity in the hair, but also the difference in pigmentation from strand to strand created by the lightening process. An oxidative toner would impart color into the highlighted strands, but may also affect the natural, or pigmented, hair causing a slight amount of lift. The result may be an uneven tonality, with the underlying warmth brought out by the oxidative color. Strand test to ensure best results.

To avoid affecting the untreated hair, several choices are available:

1. A nonoxidative toner contains no ammonia, and requires no developer (which produces no lift of the natural hair color) and is gentle on the scalp and hair. This is particularly useful for sensitive clients.
2. A semi-permanent color may be used to deposit tonality without lift. Not all colors will be delicate enough to avoid overpowering the prelightened hair. Always check the manufacturer's color chart for the base color of your chosen toner to make sure that when it combines with the contributing pigment in the hair you will have the exact tonality you wanted.
3. A deposit-only haircolor, which is an oxidative color without ammonia, can also be used to recolor hair. They do not further decolorize, but they are more permanent than nonoxidative toners. ✔

COMPOSITION OF PERMANENT HAIRCOLORS

Permanent hair dyes, on a professional level, are based almost entirely on the use of oxidative tints. Commercially these dyes are known by a variety of names: para-dyes, aniline derivative tints, permanent tints, synthetic-organic tints, penetrating tints, cream tints, and tube colors, as well as oxidative tints.

The term ***para-dye*** refers to the colorless substances, either paraphenylenediamine or paratoluenediamine, that transform into a colored material in and on the hair shaft when mixed with an oxidizer such as hydrogen peroxide. Even though some oxidation tints no longer contain either of these derivatives, para-dye has become a term that refers to all oxidation tints regardless of chemical composition.

Many permanent haircolors include ammonia in the formulation to activate the coloring process. Ammonia, as formulated into oxidative colors, has the disadvantages of a strong odor and the potential to aggressively affect melanin, causing excessive color diffusion and structural damage if not used properly.

The industry has taken strides to manufacture tint products that either replace or partially replace ammonia. However, the permanent tints containing no ammonia do not have the lifting power of those formulated with it.

Most oxidative tints contain aniline derivatives and require a ***predisposition test*** before the service. As long as the hair is of normal strength and kept in good condition, oxidative tints are compatible with other professional chemical services.

Action of Oxidative Tints

Oxidative tints are sold in bottles, canisters, and tubes in either a semi-liquid or cream form. The colorist adds the oxidizing agent, hydrogen peroxide, that activates the chemical reaction known as oxidation. This reaction, which occurs at an alkaline pH, is created to a great extent by the ammonia in the tint, and begins as soon as the two compounds are combined. For this reason, the mixed tint must be used immediately. Any leftover tint must be discarded since it deteriorates quickly.

Application of this oxidizing tint in an alkaline state causes the hair shaft to swell and the cuticle to open. The molecules of the tint base, before mixing with the oxidizer, are very small and can pass easily through the cuticle and into the cortex of the hair shaft. As the oxidation process begins, the coupling together of these small colorless tint-base molecules changes them into large chains of colored, relatively stable pigment.

These molecules become trapped beneath the cuticle as they are now too large to be shampooed out. They form acid bonds with the keratin chains in the cortex and become part of the hair structure.

Timing the application of the tint depends upon the product and the volume of peroxide selected. The general rule is the higher the working volume of hydrogen peroxide used in your formula, the longer the color has to process. Consult the manufacturer's directions and your instructor for assistance. A test strand should always be taken to ensure satisfactory results.

Single-process tints have the ability to both lighten and deposit pigment at one time to achieve the desired color. Prelightening or presoftening is not required.

Single-process tints usually contain a lightening agent, a shampoo, an aniline derivative tint, and an alkalizing agent to activate the peroxide that is added. Most color is formulated to be used with 20 volume peroxide. Color results are altered when other volumes are used.

The advantages of single-process tints are that they:

1. Can produce shades from the deepest black to the lightest blonde.
2. Can color the hair lighter or darker than the client's original shade.
3. Can blend white or gray hair to a natural hair shade.
4. Can correct streaks, off-shades, discolorations, and faded ends.
5. Are available as creams, liquids, and gels.

Types of Permanent Tints

The cosmetic chemicals that make oxidative haircoloring possible are available to salon colorists in several forms: liquids, creams, and gels. Each of these haircoloring bases has its loyal professional users and the choice of one form or the other is a matter of individual preference.

As the name implies, the viscosity of liquid haircolor is generally thinner, and may be applied with a bottle technique to better control the placement of the color formula. Liquid haircolor products may generally contain a greater amount of ammonia and less conditioning bases in their composition than creams or gels, but may also be more economically priced and have excellent penetrating ability.

Cream haircolor products may come in tube or canister form from the manufacturer, and have conditioners and thickening agents. They can sometimes be too viscous (thick) to be applied from an applicator bottle, and are generally mixed with cream developer when applying by brush-and-bowl technique.

The consistency of a gel haircolor falls between that of a liquid and a cream. It is more penetrating than a cream (but less conditioning), and the same or more penetrating than a liquid (but more conditioning). It can be applied using a bottle or brush technique.

Formulating for Lift and Deposit

The formulation for lift and deposit of a permanent oxidative haircolor is based upon the product you select. Always follow manufacturer's guidelines for their product to obtain the precise amount of lifting of natural pigment (to create the proper degree of contributing pigment) as well as the correct amount of depositing pigment (to enhance or conceal the newly created undertone) to produce your final desired result.

Manufacturers currently offer liquid haircoloring products that use an American "Shades System," and also cream or gel colors that are based on the European "Level System." If the client wants to go darker, simply select the desired level of oxidative tint (the tonal value may have to be adjusted, depending upon the client's current hair color) mixed with 10 or 20 volume developer (based on your test strand results) and proceed with the service.

If your client wants to go lighter, you will select the correct level of color for lift and deposit based upon which manufacturer's system you will be using (Shade or Level System). Remember that tint does not lift tint. A color remover product must first be used to lighten the tinted hair before applying the final color formula.

For the American Shades of Lift System, you would subtract the present level from the desired level. For example, if your client's natural color is a level 6 dark blonde, and the shade desired is a level 8 light blonde you would use an oxidative tint that is 2 levels lighter (8–6=2) than the desired color to achieve the desired lift (remember to formulate for the contributing warmth into your depositing tone). Always refer to the manufacturer's color selection chart accompanying your product for help in formulating properly.

In the European Level System, the color level you choose is the color you will use (but not necessarily the same tone). The lift is determined by the choice of developer. For example, 10 volume developer is for deposit with minimal (up to 1 level) lift; 20 volume is the most recommended strength for adequate deposit and up to 2 levels of lift; 30 volume is for approximately 3 levels of lift; and 40 volume is for 4 levels of lift. Some manufacturers offer haircoloring additives to "boost" the color an extra level, but in doing so create lift at the expense of the loss of depositing pigment, which may result in inadequate refinement of the natural underlying (contributing) pigment. This could produce considerably more warmth than desired. If a client wishes to be a color more than 2 levels lighter, the end tonal result will be warm. Beyond 4 to 5 levels from the natural hair color, most manufacturers recommend a double-process lightening product to achieve the correct balance of lift and deposit.

The more lifting ability a haircolor has, the less depositing ability of the base color. Always remember to formulate with both lift and deposit in mind, to achieve the proper balance for the desired end result. A higher lifting formula than necessary may not have enough depositing tonality to subdue the warmth of a client's natural contributing pigment. Lift and deposit can further be influenced by varying the volume of hydrogen peroxide mixed with the haircolor product. (Fig. 12.58, page 294)

Mixing Procedure

Bottle Application: Measure into a clear applicator bottle (markings for ounces or milliliters are generally provided on the side by the manufacturer) an amount of color product sufficient to saturate

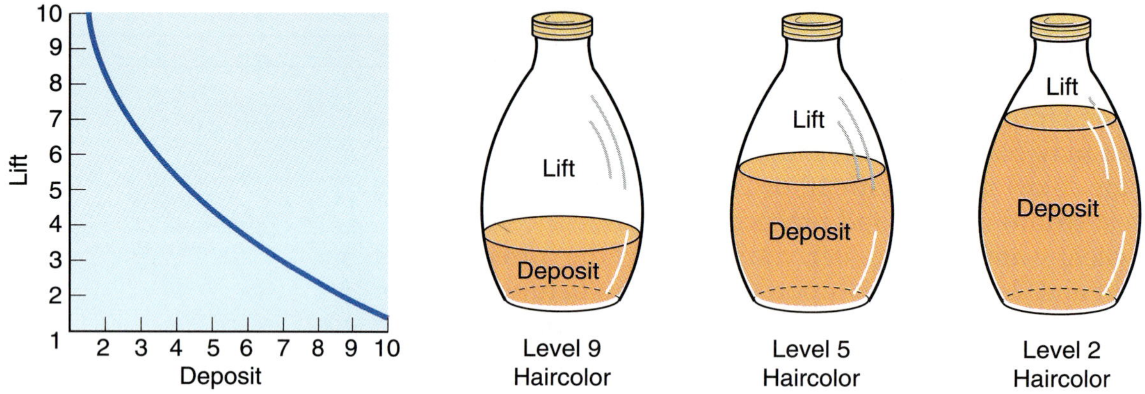

12.58—Lift and deposit ratios.

hair in the areas of the head to be colored. Add the appropriate volume and consistency of developer. Be sure to select an applicator bottle large enough to accommodate both the color product and developer, with enough "air" space to shake the bottle until mixture is thoroughly blended.

Brush-and-Bowl Application: Using a nonmetallic mixing receptacle (glass or plastic bowl will do), add the color or colors selected by your test strand in the appropriate proportions to create the lift and tonal deposit desired. Measure and slowly add the developer (generally cream consistency for added thickness and control during application). Stir into mixture using a tint applicator brush until thoroughly blended.

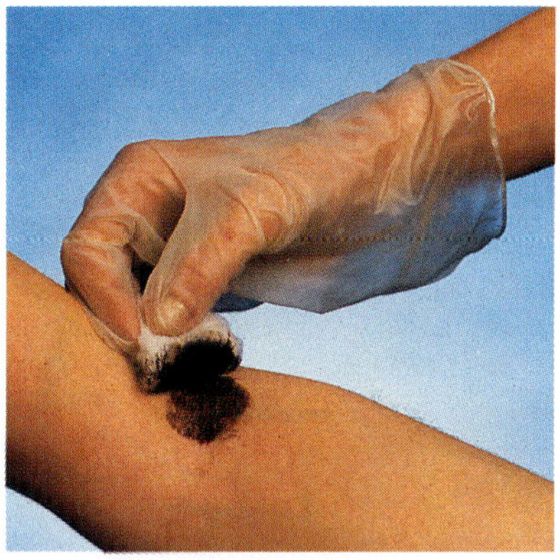

12.59—Give a patch test.

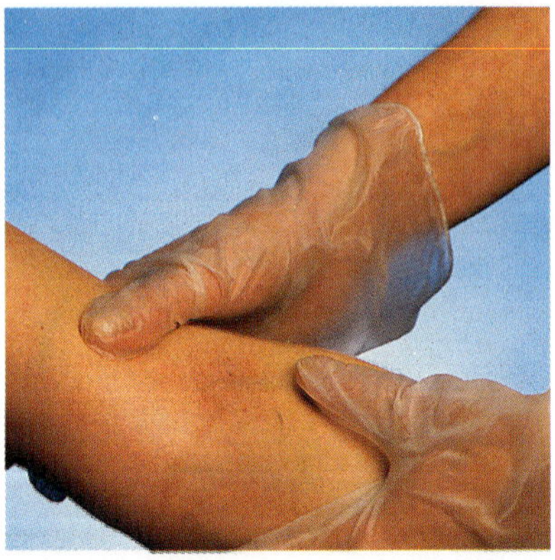

12.60—Proceed if test is negative.

Application Procedures

Virgin hair is hair that has had no chemical services and has not been damaged by natural factors such as wind and sun.

The procedure that follows is a basic single-process color procedure for virgin hair. Your instructor may have another technique just as correct for the particular color used.

Implements and Materials

Towels	Tint cape	Protective gloves
Comb	Applicator bottle or brush	Plastic or glass bowl
Timer	Mild shampoo	Selected tint
Cotton	Color chart	Finishing rinse
Record card	Hydrogen peroxide	Protective cream

Preliminary Steps

1. Give patch test 24 to 48 hours before the service. (Fig. 12.59) Proceed only if test is negative. (Fig. 12.60)
2. Thoroughly analyze scalp and hair. Perform any necessary preconditioning treatments, and record results on client's record card.
3. Assemble all necessary supplies.

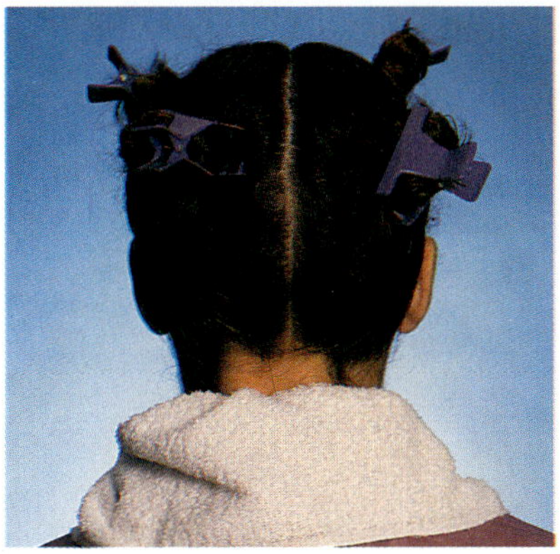
12.61—Hair sectioned into four quarters.

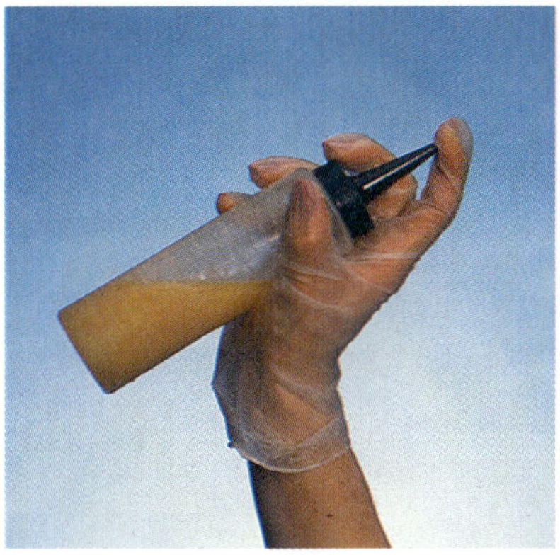
12.62—Prepare and mix tint formula.

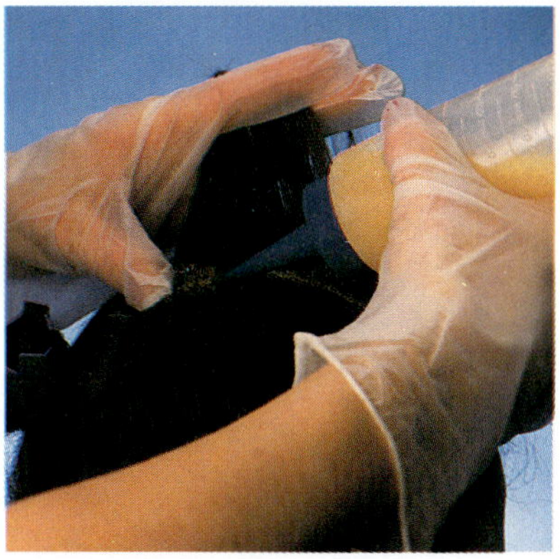
12.63—Begin applying color.

4. Prepare client. Protect clothing with a towel and tint cape. Ask client to remove all jewelry and place safely away.
5. Apply protective cream around hairline and over ears.
6. Put on protective gloves.
7. Perform a strand test.
8. Record results on record card.

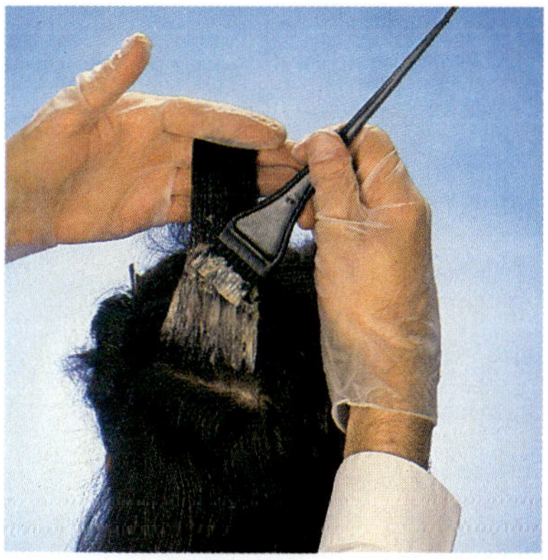
12.64—Apply tint to the hair ends.

Procedure

1. Section the hair into four quarters. (Fig. 12.61)
2. Prepare tint formula for either bottle or brush application. (Fig. 12.62)
3. Begin in section where color change will be greatest or hair is most resistant. (Fig. 12.63)
4. Part off ¼″ (.625 cm) subsection with applicator.
5. Lift subsection and apply tint to hair ½″ (1.25 cm) from scalp up to, **but not through**, the porous ends. (Fig. 12.64)

◆ NOTE: The hair at the scalp will process faster due to body heat and incomplete keratinization. For this reason the tint is applied in the scalp area after being applied to the shaft. Your strand test will determine the application procedure and timing for even color development.

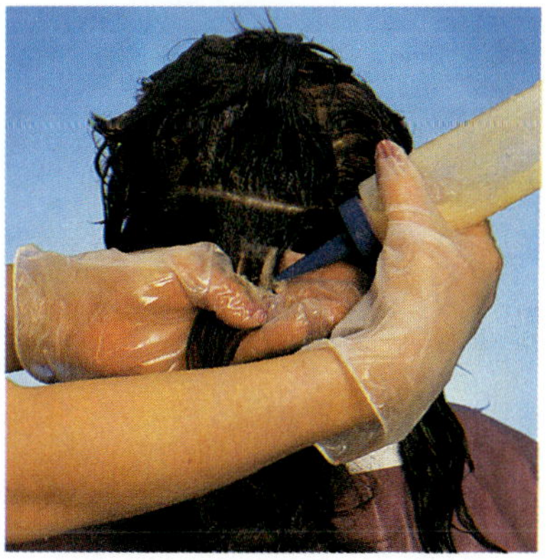
12.65—Blend tint to hair ends.

6. Process according to strand test results. Check for color development by removing color as described in the strand test procedure on page 232.
7. Apply tint mixture to hair at scalp.
8. Blend tint to hair ends. (Fig. 12.65)
9. Lightly rinse with lukewarm water. Massage color to lather and rinse thoroughly.
10. Remove any stains around hairline with remaining tint mixture, shampoo, or stain remover. Use cotton or terry towel to gently remove stains.

11. Shampoo hair thoroughly with a mild (acid-balanced) shampoo.
12. Apply an acid or a finishing rinse to close the cuticle, restore pH, and prevent fading.
13. Style hair.
14. Complete record card and file.

Cleanup

1. Discard all disposable supplies and materials.
2. Close containers tightly, wipe them off, and put them in their proper places.
3. Clean and sanitize implements.
4. Sanitize tint cape.
5. Sanitize work area.
6. Wash and sanitize hands.

When tinting close to or darker than natural hair color, follow the same preparation and procedure as for a lighter shade. Then proceed as follows:

1. Select appropriate color.
2. Application begins where the hair is the most resistant. (If gray is present, application most likely will begin in the front. If no gray is evident, then begin in the back.)
3. Apply tint from scalp to the porous ends using ¼" (.625 cm) subpartings.
4. Process according to strand test results.
5. When color has developed to desired degree, distribute the tint through the ends with a large-toothed comb to ensure complete coverage.
6. Continue processing according to strand test results.
7. Shampoo color off and complete styling and cleanup in usual manner.

The same preparation and procedure are used for long hair as for short hair. Condition the ends according to your analysis. You will probably need more color material than you used for short hair.

Single-Process Tint Retouch Application

As the hair grows, you will need to do a retouch so the hair looks attractive and not two-toned. After you assemble the materials and implements as for a virgin tint, follow the procedure below.

Preliminary Steps

1. Give a patch test 24 to 48 hours before the service. Proceed only if test is negative.
2. Assemble all necessary supplies.
3. Prepare client. Protect clothing with a towel and tint cape. Ask client to remove all jewelry and put safely away.

4. Take out client's record card. Consult with client to see if she or he liked the original color. Carefully analyze hair and condition previously tinted hair as needed.
5. Apply protective cream around hairline and over ears.
6. Perform a strand test.
7. Record all results on record card.

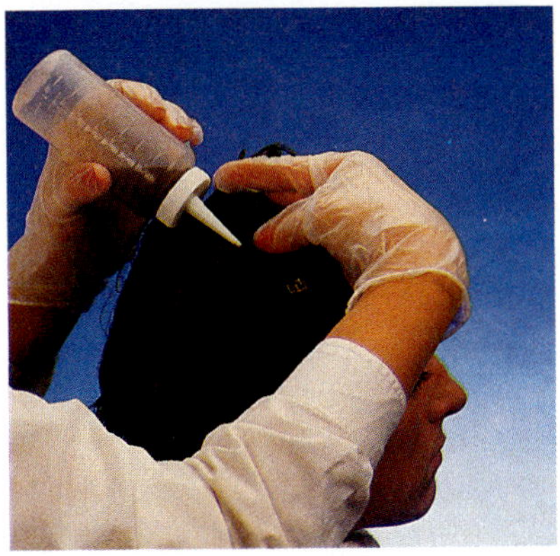

12.66—Apply tint up to new growth only.

Procedure

1. Section the hair into four quarters.
2. Prepare tint formula.
3. Begin in section where color was begun in the virgin application.
4. Part off ¼″ (.625 cm) subsection with applicator.
5. Apply tint to new growth only. (Fig. 12.66) *Do not overlap.* Overlapping of color can cause breakage and create lines of demarcation.
6. Confirm color development by strand testing.
7. Apply diluted color formula to ends according to your analysis and strand test results. Dilute the remaining tint mixture with distilled water, shampoo, or conditioner. (This step is done only if color is faded.)
8. Lightly rinse with lukewarm water. Massage color to lather and rinse thoroughly.
9. Remove any stains around hairline with remaining tint mixture, shampoo, or stain remover. Use cotton to gently remove stains.
10. Shampoo hair thoroughly with a mild (acid-balanced) shampoo.
11. Apply an acid or a finishing rinse to close the cuticle, restore pH, and prevent fading.
12. Style hair.
13. Complete record card and file.
14. Clean up in the usual manner.

Highlighting shampoo tints are prepared by combining aniline derivative tints, hydrogen peroxide, and shampoo. They are used when a very slight change in hair shade is desired, or when the client's hair processes very rapidly. These tints highlight the hair's natural color in a single application. A patch test is required.

Highlighting shampoos are a mixture of shampoo and hydrogen peroxide. The natural color is slightly lightened. No patch test is required.

Procedure

Perform consultation and analysis as for a regular color procedure. If highlighting shampoo tint is to be used, a patch test must have been performed 24 to 48 hours before.

1. Drape client and take to shampoo bowl.
2. Distribute the color over clean, damp hair. Gently lather and process for 8 to 15 minutes.
3. Complete as for a regular tint procedure.

Double-Process Tint

If the client desires a drastically lighter color, the hair should first be prelightened. It is sometimes much more efficient to use a double-process application to achieve pale or cool colors. This avoids the warm undertones the hair contributes from the lightening process, which a single-process tint may not be able to overcome. Remember, the higher the amount of lift in the tint, the less pigment deposit. By decolorizing the hair with a lightener and using a separate product to add the desired tonality, you have more control over the coloring process.

It is also possible to have the hair's contributing pigment work for you in a double-process coloring application. By prelightening the hair to the desired degree of decolorization, you can create a perfect foundation for longer lasting red colors that stay true to tone, without muddiness.

The prelightener is applied in the same manner as for a regular hair lightening treatment. After the prelightening has reached the desired shade, the hair is lightly shampooed, acidified, and towel dried. The color is then applied in the usual manner after a strand test has been taken.

Occasionally gray hair is so resistant that even when formulation, application, and timing are correct, coverage is not satisfactory and presoftening becomes necessary. Presoftening is a two-step or double-application haircoloring in which two distinct and separate applications of product are necessary to achieve the desired shade. The presoftener is applied, processed, and removed. The second step is the application of the tint to complete the two-step process.

The purpose of presoftening is twofold: to soften and open the cuticle for improved penetration of color and to create missing yellow or gold tones in the hair so that the tint with a balance of color will adhere to the hair and process on-tone.

If the client's hair is gray and resistant, the hair should be presoftened with gold-based tints or oil or cream bleaches. All will work to soften and open the cuticle. However, a gold-based tint will deposit missing yellow or gold into the hair while a bleach will only diffuse and oxidize the remaining natural pigment within the shaft.

Follow the manufacturer's recommended directions to mix either an oil bleach or a lifting tint. The ammonia in these products is required to create the desired degree of porosity for color acceptance. However, if using a cream bleach, use no protinator, activator, or catalyst. White or gray hair does not require high lift, and to do so will only cause unnecessary damage.

A gold-based tint 1 to 2 levels lighter than the desired level can be applied directly to the hair to be presoftened without mixing with developer, using only the ammonia content and staining ability in the product. Allow the tint to remain on the hair 5–10 minutes, then wipe gently with a cloth or paper towel to remove. Shampooing is not necessary as a little of the presoftening tint may remain on the hair, with the regular (desired) color formula applied directly over it.

Presoftening is also effective on nongray (pigmented) resistant hair, but care must be given to leave the presoftening mixture on the hair only long enough to open the cuticle, rendering the hair

Question & Answer

HELPING CLIENTS MAKE A CHANGE

Q *How can I convince my clients with 20 percent or more gray hair to try a haircolor change?*

A The thought of change is frightening to some women and men. They resist a change in personal appearance because they are unwilling to make a permanent commitment, especially one they are not sure they will like.

First suggest a semi-permanent color that will fade in six to eight shampoos. Explain to the client that her own natural color will be enhanced by using a formula lighter and warmer than her own. Use a product that has no ammonia and no peroxide. If the client is dissatisfied the color will disappear—without a trace.

Note: Be sure you know the product before you promise a client it will leave her hair unchanged after a few shampoos. Some types of semi-permanent haircolors must be mixed with crystallized or powdered developer at the time of use. That causes the formula to penetrate the cortex and create a chemical change in the natural pigment. Be sure to use a product that contains no ammonia, peroxide or any type of developer.

If the client wants the gray minimized, use a semi-permanent formula that matches her own color. Tell her, however, that her own dark hair will likely become darker as well as the gray hair.

If she wants the gray to appear as highlights, choose a formula lighter and warmer than the natural color. Apply the formula over the entire head, and allow it to process for approximately 25 minutes. It will not lighten the natural hair and will turn the gray into lively, warm highlights.

If the client has concentrated clumps of gray, simply spot-color the hair using two formulas—one to darken the concentrated gray areas, and one to add light color and shine to the mixed gray areas.

Clients are usually so pleased with the results they want even more highlighting. In these cases carefully foil and bleach minute strands throughout, especially around the face. Then apply a non-peroxide toner (a semi-permanent haircolor) two or three shades lighter than her own. Most clients introduced to haircolor in this manner become regular haircolor clients.

—*From* Milady's Salon Solutions *by Louise Cotter*

porous enough to accept the tint. Otherwise, you may create more underlying warmth than you desired, and will have to compensate for this added warmth in your color selection and formulation for deposit.

✔ Completed—Learning Objective No. 6

SINGLE- AND DOUBLE-PROCESS TINT APPLICATIONS

Presoftening Application Procedure

1. Mix product according to manufacturer's directions.
2. Apply with brush or bottle in most resistant areas first.
3. Process at room temperature for 5–20 minutes.
4. Rinse thoroughly and shampoo.
5. Apply tint in usual manner. ✔

SPECIAL PROBLEMS IN HAIRCOLOR/CORRECTIVE COLORING

Each haircoloring service is unique. The colorist must carefully analyze the hair and consult with the client. Strand tests must be taken to ensure good results. But even the most skilled colorist will occasionally have a haircoloring problem. This may be due to the particular structure or condition of the client's hair or to the effects of prior treatments to the hair.

DAMAGED HAIR

Blow-drying, wind, harsh shampoos, and chemical services all take their toll on the condition of the hair. Coating compounds such as hair sprays, styling agents, and some conditioners can prevent color penetration. Preventative and corrective steps that you should take include the following:

1. Incorporate reconditioning into any chemical service that you give.
2. Ensure that the client uses high-quality products at home. (Sell the best.)
3. Precondition hair if your analysis tells you it is damaged. Use a penetrating conditioner that can deposit protein, oils, and moisture regulators.
4. Complete each chemical service by normalizing the pH with a finishing rinse. This will restore the cuticle's protective capacity.
5. If hair is still unresponsive after a conditioning treatment, postpone any further chemical service until the hair is reconditioned.
6. Schedule the client for between-service conditioning.

Hair is considered damaged when the hair has one or more of the following conditions:

- Rough texture
- Over-porous
- Brittle and dry
- Breakage
- No elasticity
- Spongy, matted when wet
- Color fades or absorbs too rapidly

Any of these hair conditions will create problems during a tinting, lightening, permanent waving, or hair relaxing treatment. Therefore, damaged hair should receive reconditioning treatments prior to and after the application of these chemical processes.

Reconditioning Procedure

1. Always thoroughly analyze the hair to determine the problem. Consult with the client until you can discover the source of the damage. You can then correct the problem and avoid its recurrence.
2. Shampoo the hair with a mild shampoo. Use care to keep your hands underneath the hair, and only use gentle massage techniques to avoid tangling the fragile hair.
3. Rinse very well and towel blot gently.
4. Apply the conditioner as the manufacturer directs. If it is a liquid, use a spray bottle; if it is a cream, apply with a sanitized spatula or tint brush.
5. Blend the conditioner through the hair with a wide-toothed comb.
6. Cover the hair with a plastic cap if required, and follow the manufacturer's directions for heat application and timing.
7. Rinse well. Re-examine the hair and proceed with the coloring service only if the hair's condition indicates that the treatment will be successful.

FILLERS

Fillers are specialized preparations that are designed to help equalize porosity and deposit a base color in one application. They can be a manufacturer's preparation or a mixture of tint and conditioner that your instructor will assist you in preparing.

Fillers are absorbed by the hair shaft on the basis of porosity. The greater the porosity, the greater the absorption of the filler. Inside the cortex, the filler molecules fill in the spaces left in the shaft from prior diffusion of melanin. This creates a base to which tint molecules can now attach, as well as a smooth and even surface on the shaft, which the eye perceives as warmth and sheen. Through this process fillers help prevent the flat, dull color that can result when tinting damaged hair.

Conditioner fillers are used to recondition damaged hair before salon service. Conditioner fillers can be applied in a separate procedure, or immediately prior to color application. The conditioner and the tint are then working at the same time.

Color fillers are recommended if the hair is in a damaged condition and there is doubt that the color result will be an even shade.

Advantages of Using a Color Filler

1. Deposits color to faded ends.
2. Helps hair to hold color.
3. Helps color to develop uniformly from scalp to ends.
4. Prevents streaking.
5. Prevents off-color results.
6. Prevents dullness.
7. Produces more uniform, natural-looking color in a tint.

How to Use Color Fillers

Color fillers may be applied directly from their containers to damaged hair prior to tinting. Color fillers may be added to the tint and applied to damaged ends. They may be used full strength or diluted with distilled water.

Selection of Correct Color Filler

To obtain satisfactory results, select the color filler that will replace the missing primary in your formulation. Always remember that all three primaries—red, blue, and yellow—must be present for natural-looking hair color. If you have blonde (yellow) hair, for example, that is being tinted back to an ash (yellow and blue) brown, you will need to use an orange-red filler so that the end result will be correct.

REDS FADING

Fading is a common problem of tinted red hair. The combination of ammonia and peroxide in the tinting formula diffuses the natural pigment, resulting in smaller molecules within the hair shaft. Artificial pigments then attach to the diffused melanin to create a new color. However, with every shampooing; blow-drying; permanent waving; sun, chlorine, or salt water exposure, the artificial pigment is removed through porosity of the cuticle. This leaves behind the smaller, diffused melanin molecules and the warmth created by the oxidation process.

The first step to devising a solution to this situation is to determine the cause of the fading. A scarf, hat, or conditioner with UV absorbers all protect hair from the sun. Rinsing, preferably shampooing and conditioning, salt and chlorinated water from the hair immediately after emerging will lessen their damaging effects. Applying less heat to the hair will also help to prevent damage to the cuticle and diffusion of artificial and natural color. Also, a milder permanent waving solution should be advised for those clients who combine color and perming.

Use of a lower volume of hydrogen peroxide can also prevent excessive fading and brassiness. If the desired depth of red is of the same or deeper level than the natural color, the hue can be achieved through deposition without excessive lift. This technique can be particularly useful in achieving and retaining the violet-based reds.

For warmer or brighter (red-orange or gold) reds on darker natural levels, prelightening before application of your tint can have its advantages. The lightening process naturally brings out the warm contributing pigment, which serves as the ideal foundation for a vibrant red color. However, care must be taken to avoid over-lightening the hair, which will create the opposite reaction than you desire—dull, flat, lifeless color tonality.

Often, when using a single-process tint to achieve the desired red color tonality, a colorist may misjudge the natural hair color level and use a tint with too much lift and not enough depositing pigment to support the desired final result. This leads to the same diffusion of melanin and fading of tone.

When performing a retouch application with a red-based tint, the formula used to create the correct amount of lift at the new growth (utilizing the hair's natural contributing pigment) may produce too much lift if it is pulled through the ends to refresh the color. Better-lasting reds are created by using a separate formula with a deposit-only haircolor product for the hair ends. Your selection should correspond in tone and level to the formula used on the new growth. Strand testing will help indicate the correctness of your color choice.

CORRECTING BRASSINESS AND OTHER UNWANTED TONES IN THE HAIR

As the artificial pigment fades and brassiness becomes apparent, the natural tendency of the client is to request more frequent retouches. Scheduling retouches at closer and closer intervals causes greater porosity and diffusion of the natural pigment, leaving the hair brassier than before as the tint once again fades. A never-ending cycle begins.

The first step to camouflage excessive brassiness in either natural or tinted hair is to analyze it. Is it red, yellow, or orange? Locate the particular shade on the color wheel and use the complementary color to neutralize it. A number of options exist for solving the problem: Temporary rinses, a soap cap during retouches, fillers, and semi-permanent colors of a neutralizing shade can be effective in correcting brassiness, depending upon the situation. Your instructor will guide you in recommending the appropriate treatment for your situation.

TINT REMOVAL

Sometimes it is necessary to remove all or part of the tint from the hair in order to achieve the correct color. The client may want to change to a lighter shade (tint will not lift tint), or the present haircolor may have been a mistake. Occasionally color builds up or processes too dark due to an over-porous condition of the hair shaft.

Commercial products are used to remove penetrating tints and are known as tint, dye, or color removers. Dye removers are not generally sold for use by nonprofessionals because the process is too complex for the untrained. Therefore, color removing is a professional service that can bring new clients into the salon and convert them to loyal customers.

Composition and Action

Color removers may contain ingredients designed to diffuse pigment, both natural and artificial, and are sometimes mixed with hydrogen peroxide. Others have the option of being mixed with distilled water to create a milder color remover. Check the individual manufacturer's directions.

While bleach lightening mixtures are the most efficient products in lightening virgin hair, they are not the best product to use on hair that has been darkened or tinted red with an aniline derivative tint. Bleach locks in golds, oranges, and reds that occur as artificial haircolor decolorizes. Because bleach locks in and cannot remove brassiness in tinted hair, it often becomes impossible to lighten the hair to the desired shade without total destruction of the hair shaft.

A dye solvent is chemically formulated to diffuse and dissolve these artificial color molecules without locking in brassiness. However, as the color remover lightens the artificial color molecules, it also lifts color from the natural pigment or melanin as well.

The removal of tint is always an advanced technique that requires careful analysis of the hair's condition and color. Reconditioning is often necessary after tint removal and before corrective coloring.

Procedure

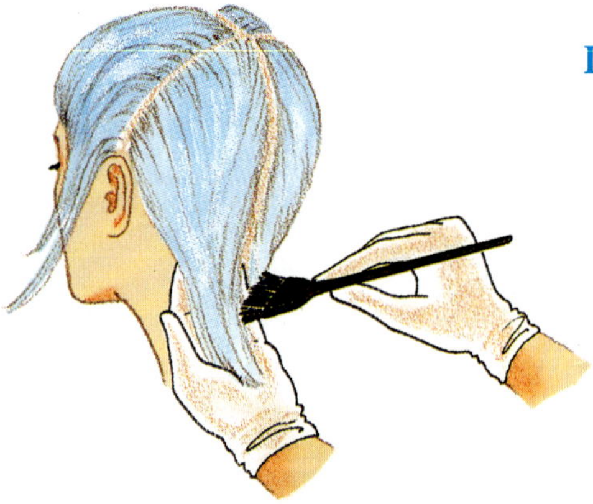

12.67—Apply mixture.

1. Prepare client.
2. Shampoo if required by manufacturer. Avoid manipulating the scalp.
3. Section hair into four quarters.
4. Wear gloves to protect your hands.
5. Mix preparation in glass or plastic bowl according to manufacturer's directions.
6. Immediately begin application where hair is darkest.
7. Apply mixture with tint brush. Saturate hair completely. (Fig. 12.67)
8. Work mixture through hair ends.

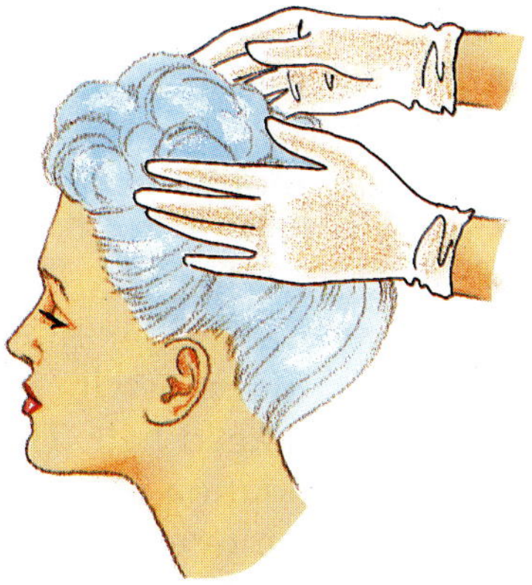

12.68—Pile hair loosely on top of head.

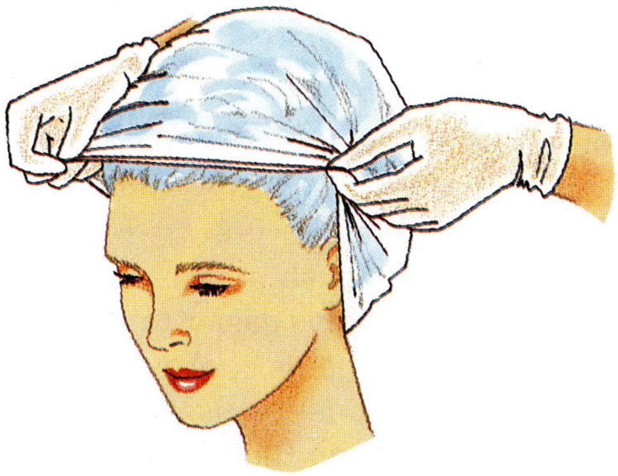

12.69—Cover head with plastic cap if required.

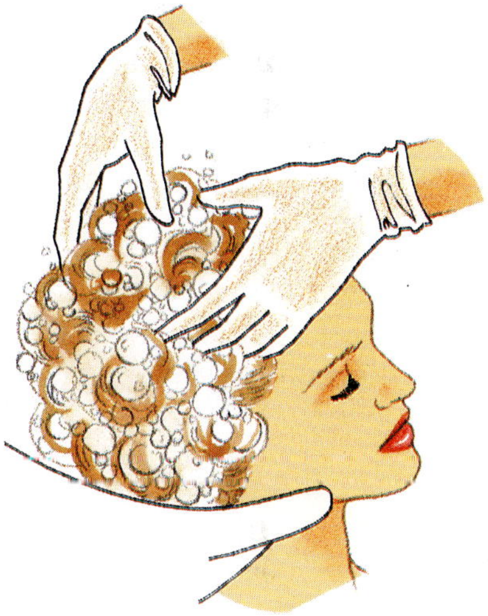

12.70—Shampoo with tepid water.

9. Pile hair loosely on top of head. (Fig. 12.68) Cover with plastic cap if required. (Fig. 12.69)
10. Strand test frequently. Lightening may happen quite rapidly.
11. When color is diffused, rinse thoroughly.
12. Shampoo gently but thoroughly to ensure all of the chemical is removed from the hair. Any tint remover that remains in the hair will continue to process. (Fig. 12.70)
13. Towel dry hair.
14. Analyze hair strength. Condition as required.
15. Perform a strand test.
16. Proceed with the application of desired tint.

If color cannot be applied, style hair in the usual manner. Schedule reconditioning treatments until the hair can withstand tinting.

Tinting After Dye Removal

The use of a color remover does not, as a general rule, create a finished result. Double-application haircoloring is almost always necessary, because the color resulting from the dye solvent is rarely even and is usually red, orange, or gold. However, before continuing, analyze the hair and scalp to decide if they can stand another chemical application.

If possible, condition the hair and wait 24 hours before proceeding. Within this time span, the sebaceous glands will secrete natural oils to protect the scalp from chemical burns. The hair also has time to return to its natural pH, and the pores in the scalp can return to normal. This 24-hour grace period is a safety precaution, but it is not mandatory or practical. If the hair is treated properly, the color service usually can be completed in one day.

Regardless of whether the new color is applied immediately or 24 hours later, the hair shaft will have a new porosity. Remember, the hair has already been treated at least twice with chemicals. Application of a tint or dye solvent causes the hair to become more porous. In this case, both chemicals have been applied to the hair.

A tint applied to porous hair will create a darker hue than on nonporous hair, so select a color at least one level lighter than desired. It's always easier to add more depth than to remove it.

Color will process cooler than it would on undamaged hair. The Law of Color must be used to add the missing foundation warmth when formulating the tint to be used after a color remover. A filler and/or a low volume developer used in tinting the hair is often desirable. Regardless of the chosen method, a strand test is a must before beginning this service.

Sometimes, the hair is so over-porous that there are insufficient protein bonds and natural melanin left within the cortex for the artificial pigment to attach to. The hair may look "gun-metal gray," and this lighter-than-expected result is a real danger sign. Hair that is this porous is very fragile and may be close to the breaking point.

TINT BACK TO NATURAL HAIR COLOR

Clients who have been either tinting or bleaching will often want to return to their natural shade. Sun, chlorinated pool water, or prior chemical services can alter the hair color.

Each tint back to natural color must be handled as an individual problem. This type of hair is porous and may absorb color quickly and process darker and cooler than expected, and may also fade faster than normal. The natural pigment may be so diffused that it will not accept color at all. Carefully record all observations and treatments on the client's record card.

Check the hair for its natural color next to the scalp. After seeing their hair lighter than their natural color for any length of time, many clients may not realize how drastic a change they may be making. Discuss with your client options such as reverse highlighting (weaving strands of darker haircolor into the existing base color), or selection of a color 1 or 2 levels lighter than their natural color. Either of these options will enable you and your client to gradually add more depth if desired, as your client adapts to the new image. A strand test will be essential to ensure desired results.

The solution to a successful tint back to natural can lie in the use of a filler to even out the porosity and achieve color correction. Formulate to create the warmth necessary to prevent a drab, unnatural-looking color in the finished product. Milder color solutions that do no lifting as they deposit are less damaging. The symptoms and solutions are similar to tinting after color removal, which we have previously discussed. Refer to this service and the use of fillers for more information.

A soap cap is used in conjunction with a tint back to natural if the tint does not exactly match the natural color. A quick soap cap, using the addition of shampoo to the tint solution to create a milder formula, will break the line of demarcation.

Procedure

1. Assemble materials.
2. Prepare client in usual manner.
3. Check results of patch test. Proceed only if results are negative.
4. Shampoo hair as directed. Give conditioning treatments according to your analysis.
5. Perform a strand test. More than one test may be necessary to determine the correct formulation and timing for desired results.
6. Section hair into four quarters.
7. Apply filler as directed by your instructor. Remember to replace the missing primary.
8. Process filler according to manufacturer's directions. Proceed directly to tint application.
9. Resection the hair into four quarters.
10. Apply color formula to ¼″ (.625 cm) subsections. Apply the tint as rapidly as possible to both sides of the subsection from the line of demarcation to the porous ends. Process according to your test strand results.
11. When correct color development has been confirmed by strand testing, apply tint to the porous ends. Continue processing.
12. A soap cap may be used after processing time is complete to blend color (optional). For a soap cap add equal amounts of shampoo to the leftover tint and mix it thoroughly. The mixture is applied quickly and worked gently through the ends of the hair.
13. Remove tint from hair with a mild shampoo.
14. Use an acid rinse to close cuticle and help prevent fading.
15. Replace moisture with a finishing rinse.
16. Style as desired, using caution to avoid excessive heat or stretching.
17. Offer the client the opportunity to purchase high-quality salon products to prevent color stripping at home, and schedule the client for conditioning treatments.
18. Complete record card and file.
19. Clean work area in the usual manner.

GRAY HAIR CHALLENGES AND SOLUTIONS

Gray, white, and salt-and-pepper hair have characteristics that create unique coloring problems. A major portion of salon coloring services are performed to either cover or enhance gray. Therefore, this section is dedicated to the study of gray, white, and salt-and-pepper hair; its structure, texture, and condition; and in particular, the characteristics that make it different from all other hair colors.

What is Gray?

The changeover from natural to gray is a gradual one. Gray hair is primarily associated with aging and heredity. Even though the loss of pigment progresses in most people throughout their lives, few become completely white. Most retain a certain percentage of pigmented hair. It can be solid or blended throughout the head, as in salt-and-pepper hair. This blending creates different shades of gray depending upon the ratio of pigmented to nonpigmented hair. Both gray and white hair contain little melanin within the cortex.

Yellowed Gray Hair

A yellow cast can occur from a variety of causes. Smoking, medication, exposure to the sun, and, to a lesser degree, hair sprays and styling aids can all cause the hair to turn yellow. Bleach and dye removers will remove yellow discoloration occurring from internal causes or the oxidation of melanin.

Undesired yellow can be overpowered by the artificial pigments deposited by tints of an equal or darker level than the yellow. Another option is to neutralize the yellow tones with a comparable level of violet.

FORMULATING FOR GRAY HAIR

Level Selection

Level selection for white hair is relatively simple because it basically accepts the level applied. However, colors that are a level 9 or lighter may not give complete coverage because of the small percentage of artificial pigment for depositing in these shades. Generally, formulations from the levels 6, 7, or 8 will give better coverage and can be used to create pastel and blonde tones if desired.

For those clients who are 80% to 100% gray, a haircolor within the blonde range is generally more flattering than a darker shade. This lighter level of artificial color may be selected to give a warm or cool finished product, depending upon the client's skin tone, eye color, and personal preference.

Another factor to consider when coloring the gray in salt-and-pepper hair to a darker level is that color on color makes a darker color. The addition of dark artificial pigment to the natural pigment (peppered hair) results in a color that the eye perceives as darker. For this reason, when attempting to cover gray in a salt-and-pepper head, a shade lighter than the naturally dark hair is generally selected.

A manufacturer's product color chart can be used in conjunction with the following formulation charts to select a color tonality within the proper level with which to perform a strand test.

Semi-Permanent Color Formulation Chart for Gray Hair

Percentage of Gray	Formulation
100–90%	Desired level
90–70%	Equal parts desired & 1 level lighter
70–50%	One level lighter than desired level
50–30%	Equal parts 1 level lighter & 2 levels lighter
30–10%	Two levels lighter than desired level

Permanent Tint Formulation Chart for Gray Hair

Percentage of Gray	Formulation
100–90%	Desired level
90–70%	Two parts desired level & 1 part lighter level
70–50%	Equal parts desired and lighter level
50–30%	Two parts lighter level & 1 part desired level
30–10%	One level lighter

The gray hair formulation chart will give you some basic general guidelines on formulating for gray hair. Of course there are other considerations, such as the client's personality and his/her own personal preferences, as well as the amount of gray and the location. You will note that in the chart there are no tones given in the formulations, only levels of haircoloring and various techniques.

Also note that in the chart there are no accommodations made for the location of the gray hair. The chart is designed so the section that indicates 30% gray presumes that the gray hair is equally distributed throughout the entire head. If, for instance, the majority of the 30% gray hair is located in the front section of the head, that section would be considered 80% gray with the back portion containing just a sprinkling of gray hair. In that instance you would have to determine what formulation would best suit the client—formulating for the 80% gray or the sprinkling of gray. If the gray hair around the face is what the client sees then you would be well advised to formulate for the 80% gray hair. The section of hair that surrounds the face is what influences the client's self-perception.

Your client is accustomed to seeing a certain percentage of gray hair. This gray hair gives the client the perception of having lighter hair. This method of formulating is a method of determining how much lighter you should make the client's hair to give the illusion of the lightness he or she is accustomed to seeing.

The client would have to have at least 10% gray before it is necessary to lighten the natural level. Once again it is the level of color, determined by the amount of gray hair, that the client is accustomed to seeing.

This is where the creativity of color mixing comes in; first using a darker haircolor that will not bring out the undesirable undertones, then achieving the level of lightness by adding some highlights.

There are any number of techniques to aid in solving your haircolor challenges. The more techniques that you have at your disposal the greater latitude you will have. Remember your knowledge and your techniques are your tools for successful haircoloring. Learning haircolor is not a destination, it is a journey that never ends.

RULES FOR EFFECTIVE COLOR CORRECTION

1. Do not panic.
2. Establish the true problem.
3. Establish what caused the problem.
4. Establish the most suitable remedy.
5. Always take one step at a time.
6. Never guarantee an exact result.
7. Always strand test for accuracy. ✔

✔ Completed—Learning Objective No. 7

CORRECTIVE HAIRCOLORING

HAIRCOLORING SAFETY PRECAUTIONS

1. Give a patch test 24 to 48 hours prior to any application of aniline derivative.
2. Apply tint only if patch test is negative.
3. Do not apply tint if abrasions are present.
4. Do not apply tint if metallic or compound dye is present.
5. Do not brush hair prior to applying color.
6. Always read and follow manufacturer's directions.
7. Use sanitized applicator bottles, brushes, combs, and towels.
8. Protect client's clothing by proper draping.
9. Perform a strand test for color, breakage, and/or discoloration.
10. Use an applicator bottle or bowl (glass or plastic) for mixing the tint.
11. Do not mix tint before you are ready to use it; discard leftover tint.
12. Wear gloves to protect your hands.
13. Do not permit the color to come in contact with the client's eyes.
14. Do not overlap during a tint retouch.
15. Do not use water that is too hot; use lukewarm water for removing color.
16. Use a mild shampoo. If an alkaline or harsh shampoo is used, it will strip the color.
17. Always wash hands before and after serving a client. ✔

✔ Completed—Learning Objective No. 8

HAIRCOLORING SAFETY PRECAUTIONS

HAIRCOLORING GLOSSARY

accelerator: (See *activator*)
accent color: (See *color additive*)
acid: An aqueous (water-based) solution having a pH less than 7.0 on the pH scale. The opposite of alkaline.
activator: An additive used to quicken the action or progress of a chemical. Another word for booster, accelerator, protenator, or catalyst.
alkaline: An aqueous (water-based) solution having a pH greater than 7.0 on a pH scale. The opposite of acid.
allergy: A reaction due to extreme sensitivity to certain foods or chemicals.
allergy test: A test to determine the possibility or degree of sensitivity. Also known as a patch test, predisposition test, or skin test.
amino acids: The group of molecules the body uses to synthesize protein. There are some 22 different amino acids found in living protein that serve as units of structure in protein.
ammonia: A colorless pungent gas composed of hydrogen and nitrogen; in water solution it is called ammonia water. Used in haircolor to swell the cuticle. When mixed with hydrogen peroxide, activates the oxidation process on melanin and allows the melanin to decolorize.
analysis (hair): An examination of the hair to determine its condition and natural color. (See *condition; consultation*)
ash: A tone or shade dominated by greens, blues, violets, or grays. May be used to counteract unwanted warm tones.
base color: The predominant tonality of an existing color, i.e., gold-based brown or blonde with a neutral base.
bleeding: Seepage of tint/lightener from foil or cap due to improper application.
blending: A merging of one tint or tone with another.
blonding: A term applied to lightening the hair.
booster: (See *activator*)
brassy tone: Red, orange, or gold tones in the hair.
build-up: Repeated coatings on the hair shaft.
catalyst: A substance used to alter the speed of a chemical reaction.
certified color: A color that meets certain standards for purity and is certified by the FDA.
chemical change: Alteration in the chemical composition of a substance.
coating: Residue left on the outside of the hair shaft.
color: Visual sensation caused by light.
color additive: A concentrated color product that can be added to haircolor to intensify or tone down the color. Another word for concentrate.
color base: The combination of dyes that make up the tonal foundation of a specific haircolor.

color lift: The amount of change natural or artificial pigment undergoes when lightened by a substance.
color mixing: Combining two or more shades together for a custom color.
color priming: The process of adding pigments to prepare the hair for the application of a final color formula.
color refresher: 1. Color applied to midshaft and ends to give a more uniform color appearance to the hair. 2. Color applied by a shampoo-in method to enhance the natural color. Also called color wash, color enhancer.
color remover: A product designed to remove artificial pigment from the hair.
color test: The process of removing product from a hair strand to monitor the progress of color development during tinting or lightening.
color wheel: The arrangement of primary, secondary, and tertiary colors in the order of their relationships to each other. A tool for formulating.
complementary colors: A primary and secondary color positioned opposite each other on the color wheel. When these two colors are combined, they create a neutral color. Combinations are as follows: blue/orange, red/green, yellow/violet.
concentrate: (See *color additive*)
condition: The existing state of the hair; elasticity, strength, texture, porosity, and evidence of previous treatments.
consultation: Verbal communication with a client to determine desired result. [See *analysis* (*hair*)]
contributing pigment: The current level and tone of the hair. Refers to both natural contributing pigment and decolorized (or lightened) contributing pigment. (See *undertone*)
cool tones: (See *ash*)
corrective coloring: The process of correcting an undesirable color.
cortex: The second layer of hair. A fibrous protein core of the hair fiber containing melanin pigment.
coverage: Reference to the ability of a color product to color gray, white, or other colors of hair.
cuticle: The translucent protein outer layer of the hair fiber.
cysteine: The naturally occurring amino acid responsible for the development of pheomelanin.
D & C colors: Colors selected from a certified list approved by the FDA for use in drug and cosmetic products.
decolorize: A chemical process involving the lightening of the natural pigment or artificial color from the hair.
degree: Term used to describe various units of measurement. (See *stage*)
dense: Thick, compact, or crowded.
deposit: Describes the color product in terms of its ability to add color pigment to the hair. Color added equals deposit.
deposit-only color: A category of color products between permanent and semi-permanent colors. Formulated to only deposit color, not

lift. They contain oxidation dyes and utilize low-volume developer.
depth: The lightness or darkness of a specific hair color. (See *level*)
developer: An oxidizing agent, usually hydrogen peroxide, that reacts chemically with coloring material to develop color molecules and create a change in natural hair color.
development time (oxidation period): The time required for a permanent color or lightener to completely develop.
diffused: Broken down, scattered; not limited to one spot.
direct dye: A pre-formed color that dyes the fiber directly without the need for oxidation.
discoloration: The development of undesired shades through chemical reaction.
double process: A technique requiring two separate procedures in which the hair is decolorized or prelightened with a lightener before the depositing color is applied.
drab: Term used to describe hair color shades containing no red or gold. (See *ash; dull*)
drabber: Concentrated color, used to reduce red or gold highlights.
dull: A word used to describe hair or hair color without sheen.
dye: Artificial pigment.
dye intermediate: A material that develops into color only after reaction with developer (hydrogen peroxide). Also known as oxidation dyes.
dye solvents or **dye remover:** (See *color remover*)
elasticity: The ability of the hair to stretch and return to normal.
enzyme: A protein molecule found in living cells that initiates a chemical process.
fade: To lose color through exposure to the elements or other factors.
fillers: 1. Color product used as a color refresher or to fill damaged hair in preparation for haircoloring. 2. Any liquid-like substance to help fill a void. (See *color refresher*)
formulas: Mixtures of two or more ingredients.
formulate: The art of mixing to create a blend or balance of two or more ingredients.
granule: A minute particle in the hair containing melanin.
gray hair: Hair with decreasing amounts of natural pigment. Hair with no natural pigment is actually white. White hairs look gray when mingled with the still-pigmented hair.
hair: A slender thread-like outgrowth of the skin of the head and body.
haircolor: (one word) An industry-coined term referring to artificial haircolor products.
hair color: (two words) The color of hair created by nature.
hair root: That part of the hair contained within the follicle, below the surface of the scalp.
hair shaft: Visible part of each strand of hair. It is made up of an outer layer called the cuticle, an innermost layer called the medulla, and an in-between layer called the cortex. The cortex layer is where color changes are made.

hard water: Water that contains minerals and metallic salts as impurities.
henna: A plant-extracted coloring that produces bright shades or red. The active ingredient is lawsone. Henna permanently colors the hair by coating and penetrating the hair shaft. (See *progressive dye*)
high-lift tinting: A single-process color with a higher degree of lightening action and a minimal amount of color deposit.
highlighting: The introduction of a lighter color in small selected sections to increase lightness of hair. Generally not strongly contrasting from the natural color.
hydrogen peroxide: An oxidizing chemical made up of 2 parts hydrogen and 2 parts oxygen (H_2O_2), used to aid the processing of permanent haircolor and lighteners. Also referred to as developer; available in liquid or cream.
intensity: Used in haircoloring to describe the "strength" of the color's tonality. A tonality can be mild, medium, or strong in intensity.
keratin: The insoluble protein material that is the substance of hair.
level: A unit of measurement, used to evaluate the lightness or darkness of a color, excluding tone.
level system: A system colorists use to analyze the lightness or darkness of a hair color.
lift: The lightening action of a haircolor or lightening product on the hair's natural pigment.
lightener: The chemical compound that lightens the hair by dispersing, dissolving, and decolorizing the natural hair pigment. (See *prelighten*)
lightening: (See *decolorize*)
line of demarcation: An obvious difference between two colors on the hair shaft.
medulla: The center structure of the hair shaft, which may not be present in every hair fiber. Very little is known about its actual function.
melanin: The tiny grains of pigment in the hair cortex that create natural hair color.
melanocytes: Cells in the hair bulb that manufacture melanin.
melanoprotein: The protein coating of a melanosome.
melanosome: Protein-coated granule containing melanin.
metallic dyes: Soluble metal salts such as lead, silver, and bismuth that produce colors on the hair fiber by progressive build-up and exposure to air.
molecule: Two or more atoms chemically joined together; the smallest part of a compound.
neutral: 1. A color balanced between warm and cool, which does not reflect a highlight of any primary or secondary color. 2. Also refers to a pH of 7.
neutralization: The process that counterbalances or cancels the action of an agent or color.

neutralize: Render neutral; counterbalance of action or influence. (See *neutral*)
new growth: The part of the hair shaft that is between previously chemically treated hair and the scalp.
nonalkaline: (See *acid*)
off-the-scalp lightener: Generally a stronger lightener usually in powder form, not to be used directly on the scalp.
on-the-scalp lightener: A liquid, cream, or gel form of lightener that can be used directly on the scalp.
opaque: Allowing no light to shine through.
outgrowth: (See *new growth*)
overlap: Occurs when the application of color or lightener goes beyond the line of demarcation.
over-porosity: The condition where hair reaches an undesirable stage of porosity, requiring correction.
oxidation: 1. The reaction of dye intermediates with hydrogen peroxide found in haircoloring developers. 2. The interaction of hydrogen peroxide on the natural pigment.
oxidative haircolor: A product containing oxidation dyes that require hydrogen peroxide to develop the permanent color.
para tint: A tint made from oxidation dyes.
para-phenylenediamine: An oxidation dye used in most permanent haircolors, often abbreviated as P.P.D.
patch test: A test required by the Food and Drug Act, made by applying a small amount of the haircoloring preparation to the skin of the arm or behind the ear to determine possible allergies (hypersensitivity). Also called predisposition or skin test.
penetrating haircolor: Color that enters or penetrates the cortex or second layer of the hair shaft.
permanent haircolor: A category of haircolor products mixed with developer that create a lasting color change.
peroxide: (See *hydrogen peroxide*)
peroxide residue: Traces of peroxide left in the hair after treatment with lightener or tint.
persulfate: In haircoloring, a chemical ingredient commonly used in activators. It increases the speed of the decolorization process. (See *activator*)
pH: The degree of acidity or alkalinity of any water solution. The pH scale is a numerical scale from 0 (very acidic) to 14 (very alkaline). A pH of 7 is neutral.
pheomelanin: Naturally occurring red/yellow pigment.
pigment: Any substance or matter used as coloring; natural or artificial hair color.
porosity: Ability of the hair to absorb water or other liquids.
powder lightener: (See *off-the-scalp lightener*)
prebleach: (See *prelighten*)
predisposition test: (See *patch test*)

prelighten: Generally the first step of double-process haircoloring, used to lift or lighten the natural pigment. (See *decolorize*)
presoften: The process of treating gray or very resistant hair to allow for better penetration of color.
primary colors: Pigments or colors that are fundamental and cannot be made by mixing colors together. Red, yellow, and blue are the primary colors.
prism: A transparent glass or crystal solid that breaks up white light into its component colors, the spectrum.
processing time: The time required for the chemical treatment to react on the hair.
progressive dye or **progressive dye system:** 1. A coloring system that produces increased absorption with each application. 2. Color products that deepen or increase absorption over a period of time during processing.
regrowth: (See *new growth*)
resistant hair: Hair that is difficult to penetrate with moisture or chemical solutions.
retouch: Application of color or lightening mixture to new growth of hair.
salt-and-pepper: The descriptive term for a mixture of pigmented and gray or white hair.
secondary color: Colors made by combining two primary colors in equal proportion; green, orange, and violet are secondary colors.
semi-permanent haircolor: Haircolor that lasts through several shampoos. It penetrates the hair shaft and stains the cuticle layer, slowly fading with each shampoo.
sensitivity: A skin highly reactive to the presence of a specific chemical. Skin reddens or becomes irritated shortly after application of the chemical. On removal of the chemical, the reaction subsides.
shade: 1. A term used to describe a specific color. 2. The visible difference between two colors.
sheen: The ability of the hair to shine, gleam, or reflect light.
single-process haircolor: Refers to an oxidative tint solution that lifts or lightens while also depositing color in one application. (See *oxidative haircolor*)
softening agent: A mild alkaline product applied prior to the color treatment to increase porosity, swell the cuticle layer of the hair, and increase color absorption. Tint that has not been mixed with developer is frequently used. (See *presoften*)
solution: A blended mixture of solid, liquid, or gaseous substances in a liquid medium.
solvent: Carrier liquid in which other components may be dissolved.
specialist: One who concentrates on only one part or branch of a subject or profession.
spectrum: The series of colored bands diffracted and arranged in the order of their wavelengths by the passage of white light through a prism. Shading continuously from red (produced by the longest

wave visible) to violet (produced by the shortest): Red, orange, yellow, green, blue, indigo, and violet.
spot lightening: Color correcting using a lightening mixture to lighten up darker areas.
stabilizer: General name for ingredient that prolongs lifetime, appearance, and performance of a product.
stage: A term used to describe a visible color change that natural hair color goes through while being lightened. (See *degree*)
stain remover: Chemical used to remove tint stains from skin.
strand test: Test given before treatment to determine development time, color result, and the ability of the hair to withstand the effects of chemicals.
stripping: (See *color remover*)
tablespoon: ½ of an ounce, 3 teaspoons, 15 milliliters.
teaspoon: ⅙ of an ounce, ⅓ of a tablespoon, 5 milliliters.
temporary haircolor or **temporary rinses:** Color made from preformed dyes that are applied to the hair, but are readily removed with shampoo.
terminology: The special words or terms used in science, art, or business.
tertiary colors: The mixture of a primary and an adjacent secondary color on the color wheel. Red-orange, yellow-orange, yellow-green, blue-green, blue-violet, red-violet. Also referred to as intermediary colors.
texture, hair: The diameter of an individual hair strand. Termed: coarse, medium, or fine.
tint: Permanent oxidizing haircolor product having the ability to lift and deposit color in the same process.
tint back: To return hair back to its original or natural color.
tone or **tonality:** A term used to describe the warmth or coolness in color.
toner: A pastel color to be used after prelightening.
toning: Adding color to modify the end result.
touch-up: (See *retouch*)
translucent: The property of letting diffused light pass through.
tyrosinase: The enzyme (tyrosinase) that reacts together with the amino acid (tyrosine) to form the hair's natural melanin pigment.
tyrosine: The amino acid (tyrosine) that reacts together with the enzyme (tyrosinase) to form the hair's natural melanin pigment.
undertone: The underlying color that emerges during the lifting process of melanin, which contributes to the end result. When lightening hair, a residual warmth in tone always occurs. Also referred to as contributing pigment.
urea peroxide: A peroxide compound occasionally used in haircolor. When added to an alkaline color mixture, it releases oxygen.
value: (See *depth; level*)
vegetable color: A color derived from plant resources.
virgin hair: Natural hair that has not undergone any chemical or physical treatment.

viscosity: A term referring to the thickness of the solution.
volume: The concentration of hydrogen peroxide in water solution. Expressed as volumes of oxygen liberated per volume of solution; 20 volume peroxide would thus liberate 20 pints (9.4 liters) of oxygen gas for each pint (liter) of solution.
warm: Containing red, orange, yellow, or gold tones.

REVIEW QUESTIONS

HAIRCOLORING

1. What is the difference between primary, secondary, and tertiary colors?
2. What are the classifications of haircolor? How do they act on the hair?
3. What is the correct procedure for giving a haircoloring consultation? A strand test?
4. How is temporary haircolor applied?
5. What are some advantages of semi-permanent haircoloring?
6. What is the procedure for a single-process tint?
7. How does the procedure vary for a tint retouch?
8. What are the safety precautions to follow during the haircoloring process?
9. What is the activity of hydrogen peroxide during haircoloring?
10. For what two purposes are hair lighteners used?
11. Name the types of lighteners and the uses of each.
12. What methods are available to achieve special effects highlighting?
13. What preventative and corrective steps avoid or solve haircoloring problems?

CHEMICAL HAIR RELAXING AND SOFT CURL PERMANENT

13

LEARNING OBJECTIVES

AFTER COMPLETING THIS CHAPTER, YOU SHOULD BE ABLE TO:

1. Define the purpose of chemical hair relaxing.
2. List the different products used in chemical hair relaxing.
3. Explain the difference between sodium hydroxide relaxers and thio relaxers.
4. Describe the three basic steps of chemical hair relaxing.
5. Explain client analyzation for a chemical hair relaxing treatment.
6. Demonstrate the procedures used for a sodium hydroxide hair relaxing process.
7. Demonstrate the procedures used for an ammonium thioglycolate hair relaxing process.
8. Demonstrate the procedures used for a chemical blow out.
9. Demonstrate the procedures used for a soft curl permanent.

INTRODUCTION

✔ Completed—Learning Objective No. 1

DEFINE PURPOSE OF CHEMICAL HAIR RELAXING

Chemical hair relaxing is the process of permanently rearranging the basic structure of overly curly hair into a straight form. When done professionally, it leaves the hair straight and in a satisfactory condition, to be set into almost any style. ✔

CHEMICAL HAIR RELAXING PRODUCTS

✔ Completed—Learning Objective No. 2

LIST CHEMICAL HAIR RELAXING PRODUCTS

The basic products that are used in chemical hair relaxing are a chemical hair relaxer, a neutralizer, and a petroleum cream, which is used as a protective base to protect the client's scalp during the sodium hydroxide chemical straightening process. ✔

CHEMICAL HAIR RELAXERS

The two general types of hair relaxers are ***sodium hydroxide,*** which does not require pre-shampooing, and ***ammonium thioglycolate,*** which may require pre-shampooing.

Sodium hydroxide (caustic type hair relaxer often called a hair straightener) both softens and swells hair fibers. As the solution penetrates into the cortical layer, the cross-bonds (sulfur and hydrogen) are broken. The action of the comb, the brush, or the hands in smoothing the hair and distributing the chemical straightens the softened hair.

Manufacturers vary the sodium hydroxide content of the solution from 5% to 10%, and the pH factor between 10 and 14. In general, the more sodium hydroxide used and the higher the pH, the quicker the chemical reaction will take place on the hair, and the greater the danger will be of hair damage.

CAUTION

Because of the high alkaline content of sodium hydroxide, great care must be taken in its use.

✔ Completed—Learning Objective No. 3

SODIUM HYDROXIDE VS. THIO RELAXERS

Although ammonium thioglycolate (thio type relaxer often called a relaxer) is less drastic in its action than sodium hydroxide, it softens and relaxes overly curly hair in somewhat the same manner. You may recall that this is the same solution used in permanent waving. ✔

NEUTRALIZER

The ***neutralizer*** also is called a ***stabilizer*** or ***fixative.*** The neutralizer stops the action of any chemical relaxer that may remain in the hair after rinsing. The neutralizer for a thio type relaxer reforms the cysteine (sulfur) cross-bonds in their new position and rehardens the hair.

BASE AND "NO BASE" FORMULAS

When using sodium hydroxide, there are two types of formulas, base and no base. The base formula is a petroleum cream that is designed to protect the client's skin and scalp during the sodium hydroxide chemical straightening process. This protective base also is important during a chemical straightening retouch. It is applied to protect hair that has been straightened previously, and to prevent over-processing and hair breakage.

Petroleum cream has a lighter consistency than petroleum jelly, and is formulated to melt at body temperature. The melting process ensures complete protective coverage of the scalp and other areas with a thin, oily coating. This helps to prevent burning and/or irritation of the scalp and skin. Previously treated hair should be protected with cream conditioner during the straightening process.

"No base" relaxers are also available. These relaxers have the same chemical reaction on the hair, although usually the reaction is milder. The procedure for the application of a "no base" relaxer is the same as for a regular relaxer except that the base cream is not applied. It is advisable to use a protective cream around the hairline and over the ears.

STEPS IN CHEMICAL HAIR RELAXING

All chemical hair relaxing involves three basic steps: ***processing, neutralizing,*** and ***conditioning.***

PROCESSING

As soon as the chemical relaxer is applied, the hair begins to soften so that the chemical can penetrate to loosen and relax the natural curl.

NEUTRALIZING

As soon as the hair has been sufficiently processed, the chemical relaxer is thoroughly rinsed out with warm water, followed by either a built-in shampoo neutralizer or a prescribed shampoo and neutralizer.

CONDITIONING

Depending on the client's needs, the conditioner may be part of a series of hair treatments, or it may be applied to the hair before or after the relaxing treatment. ✔

✔ Completed—Learning Objective No. 4

THREE BASIC STEPS IN CHEMICAL HAIR RELAXING

CAUTION

Overly curly hair that has been damaged from heat appliances or other chemicals must be reconditioned before a relaxer service is performed.

Hair treated with lighteners or metallic dyes must not be given a chemical hair relaxer, because it might cause excessive damage or breakage.

RECOMMENDED STRENGTH OF RELAXER

The strength of relaxer used is determined by the strand test. The following guidelines can help in determining which strength relaxer to use for the test.

1. Fine, tinted, or lightened hair—Use mild relaxer.
2. Normal, medium-textured virgin hair—Use regular relaxer.
3. Coarse virgin hair—Use strong or super relaxer.

ANALYSIS OF CLIENT'S HAIR

It is essential that the cosmetologist have a working knowledge of human hair, particularly when giving a relaxing treatment. You will learn to recognize the qualities of hair by visible inspection, feel, and special tests. Before attempting to give a relaxing treatment to overly curly hair, the cosmetologist must judge its texture, porosity, elasticity, and the extent, if any, of damage to the hair. (For more complete information on hair analysis, refer to the chapter on permanent waving.)

CLIENT'S HAIR HISTORY

To help ensure consistent, satisfactory results, records should be kept of each chemical hair relaxing treatment. These records should include the client's hair history, products and conditioners used (see sample form on page 285), and the client's release statement. The release statement is used to protect the cosmetologist, to some extent, from the responsibility for accidents or damages. You should be sure to find out if the client has ever had a hair relaxing. If so, was there any reaction? You must not chemically relax hair that has been treated with a metallic dye. To do so damages or destroys the hair. In addition, it is not advisable to use chemical relaxers on hair that has been bleached lighter.

Before starting to process the hair, you must know how the client will react to the relaxer. Therefore, the client must receive: (1) a thorough scalp and hair examination and (2) a hair strand test.

RELAXER RECORD

Name .... Tel. ....

Address .... City .... State .... Zip ....

DESCRIPTION OF HAIR

Form	**Length**	**Texture**		**Porosity**	
☐ wavy	☐ short	☐ coarse	☐ soft	☐ very porous	☐ less porous
☐ curly	☐ medium	☐ medium	☐ silky	☐ moderately porous	☐ least porous
☐ extra-curly	☐ long	☐ fine	☐ wiry	☐ normal	☐ resistant

Condition

☐ virgin ☐ retouched ☐ dry ☐ oily ☐ lightened

Tinted with ....

Previously relaxed with (name of relaxer) ....

☐ Original sample of hair enclosed ☐ not enclosed

TYPE OF RELAXER OR STRAIGHTENER

☐ whole head ☐ retouch

☐ relaxer .... strength .... ☐ straightener .... strength ....

Results

☐ good ☐ poor ☐ sample of relaxed hair enclosed ☐ not enclosed

Date	Operator	Date	Operator
....	....	....	....
....	....	....	....
....	....	....	....

SCALP EXAMINATION

Inspect the scalp carefully for eruptions, scratches, or abrasions. To obtain a clearer view of the scalp, part the hair into ½" (1.25cm) sections. Hair parting may be done with the index and middle fingers or with the handle of a rat-tail comb. In either case, you must exercise great care not to scratch the scalp. Such scratches may become seriously infected when aggravated by the chemicals in the relaxer. (Fig. 13.1)

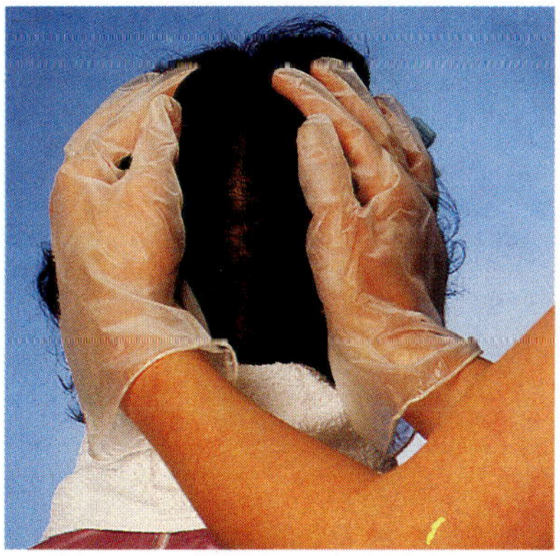

13.1—Examining the scalp.

If the client has scalp eruptions or abrasions, do not apply the chemical hair relaxer until the scalp is healthy. If the hair is not in a healthy condition, prescribe a series of conditioning treatments to return it to a more normal condition. Then you may give a strand test.

STRAND TESTS

To help you estimate the results you may expect to get from a chemical relaxing, it is advisable to test the hair for porosity and elasticity. This can be done using one of the following strand tests:

Finger test determines the degree of porosity in the hair. Grasp a strand of hair and run it between the thumb and index finger of the right hand, from the end toward the scalp. If it ruffles or feels bumpy, the hair is porous and can absorb moisture.

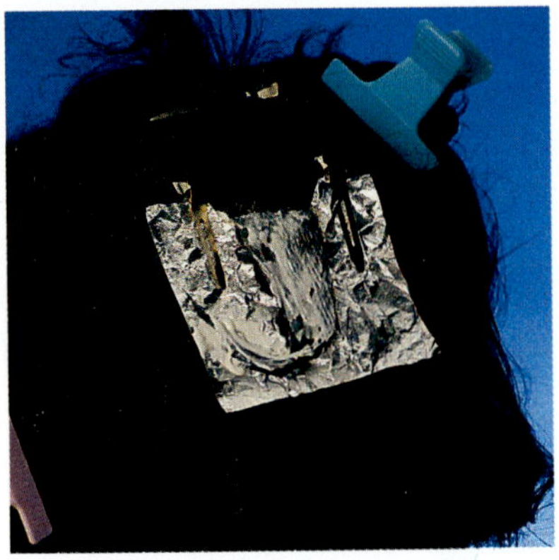
13.2—Relaxer strand test.

✔ Completed—Learning Objective No. 5

CLIENT ANALYZATION FOR CHEMICAL HAIR RELAXING

Pull test. This test determines the degree of elasticity in the hair. Normally, dry, curly hair will stretch about one-fifth its normal length without breaking. Grasp half a dozen strands from the crown area and pull them gently. If the hair appears to stretch, it has elasticity and can withstand the relaxer. If not, conditioning treatments are recommended prior to a chemical relaxing treatment.

Relaxer test. Application of the relaxer to a hair strand will indicate the reaction of the relaxer on the hair. Take a small section of hair from the crown or another area where the hair is wiry and resistant. Pull it through a slit in a piece of aluminum foil placed as close to the scalp as possible. Apply relaxer to the strand in the same manner as you would apply it to the entire head. Process the strand until it is sufficiently relaxed, checking the strand every 3 to 5 minutes. Make careful note of the timing, the smoothing required, and the hair strength. Shampoo the relaxer from the strand only, towel dry, and cover with protective cream to avoid damage during the relaxing service. If breakage has occurred, you should do another strand test using a milder solution. (Fig. 13.2) ✔

CHEMICAL HAIR RELAXING PROCESS (WITH SODIUM HYDROXIDE)

The procedure outlined below is based primarily on products containing sodium hydroxide. For this, or any other kind of product, follow the manufacturer's directions and be guided by your instructor.

EQUIPMENT, IMPLEMENTS, AND MATERIALS

Chemical relaxer
Neutralizer or neutralizing shampoo
Shampoo and cream rinse
Shampoo cape
Protective base
Conditioner-filler
Protective gloves
Towels
Rollers
Comb and brush
Spatula
Timer
Conditioner
Absorbent cotton
Neck strip
Clips and picks
End papers
Setting lotion
Record card

PREPARATION

1. Select and arrange the required equipment, implements, and materials.
2. Wash and sanitize your hands.

3. Seat client comfortably. Remove earrings and neck jewelry; adjust towel and shampoo cape.
4. Examine and evaluate the scalp and hair.
5. Give a strand test and check results.
6. Do not shampoo hair. (Hair ends may be trimmed after the application of the chemical relaxer.)
7. Have client sign release card.

PROCEDURE

1. Part hair into four or five sections, as recommended by your instructor. (Figs. 13.3, 13.4)

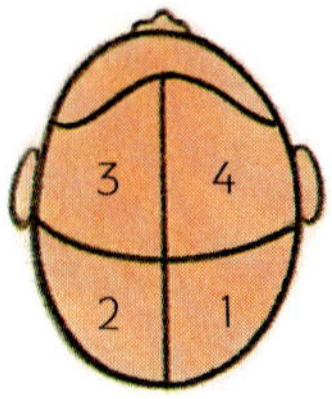

13.3—Part hair into four sections.

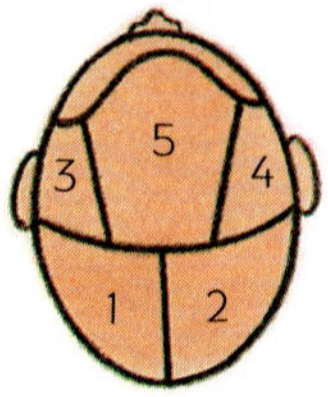

13.4—Part hair into five sections; three sections in front area, two sections in back area.

2. Dry hair. If moisture or perspiration is present on the scalp because of excessive heat or humidity, place the client under a cool dryer for several minutes.
3. Apply protective base. Manufacturers recommend the use of a protective base to protect the scalp from the strong chemicals in the relaxer. To apply it properly, subdivide each of the four or five major sections into ½″ to 1″ (1.25 to 2.5 cm) partings, to permit thorough scalp coverage. (Fig. 13.5)

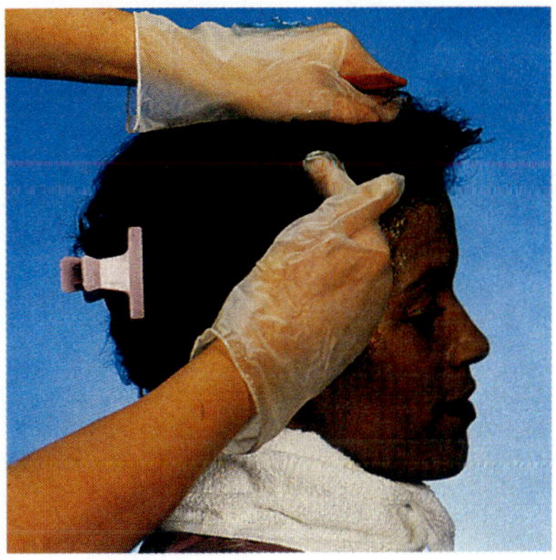

13.5—Applying protective base.

Apply the base freely to the entire scalp with the fingers. The hairline around the forehead, nape of the neck, and area over and around the ears must be completely covered. Complete coverage is important to protect the scalp and hairline from irritation.

◆ NOTE: When using a "no base" relaxer, a protective base is not necessary. It is recommended that a protective cream be used on the hairline and around the ears.

APPLYING THE CONDITIONER-FILLER

In many cases a conditioner-filler is required before the chemical relaxer can be used. The conditioner-filler, usually a protein product, is applied to the entire head of hair when dry. It protects over-porous or slightly damaged hair from being over-processed on any part of the hair shaft. It evens out porosity of the hair shaft, and permits uniform distribution and action of the chemical relaxer.

To give complete benefits from the conditioner-filler, rub it gently onto the hair from the scalp to the hair ends, using either the hands or a comb. Then towel dry the hair or use a cool dryer to completely dry the hair.

CAUTION

Avoid the use of heat, which will open the pores of the scalp and cause irritation or injury to the client's scalp.

Protective gloves must be worn by the cosmetologist to prevent damage to hands.

APPLYING THE RELAXER

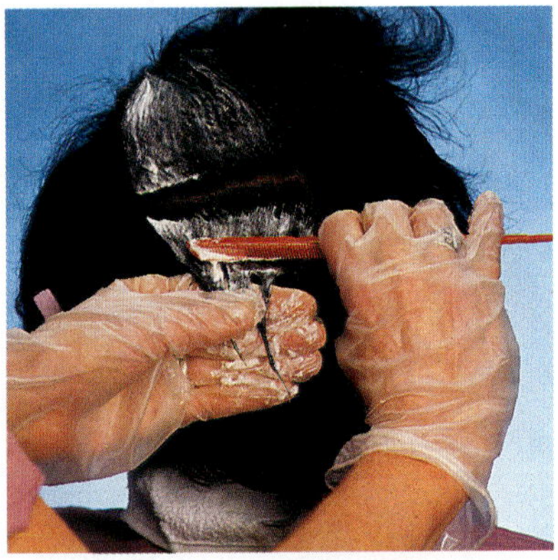

13.6—Applying relaxer on top of strand.

Divide the head into four or five sections, in the same manner as for the application of the protective base.

The processing cream is applied last to the scalp area and hair ends. The body heat will speed up the processing action at the scalp. The hair is more porous at the ends and may be damaged. In both these areas, less processing time is required, and, therefore, the relaxer is applied last.

There are three methods in general use for the application of the chemical hair relaxer: the comb method, the brush method, and the finger method.

COMB METHOD

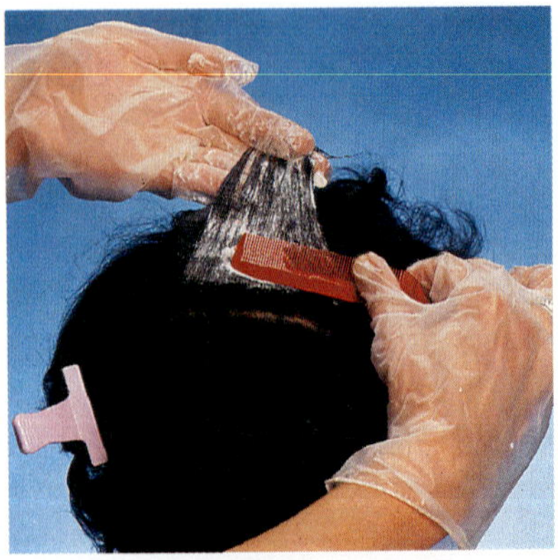

13.7—Applying relaxer underneath strand.

Remove a quantity of relaxing cream from the jar. Beginning in the back right section of the head, carefully part off ¼″ to ½″ (.66 to 1.25 cm) of hair, depending on its thickness and curliness. Apply the relaxer with the back of the comb, starting ½″ to 1″ (1.25 to 2.5 cm) from the scalp, and spread to within ½″ (1.25 cm) of the hair ends. First apply the relaxer to the top side of the strand. (Fig. 13.6) Then, raise the subsection and apply the relaxer underneath. (Fig. 13.7) Gently lay the completed strand up, out of the way.

Complete the right back area and, moving in a clockwise direction, cover each section of the head in the same manner. Then, go back over the head in the same order, applying additional relaxing cream, if necessary, and spreading the relaxer close to the scalp and up to the hair ends. Avoid excessive pressure or stretching of the hair.

Smoothing the cream through the hair not only spreads the cream, but also gently stretches the hair into a straight position.

An alternate technique is to begin application at the nape, approximately 1" (2.5 cm) from the hairline, and continue toward the crown. The last place to apply relaxer is at the hairline. Be guided by your instructor's and the manufacturer's instructions.

BRUSH OR FINGER METHOD

The brush or finger method of applying the relaxer to the hair is the same as the comb method, except the brush or the fingers and palms are used instead of the back of the comb. ***Wear protective gloves.***

PERIODIC STRAND TESTING

While spreading the relaxer, inspect its action by stretching the strands to see how fast the natural curls are being removed. Another method of testing is to press the strand to the scalp using the back of the comb or your finger. Examine the strand after your finger is removed. If it lies smoothly, the strand is sufficiently relaxed; if the strand reverts or "beads" back away from the scalp, continue processing.

RINSING OUT THE RELAXER

When the hair has been sufficiently straightened, rinse the relaxer out rapidly and thoroughly. (Fig. 13.8) The water must be warm, not hot. If the water is too hot, it may burn the client and cause discomfort because of the very sensitive condition of the scalp. If the water is too cold, it will not stop the processing action. The direct force of the rinse water should be used to remove the relaxer and avoid tangling the hair. Part hair with fingers to make sure no traces of the relaxer remain. Unless the relaxer is completely removed, its chemical action continues on the hair. The stream of water should be directed from the scalp to the hair ends.

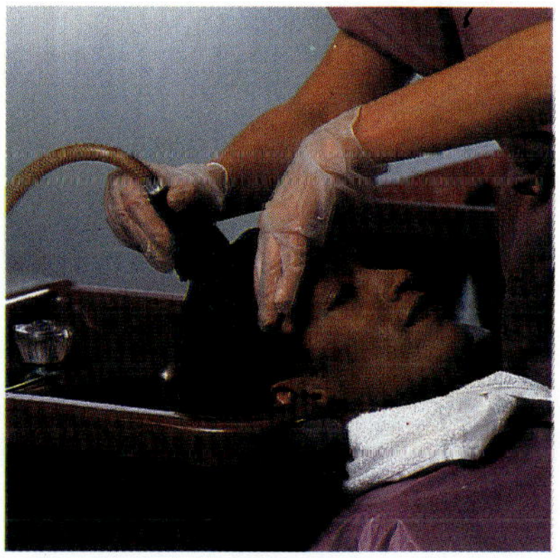

13.8—Rinsing out relaxer.

CAUTION

Do not get relaxer or rinse water into the eyes or on unprotected skin. If the relaxer or rinse water gets into the client's eyes, wash it out immediately, and refer the client to a doctor without delay.

SHAMPOOING/NEUTRALIZING

When the hair is thoroughly rinsed, neutralize the hair as directed by your instructor. Most manufacturers provide a neutralizing shampoo that is applied to the hair after rinsing. Others prescribe the use of a nonalkaline or a cream shampoo followed by a neutralizer.

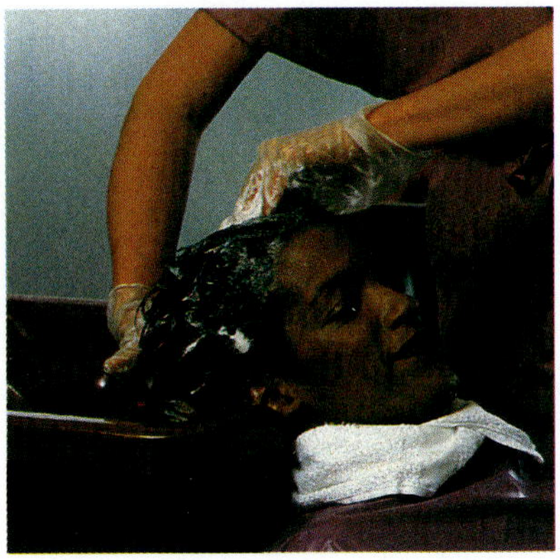
13.9—Shampooing the hair.

Gently work the shampoo into the hair. Use care to avoid tangling the hair or breaking any fragile ends. Manipulate the shampoo by working with the fingers underneath the hair, not on top. Rinse with warm water, making sure to keep the hair straight. Repeat the shampoo until the hair lathers well and all the relaxer is removed. (Fig. 13.9)

After shampooing, completely saturate the hair with the neutralizer if it is required by the manufacturer. Beginning at the nape, carefully comb with a wide-tooth comb, working upward, toward the forehead. Use the comb to:

1. Keep the hair straight.
2. Ensure complete saturation with the neutralizer.
3. Remove any tangles without pulling.

Time the neutralizer as directed and rinse thoroughly. Towel blot gently. Condition hair as necessary and proceed with styling. Discard used supplies. Cleanse and sanitize equipment. Wash and sanitize hands. Complete record of all timings and treatments during the service, and file the record card.

◆ NOTE: Different products used for relaxing require different methods. Always follow the manufacturer's directions.

APPLYING THE CONDITIONER

Many manufacturers recommend that you apply a conditioner before setting the hair, to offset the harshness of the sodium hydroxide in the relaxer and to help restore some of the natural oils to the scalp and hair.

Two types of conditioners available are:

1. ***Cream-type conditioners*** are applied to the scalp and hair, then carefully rinsed out. The hair is then towel dried. Apply setting lotion; set the hair on rollers; dry and style the hair in the usual manner.
2. ***Protein-type (liquid) conditioners*** are applied to the scalp and hair prior to hairsetting and allowed to remain in the hair to serve as a setting lotion. Set the hair on rollers, dry, and style in the usual manner.

◆ NOTE: Because of the fragile condition of the hair, it is advisable to wind the hair on the roller without extreme tension.

HOT THERMAL IRONS

To avoid hair breakage, excessive heat and excessive stretching should be avoided. Thermal curling with warm heat can be used to curl chemically relaxed hair. Conditioning treatments should be recommended and the hair dried completely before thermal curling. (See chapter on thermal hairstyling for a discussion of thermal irons.)

Question & Answer

RELAXING TWO DEGREES OF CURL

Q *Is it advisable to relax only half the head if excessive curl is in the front only?*

A It is not unusual for a person to have mixed hair textures. If you closely examine most Caucasian heads you'll find areas that are fine and straight while others are wavy to curly. It is no different with the hair of African-American clients. The reason for this is not thoroughly understood except to say each hair follicle controls the size, shape, and growth pattern of the hair growing from that particular root. Just as hair on different parts of the body differs in strength and structure, so can the hair on various portions of one's head.

It is not advisable to chemically re-structure only a portion of the hair on one head. Hair that has been chemically treated does not react the same as virgin hair and will make styling noticeably difficult.

Use a relaxer formulated with an ammonium thioglycolate base—widely called a curl re-arranger. The thio-based relaxer has a lower pH factor than sodium hydroxide relaxers; therefore they are not formulated to be used on kinky or wool-like hair. They are great for use on virgin hair with moderate curls or hair that must be relaxed for style control.

Inasmuch as the relaxer is thio-based, it is compatible with liquid thio-perm solution. The best solution for chemically treating hair that is only partially curly is to first apply a thio relaxer to the curly portion, then process and rinse. Then perm the entire head using large perm rods to relax and widen the original wave pattern for easier styling. All the hair, having been chemically treated, will react the same when dry.

—*From* Milady's Salon Solutions *by Louise Cotter*

SODIUM HYDROXIDE RETOUCH

✔ Completed—Learning Objective No. 6

PROCEDURE FOR SODIUM HYDROXIDE HAIR RELAXING PROCESS

Hair grows about ¼″ to ½″ (.66 to 1.25 cm) per month. A retouch should probably be done every 6 weeks to 2 months, depending on how quickly the client's hair grows.

Follow all the steps for a regular chemical hair relaxing treatment, with one exception: ***apply the relaxer only to the new growth.*** In order to avoid breakage of previously treated hair, apply a cream conditioner over the hair that received the earlier treatment, thus avoiding overlapping and damage. ✔

CHEMICAL HAIR RELAXING PROCESS (WITH AMMONIUM THIOGLYCOLATE)

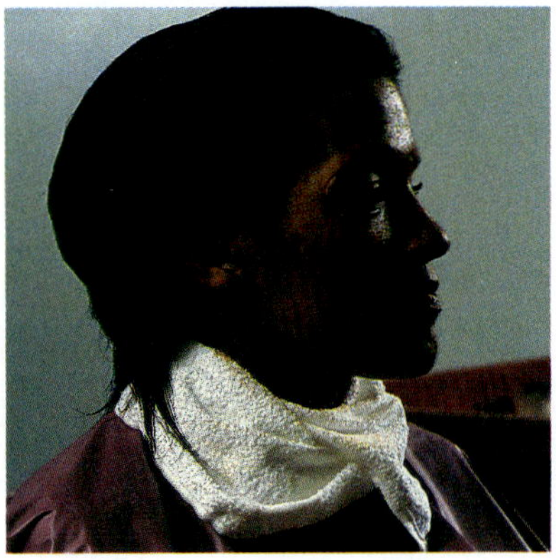

13.10—Relaxed hair.

Ammonium thioglycolate (also called thio relaxer) is the same type of product used in cold waving, with a heavy cream or gel added to the formula in order to keep the hair in a straightened position. (Fig. 13.10)

As in cold waving, the relaxer breaks the sulfur and hydrogen bonds, softening and swelling the hair. The mechanical action of the hands, brush, or fingers smooths the hair and holds it in a straightened position.

Once the hair is straightened, the neutralizer is applied (serving the same purpose as the neutralizer in cold waving). It re-forms the sulfur and hydrogen bonds and rehardens the hair in its newly straightened position.

Manufacturers vary their products according to the texture and condition of the hair. Tinted and lightened hair require a weaker formula than virgin hair.

Thio relaxers have a milder relaxing action on curly hair. You may choose to use them on fine-textured hair, or when it is desirable to remove less curl from the hair. Thio relaxers can also be used to reduce excessive curl formed in a permanent wave. Consult your instructor for directions and precautions for this specialized service.

Techniques for thio relaxers vary. The general procedure involves preparing the hair (gently shampooing if required), applying a base if necessary, applying the relaxer in the manner outlined under "Chemical Hair Relaxing Process (with Sodium Hydroxide)," and periodic strand testing. Directions at this point may vary greatly, so follow the manufacturer's directions *carefully.* Remove the relaxer from the hair and neutralize as directed, condition, and proceed with styling of the hair. As with any chemical service, exercise caution so that the hair is not excessively heated or stretched during styling as this may cause damage to both the hair and the desired curl formation.

THIO RETOUCH

As noted earlier, hair grows at the rate of ¼" to ½" (.66 to 1.25 cm) per month. A thio retouch should be given when there is a noticeable regrowth. Follow all steps for a regular thio hair relaxing treatment, with the exception of the relaxer, which is applied only to the new growth. A conditioner should be applied to the previously relaxed hair to protect it from damage.

OTHER RELAXERS

Researchers have also developed acid-based relaxers for the treatment of overly curly hair. Like acid permanent waves, the relaxer works with bisulfites rather than with thioglycolate acid. This type of relaxer is designed as a milder-acting one, much like the thio. Some can also be used as a pre-wrap preparation for performing a permanent wave on excessively curly hair. ✔

✔ Completed—Learning Objective No. 7

PROCEDURE FOR AMMONIUM THIOGLYCOLATE HAIR RELAXING PROCESS

CHEMICAL BLOW OUT

To meet the needs of salon clients, great versatility in hairstyling may be achieved with the chemical blow out. This technique removes only a small amount of the curl, leaving the hair in a more manageable condition. A chemical blow out is a combination of chemical hair straightening and hairstyling, which creates a well-groomed style in the African-American tradition.

The chemical blow out may be done with either the thio hair relaxer or the sodium hydroxide relaxer. The important consideration with either method is not to over-relax the hair to the point where the blow out process becomes impossible to perform. Usually, when the thio relaxer is used, the hair is shampooed first. When the sodium hydroxide relaxer is used, the hair is shampooed after the hair is relaxed. (Follow the manufacturer's or your instructor's directions.)

EQUIPMENT, IMPLEMENTS, AND MATERIALS

Use the same equipment, implements, and materials as for a regular chemical relaxing, plus a wide-tooth comb (hair lifter or pick), scissors, clippers, and hand blower.

PROCEDURE

1. Prepare and drape client as for a regular hair relaxing treatment.
2. Apply scalp conditioner and/or base to the scalp.
3. Wear protective gloves; apply relaxer in the usual manner.

4. Stop the relaxing procedure by rinsing the relaxer from the hair with warm water before it is straightened and while it still shows a wave or curl formation.
5. Apply neutralizer or neutralizing shampoo.
6. Rinse out neutralizer and towel blot the hair.
7. Apply a conditioner to scalp and hair to help restore the natural oils removed by the relaxer.

✔ Completed—Learning Objective No. 8

CHEMICAL BLOW OUT PROCEDURE

If the blow out style is desired, dry the hair with a hand dryer while lifting the hair with a hair lifter or pick. Dry from the scalp out to the ends. Distribute the dry hair evenly around the head and shape with clippers or shears. Continue to lift the hair out from the head to check progress of cut.

The hair can also be shaped while wet, then combed into place to let it dry naturally. For a softer look, the hair can be picked or combed when dry. ✔

REVIEW OF SAFETY PRECAUTIONS

When giving a chemical relaxing treatment, you can never be too cautious. Here is a review of the safety measures that will ensure a comfortable and safe treatment for your client.

1. Examine the scalp for abrasions; if any are present, do not give a hair relaxing treatment.
2. Analyze the hair; give a strand test.
3. Do not relax damaged hair. Suggest a series of conditioning treatments.
4. Do not shampoo the hair prior to the application of a sodium hydroxide product.
5. Do not apply a sodium hydroxide relaxer over a thio relaxer.
6. Do not apply a thio relaxer over a sodium hydroxide relaxer.
7. Never use a strong relaxer on fine hair, as it may cause breakage.
8. Cool or warm irons may be used on chemically relaxed hair. Do not use excessive heat, as it may cause damage to relaxed hair.
9. Apply a protective base, to avoid burning or irritating the scalp with the sodium hydroxide relaxer.
10. Wear protective gloves.

11. Protect client's eyes.
12. Use extreme care when applying the relaxer to avoid accidentally spreading it on the ears, scalp, or skin.
13. Strand test the action of the relaxer frequently to determine how fast the natural curl is being removed.
14. Be sure to thoroughly rinse the relaxer from the hair. Failure to do so permits the relaxer to continue to process, resulting in hair damage. Direct stream of warm water from scalp to hair ends.
15. Wear protective gloves until all the relaxer has been removed. When rinsing the shampoo from the hair, always work from the scalp to the ends, to prevent tangling the hair.
16. Use a wide-tooth comb and avoid pulling when combing the hair after the relaxation process is complete. Avoid scratching the scalp with comb or fingernails.
17. Apply a conditioner to the scalp and hair before setting the hair.
18. When retouching the new growth, do not allow the relaxer to overlap onto the hair already straightened.
19. Do not give a hair relaxing treatment to hair treated with a metallic dye.
20. At the completion of each treatment, fill out a complete record card.
21. Have the client sign a release statement to protect the salon and the cosmetologist.
22. It is not advisable to use chemical relaxers on lightened hair.

SOFT CURL PERMANENT

Soft curl permanent waving is a method of permanently waving overly curly hair. It is known by various names given by the manufacturers of the products.

CAUTION

The product used contains ammonium thioglycolate (thio).

1. *Do not use on hair that has been treated with sodium hydroxide products.*
2. *Do not use on hair that has been treated with metallic dye or compound henna.*

IMPLEMENTS AND MATERIALS

Shampoo cape
Neck strips and towels
Mild shampoo
Combs
Gloves
Protective cream
Thio gel, cream, or lotion
Applicators
Curling rods
Porous end papers
Pre-wrap solution
Waving lotion
Cotton or neutralizing bands
Plastic cap
Neutralizer
Styling lotion (curl activator)
Finishing rinse
Hair clips
Scissors or razor
Record cards

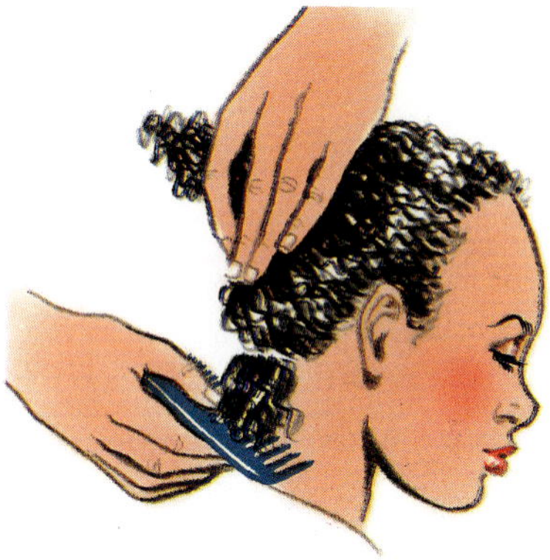

13.11—Remove tangles from hair.

PROCEDURE

This procedure can be used for both men and women.

1. Examine the client's scalp. Do not use permanent waving gel or cream if the scalp shows signs of abrasions or lesions, or if the client has experienced an allergic reaction to a previous perm.
2. Shampoo and rinse hair thoroughly. Towel dry, leaving hair damp.
3. Remove tangles with a large-tooth comb. (See Fig. 13.11)
4. Part hair into four to five sections, as recommended by your instructor. *(If the manufacturer requires it, put a protective cream on the entire scalp, including around the hairline.)*
5. Wear protective gloves.
6. Apply thio gel or cream to one section at a time, using the back of a comb, a haircoloring brush, or fingers. Use a tail comb to part hair and begin the application of thio gel or cream to the hair nearest the scalp, preferably starting at the nape area. Work the thio gel or cream to the ends of the hair. (See Fig. 13.12)
7. Comb the thio gel or cream through the entire head, first with a wide-tooth comb, then with a smaller-tooth comb. (See Fig. 13.13)
8. When the hair becomes supple and flexible, rinse with tepid water and towel dry. Do not tangle the hair.

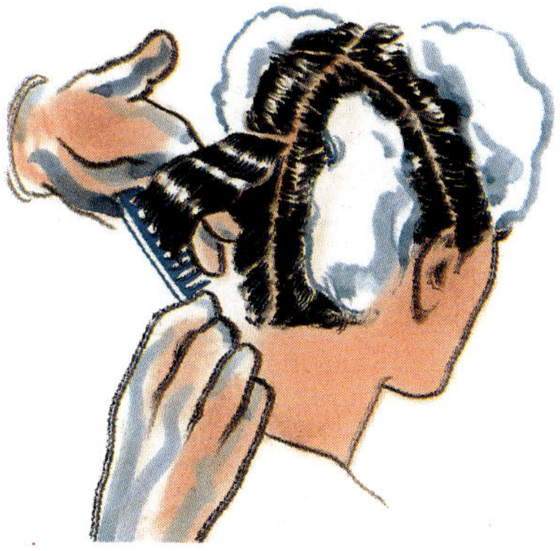

13.12—Part hair into sections and coat with thio gel.

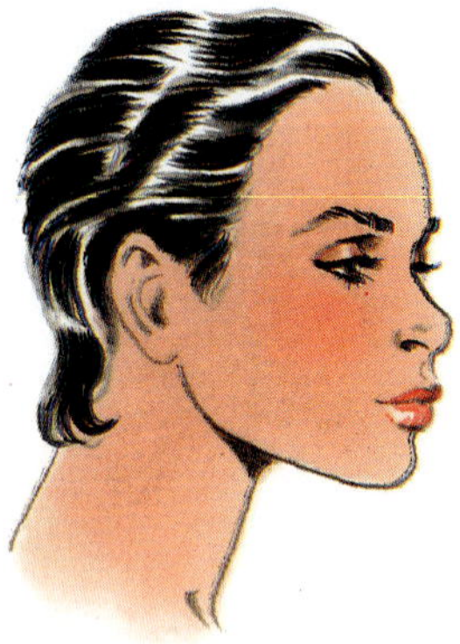

13.13—Comb thio gel through hair.

◆**NOTE:** Always follow the manufacturer's instructions on the recommended procedure for rinsing off the chemical.

9. Divide the hair into eight sections. (See Fig. 13.14) Subsection as you wrap the hair. (See Fig. 13.15)

10. Wrap hair as desired on curling rods. In order to rearrange the curl pattern of the hair, the rod selected must be at least two times larger than the natural curl. In order to achieve a good curl formation, the hair should encircle the rod at least 2½ times.

11. After the wrap has been completed, protect the client's skin by placing cotton around the hairline and neck. (See Fig. 13.16)

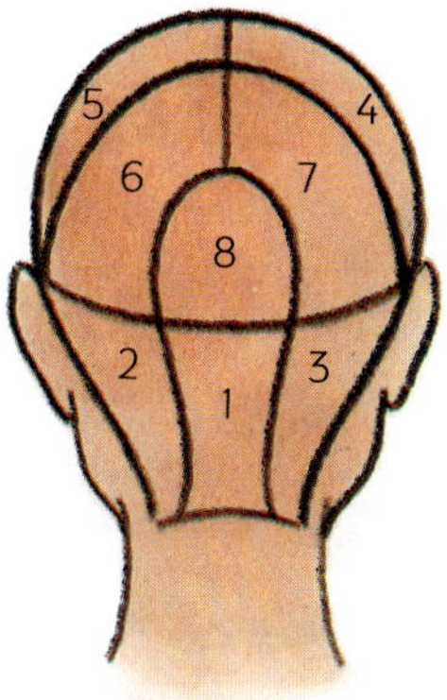

13.14—Divide the hair into eight sections.

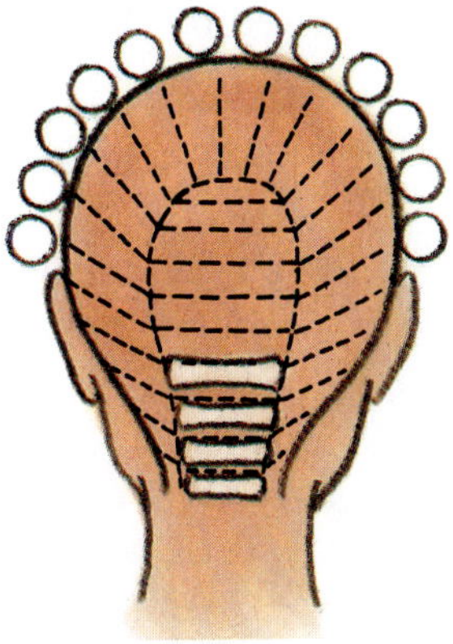

13.15—Subsection as you wrap.

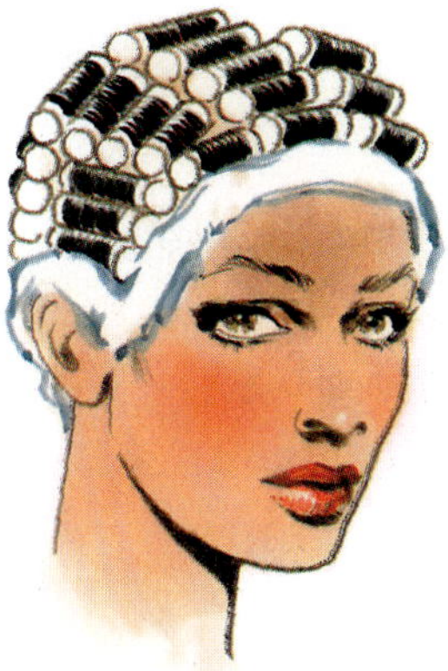

13.16—Protect client's skin with cotton around hairline.

12. Apply thio gel, cream, or lotion to all the curls until they are thoroughly saturated. (See Fig. 13.17) Replace saturated cotton.

13. Cover the client's head with a plastic cap.

14. Have the client sit under a pre-heated dryer for 15 to 25 minutes, or as recommended by the manufacturer. (See Fig. 13.18)

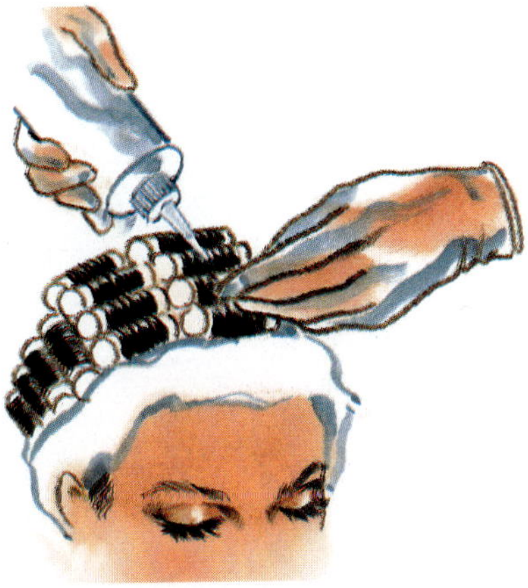

13.17—Apply thio gel to curls.

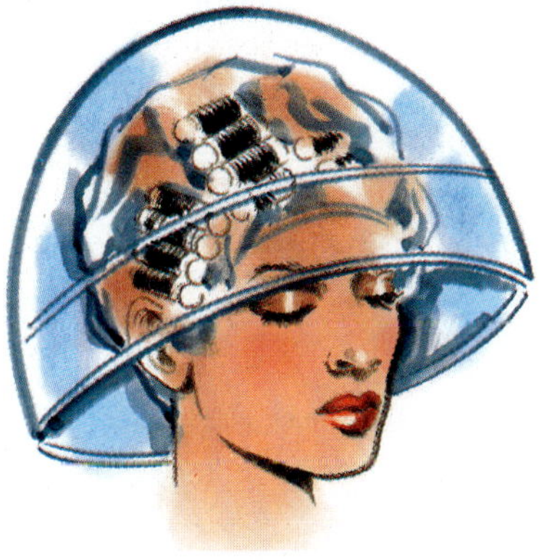

13.18—Process under pre-heated dryer.

15. Take a test curl (See Fig. 13.19), and if the desired curl pattern has not developed, have the client sit under the dryer for another 10 minutes or until a curl pattern develops.
16. When the desired curl pattern has been reached, rinse the hair thoroughly with warm (not hot) water. (See Fig. 13.20) Blot each curl with a towel.
17. Use a prepared neutralizer, or mix neutralizer as directed by the manufacturer, and saturate each curl twice. (See Fig. 13.21) Allow neutralizer to remain on the curls for 5 to 10 minutes, or as directed by the manufacturer.

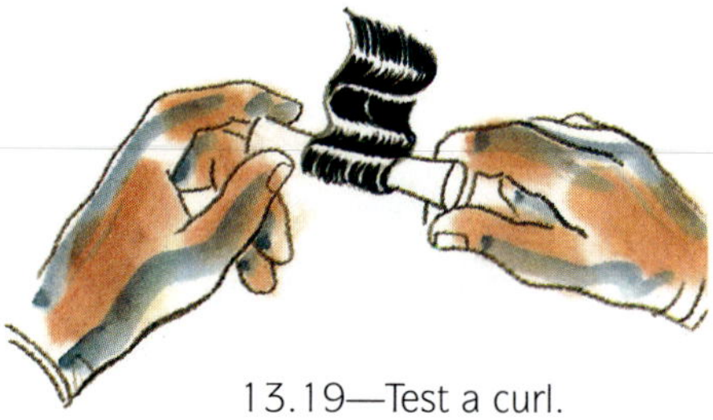

13.19—Test a curl.

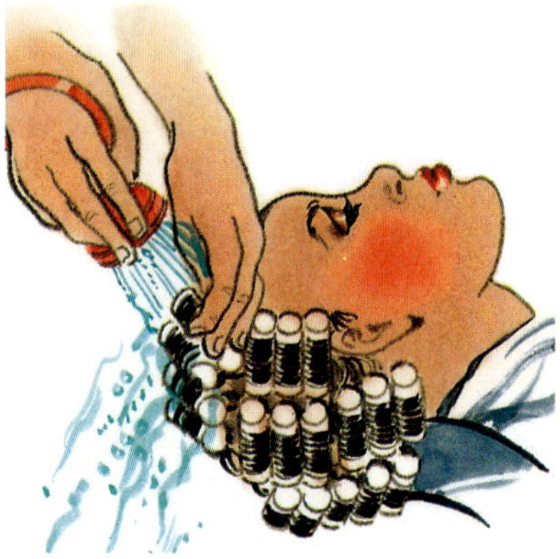

13.20—Rinse the hair.

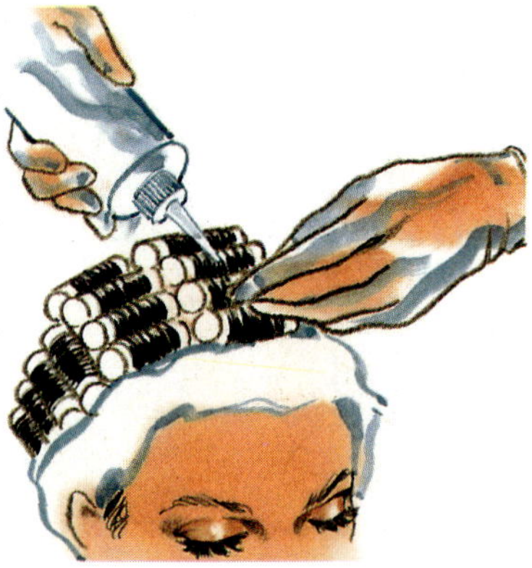

13.21—Apply neutralizer.

18. Carefully remove rods and apply balance of neutralizer to the hair. Work neutralizer through with fingers for thorough distribution (See Fig. 13.22), and allow it to remain on the hair for another 5 minutes.
19. Rinse hair thoroughly with cool water and towel blot.
20. Trim uneven hair ends. (See Fig. 13.23)
21. Apply conditioner as directed by the manufacturer.

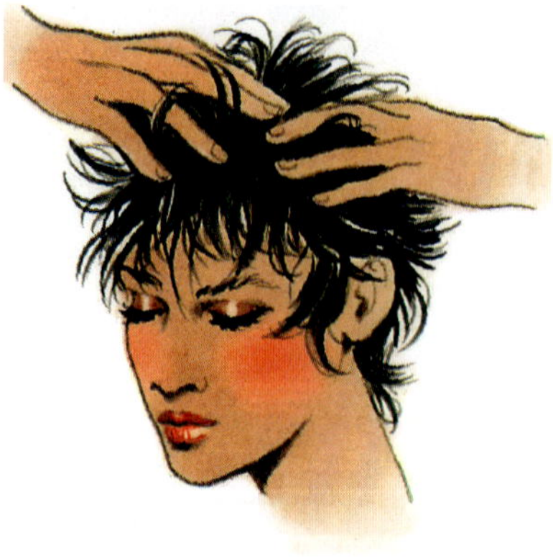

13.22—Work neutralizer through hair.

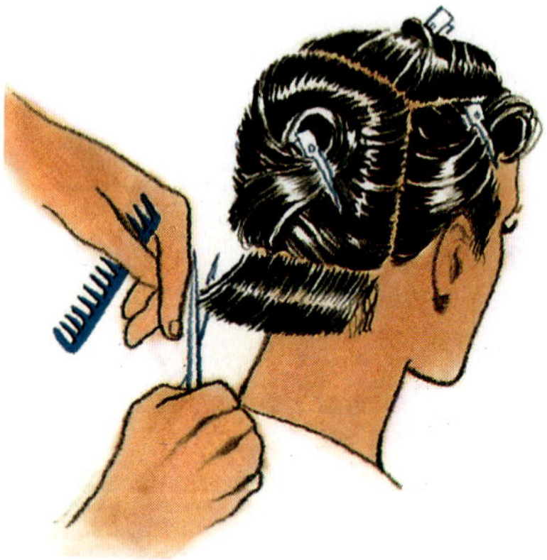

13.23—Trim hair ends.

22. Air dry hair or style as directed. (See Fig. 13.24) ✔

✔ Completed—Learning Objective No. 9

SOFT CURL PERMANENT PROCEDURE

Fig. 13.25 illustrates hairstyle *after* a soft curl permanent was given.

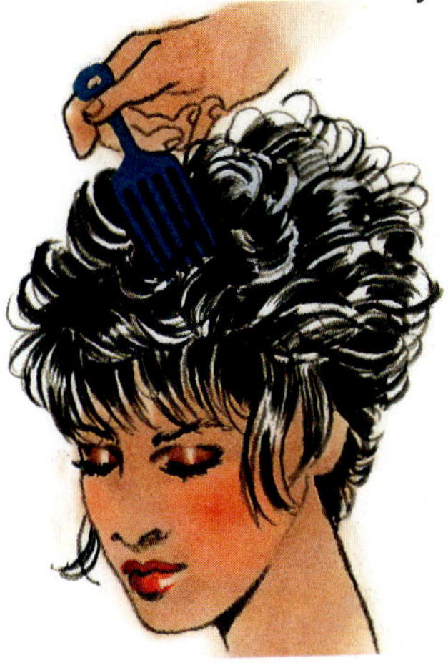

13.24—Style hair.

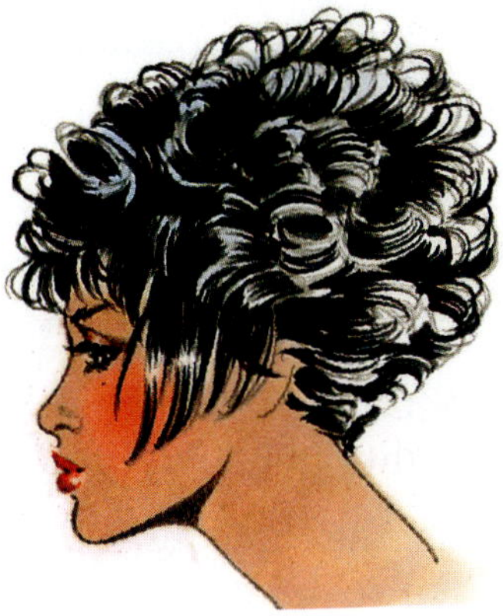

13.25—Finished hairstyle.

AFTERCARE

1. Do not comb or brush the curls when wet; use a lifting pick instead.
2. Shampoo as often as necessary, using a mild (acid-balanced) shampoo.
3. Conditioner or curl activator should be used daily to maintain flexibility, sheen, and proper moisture balance of the hair.

REVIEW OF SAFETY PRECAUTIONS

1. Do not give a soft curl permanent to hair treated with sodium hydroxide.
2. Do not give a soft curl permanent to hair that has been colored with a metallic dye or compound henna.
3. Thoroughly analyze the hair and scalp and record the information prior to giving a soft curl permanent.
4. Bleached, tinted, or damaged hair must be reconditioned until the hair is of sufficient strength to ensure that the soft curl service will not cause further damage.
5. If permanent waving lotion or neutralizer accidentally gets into the client's eye, flush the eye immediately with water and refer the client to a doctor.
6. Test curl frequently to ensure proper curl formation without damage.
7. Use protective cream around client's hairline and neck.
8. Complete client's record card carefully and accurately.

REVIEW QUESTIONS

CHEMICAL HAIR RELAXING AND SOFT CURL PERMANENT

1. What are the basic products used for chemical hair relaxing?
2. What are the two types of chemical hair relaxers?
3. What are the three steps of chemical hair relaxing?
4. What is the most important point to remember when performing a chemical service?
5. What type of hair relaxing technique achieves the greatest versatility in hairstyling?
6. List the three most important safety precautions for chemical hair relaxing.
7. What is the method of permanently waving overly curly hair?
8. If hair were treated with sodium hydroxide, what service could not be done?
9. If hair is damaged by an appliance or a chemical, what must you do before applying a chemical hair relaxer?

THERMAL HAIR STRAIGHTENING (HAIR PRESSING)

14

LEARNING OBJECTIVES

AFTER COMPLETING THIS CHAPTER, YOU SHOULD BE ABLE TO:

1. Discuss the purpose served by hair pressing.
2. Explain how to analyze the client's hair and scalp condition prior to a hair pressing.
3. List the products required for a successful hair pressing.
4. Demonstrate the procedures involved in both soft pressing and hard pressing.
4. List the safety precautions that must be observed in hair pressing.

INTRODUCTION

Hair straightening, or ***pressing,*** is a profitable service that is popular in the beauty salon. When properly done, hair pressing temporarily straightens overly curly or unruly hair. A pressing generally lasts until the hair is next shampooed. (Permanent hair straightening is covered in the chapter on chemical hair relaxing.)

✔ Completed—Learning Objective No. 1

PURPOSE OF HAIR PRESSING

Hair pressing prepares the hair for additional services, such as thermal roller curling and croquignole thermal curling (the two-loop or "Figure 8" technique). A good hair pressing leaves the hair in a natural and lustrous condition and is not harmful to the hair. ✔

There are three types of hair pressing:

1. *Soft press,* which removes about 50% to 60% of the curl and is accomplished by applying the thermal pressing comb once on each side of the hair.
2. *Medium press,* which removes about 60% to 75% of the curl and is accomplished by applying the thermal pressing comb once on each side of the hair using slightly more pressure.
3. *Hard press,* which removes 100% of the curl and is accomplished by applying the thermal pressing comb twice on each side of the hair.

ANALYSIS OF HAIR AND SCALP

Before the cosmetologist undertakes to press the client's hair, there should be an analysis of the condition of the hair and scalp in order to evaluate the client's needs.

CAUTION

Under no circumstances should hair pressing be given to a client who has a scalp abrasion, contagious scalp condition, scalp injury, or chemically treated hair.

If the client's hair and scalp are not normal, the cosmetologist should give appropriate advice concerning preliminary corrective treatments. If the hair shows signs of neglect or abuse caused by faulty pressing, lightening, or tinting, the cosmetologist should recommend a series of conditioning treatments. Failure to correct dry and brittle hair can result in hair breakage during hair pressing. ***Burnt hair strands cannot be conditioned.***

You should also remember to check the elasticity and porosity of your client's hair. Under normal conditions, if a client's hair has good elasticity, it can be safely stretched about one-fifth of its length. If the ability of the hair to absorb water (porosity) is normal, then the hair returns to its normal curly appearance when it is wet or moistened.

A careful analysis of the client's hair and scalp should cover the following points:

1. Form of hair (curly or overly curly)
2. Length of hair (long, medium, or short)
3. Texture of hair (coarse, medium, fine, or very fine)
4. Feel of hair (wiry, soft, or silky)
5. Elasticity of hair (normal or poor)
6. Shade of hair (natural, faded, streaked, or gray)
7. Condition of hair (normal, brittle, dry, oily, damaged, or chemically treated)
8. Condition of scalp (normal, flexible, or tight)

It is important that the cosmetologist be able to recognize individual differences in hair texture, hair porosity, hair elasticity, and scalp flexibility. Guided by this knowledge, the cosmetologist can determine how much pressure the hair and scalp can tolerate without breakage, hair loss, or burning from a pressing comb that is not adjusted to the right temperature.

HAIR TEXTURE

Variations in hair texture can be traced to the following factors:

1. Diameter of the hair (coarse, medium, or fine). Coarse hair has the greatest diameter. Fine hair has the smallest diameter.
2. Feel of the hair (wiry, soft, or silky).

The client's hair texture also depends on how dry, oily, gray, tinted, lightened, or curly it is. Touching the client's hair and asking specifically about hair characteristics will help you know how to treat the client's hair.

Coarse Hair

Coarse, overly curly hair has qualities that make it difficult to press. Coarse hair has the greatest diameter, and during the pressing process it requires more heat and pressure than medium or fine hair.

Medium Hair

Medium curly hair is the normal type of hair cosmetologists deal with in the beauty salon. No special problem is presented by this type of hair, and it is the least resistant to hair pressing.

Fine Hair

Fine hair requires special care. To avoid hair breakage, less heat and pressure should be applied than for other hair textures. Whereas coarse and medium hair have three layers (cuticle, cortex, and medulla), fine hair has only two layers (cortex and cuticle).

Wiry, Curly Hair

Wiry, curly hair may be coarse, medium, or fine. It feels stiff, hard, and glassy. Because of the compact construction of the cuticle cells, it is very resistant to hair pressing and it requires more heat and pressure than other types of hair.

SCALP CONDITION

✔ Completed—Learning Objective No. 2

ANALYZING HAIR AND SCALP CONDITION

The condition of the client's scalp can be classified as normal, tight, or flexible. If the scalp is normal, proceed with an analysis of the texture and elasticity of the hair. If the scalp is tight and the hair coarse, press the hair in the direction in which it grows to avoid injury to the scalp.

The main difficulty with a flexible scalp is that the cosmetologist might not apply enough pressure to press the hair satisfactorily. ✔

RECORD CARD

You should be sure to keep a record of all pressing treatments performed on a client. It also is advisable to question the client about any lightener, tint, color restorer (metallic), or other chemical treatment that was used on his or her hair.

CONDITIONING TREATMENTS

Effective conditioning treatments require special cosmetic preparations for the hair and scalp, thorough brushing, and scalp massage. These treatments usually help get better results from hair pressing. The use of an infrared lamp is optional, depending on the type of treatment being given.

A tight scalp can be rendered more flexible by the systematic use of scalp massage, hair brushing, and direct high-frequency current. The client benefits because there is better circulation of blood to the scalp.

PRESSING COMBS

There are two types of pressing combs: regular and electric. They are both constructed of either good quality stainless steel or brass. The handle is usually made of wood since wood does not readily absorb heat. The space between the teeth of the comb varies with the size and style of the comb. A comb with more space between the teeth produces a coarse-looking press. A comb with less space produces a smoother press. Pressing combs vary in size; some are short, to be used with short hair, while long combs are used with long hair. (Fig. 14.1)

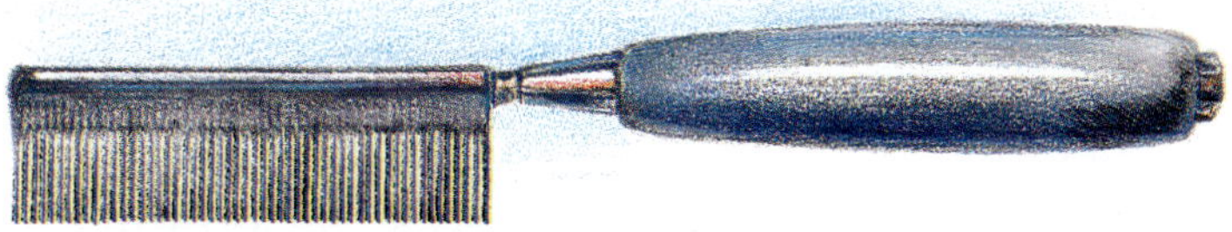

14.1—Regular pressing comb.

Heating the Comb

Depending on their composition, combs vary in their ability to accept and retain heat. Regular pressing combs may be heated on gas stoves or electric heaters. (Fig. 14.2) While the comb is being heated, its teeth should face upward and the handle should be kept away from the fire. After heating the comb to the proper temperature, test it on a piece of light paper. If the paper becomes scorched, allow the comb to cool slightly before applying it to the hair.

Electric pressing combs are available in two forms: one comes with an "on" and "off" switch; the other is equipped with a thermostat, which has a control switch that indicates high or low degrees of heat.

There is also a straightening comb attachment that fits the nozzle of a standard hand-held dryer and is less damaging than an electric comb or an oven-heated comb.

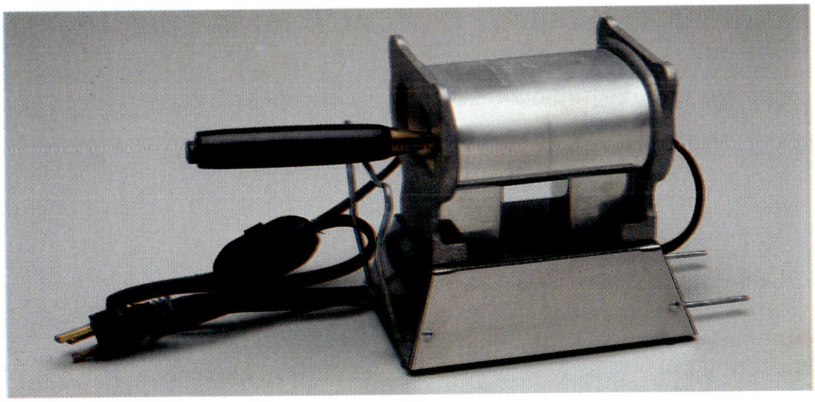

14.2—Electric heater.

Cleaning the Comb

The pressing comb will perform more efficiently if it is kept clean and free of carbon. Wipe the comb clean of loose hair, grease, and dust before and after each use. The intense heat keeps the comb sterile when all loose hair or clinging dirt is removed. Remove the carbon from the comb by rubbing its outside surface and between its teeth with one of the following: emery board, fine steel wool pad, or fine sandpaper. After using any of these cleaning methods, immerse the metal portion of the comb in a hot baking soda solution for about 1 hour; then rinse and dry. The metal will acquire a smooth and shiny appearance.

PRESSING OIL OR CREAM

Applying pressing oil or cream prior to a hair pressing treatment helps prepare the hair for pressing. Both of these products have the following beneficial effects:

1. Make hair softer
2. Prepare and condition hair for pressing
3. Help prevent hair from burning or scorching
4. Help prevent hair breakage
5. Help condition the hair after pressing
6. Add sheen to pressed hair ✔

✔ Completed—Learning Objective No. 3

PRODUCTS REQUIRED FOR SUCCESSFUL HAIR PRESSING

HAIR SECTIONING

Divide the head into four main sections. Then subdivide these sections into 1″ to 1½″ (2.5 to 3.75 cm) partings. The size of the subsections depends on the texture and density of the hair.

1. For medium textured hair of average density, use subsections of average size.
2. For coarse hair with greater density, use smaller sections to ensure complete heat penetration and effectiveness.
3. For thin or fine hair with sparse density, use larger sections.

SOFT PRESSING PROCEDURE FOR NORMAL CURLY HAIR

The following procedure is one of several ways to give a hair pressing treatment and can be changed to meet your instructor's method.

Equipment, Implements, and Materials

Pressing comb
Heating appliance (gas or electric heater or attachment)
Pressing oil
Hairbrush and comb
Grease or pomade
Shampoo
Towels and cape
Spatula
Neck strips
Thermal irons

Professional Prep

THE JOB INTERVIEW

Salon owners are looking for employees with good people skills, and you can demonstrate your attributes in this area during the job interview. Here are some tips for making the best impression:

- Call to confirm your interview. This establishes you as a professional who cares about keeping appointments.
- Pay particular attention to your appearance. After all, this is the beauty industry. Don't neglect one single aspect of your grooming or dress.
- Arrive 15 minutes early. This allows plenty of time for mishaps and eliminates rushing in at the last minute or, even worse, being late.
- Remain upbeat and positive. To most salon owners and managers, a positive attitude and pleasing personality are more important than technical skills.
- Answer the interviewer's questions honestly. If you are asked to name one of your weaknesses, admit what it is, but put yourself in a positive light by explaining how you are overcoming it.
- Ask questions of the interviewer. Take a list of questions and jot down the answers; this makes you appear organized and professional. Ask questions that display interest in the prospective employer, in the salon, and in your role, should you be hired.
- At the end of the interview, ask the interviewer for his or her business card, smile, shake hands, thank him or her, and leave promptly.

—*From* Communication Skills for Cosmetologists *by Kathleen Ann Bergant*

Preparation

1. Select and arrange required materials.
2. Wash and sanitize hands.
3. Drape client.
4. Shampoo, rinse, and towel dry client's hair.
5. Apply pressing oil or cream. (Note: Some cosmetologists prefer to apply pressing oil or cream to the hair after it has been completely dried.)
6. Dry hair thoroughly.
7. Comb and divide hair into four main sections. Pin up four sections.
8. Place pressing comb in heater.

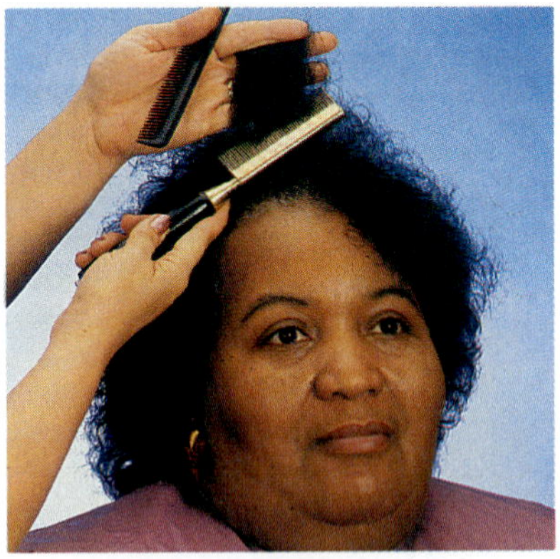

14.3—Proper handling of pressing comb.

Procedure

1. Unpin one section of hair at a time and subdivide into small hair sections. Beginning at the right side of the head, work from front to back. (Some cosmetologists prefer to start at the back of the head and work forward.)
2. If necessary, apply pressing oil evenly and sparingly over the small hair sections.
3. Test the temperature of the heated pressing comb on a white cloth or white paper to determine heat intensity before you place it on the hair.
4. Lift the end of a small hair section with the index finger and thumb of the left hand and hold it upward away from the scalp.
5. Holding the pressing comb in the right hand, insert the teeth of the comb into the top side of the hair section. (Fig. 14.3)
6. Draw out the pressing comb slightly; make a quick turn so that the hair strand wraps itself partly around the comb. The back rod of the comb actually does the pressing.
7. Press the comb slowly through the hair strand until the ends of the hair pass through the teeth of the comb.
8. Bring each completed hair section over to the opposite side of the head.
9. Continue steps 4 to 8 on both sections on the right side of the head; then do the same on both sections on the left side.

Completion

1. Apply a little pomade to the hair near the scalp and brush it through the hair.
2. If desired, thermal roller or croquignole curling can be given at this time. (The procedures and techniques are found in the chapter on thermal hairstyling.)
3. Style and comb the hair according to the client's wishes.
4. Place supplies in their proper places.
5. Sanitize implements and clean equipment.

HARD PRESS

A hard press is recommended when the results of a soft press are not satisfactory. The entire comb press procedure is repeated. Pressing oil may be added to hair strands only if necessary. A hard press is also known as a *double comb press.*

TOUCH-UPS

Touch-ups are sometimes necessary when the hair becomes curly again due to perspiration, dampness, or other conditions. The process is the same as for the original pressing treatment, with the shampoo omitted. ✔

✔ Completed—Learning Objective No. 4

SOFT PRESSING AND HARD PRESSING PROCEDURES

SAFETY PRECAUTIONS

The injuries that can occur in hair pressing are of two types:

1. Injuries that are the immediate results of hair pressing and cause physical damage, such as:
   a) Burnt hair that breaks off
   b) Burnt scalp that causes either temporary or permanent loss of hair
   c) Burns on ears and neck that form scars
2. Injuries that are not immediately evident but can subsequently cause physical damage, such as:
   a) Skin rash if the client is allergic to pressing oil
   b) Progressive breaking and shortening of the hair because of too frequent hair pressings

CAUTION

In case of a scalp burn, immediately apply 1% gentian violet jelly.

Good judgment should be used to avoid damage, with consideration always given to the texture of the hair and condition of the scalp. The client's safety is assured only when the cosmetologist observes every precaution and is especially careful during the actual hair pressing. The cosmetologist should avoid using the following:

1. Excessive heat or pressure on the hair and scalp
2. Too much pressing oil on the hair
3. Perfumed pressing oil near the scalp if the client is allergic
4. Too frequent hair pressing

RELEASE STATEMENT

A release statement should be used for hair pressing, permanent waving, hair tinting, or any other service that might require the cosmetologist's release from responsibility for accidents or damages.

REMINDERS AND HINTS ON SOFT PRESSING

1. Keep the comb clean and free from carbon at all times.
2. Avoid overheating the pressing comb.
3. Test the temperature of the heated comb on a white cloth or white paper before applying it to the hair.
4. Adjust the temperature of the pressing comb to the texture and condition of the client's hair.
5. Use the heated comb carefully to avoid burning the skin, scalp, or hair.
6. Prevent the smoking or burning of hair during the pressing treatment by:
   a) Drying the hair completely after it is shampooed.
   b) Avoiding excessive application of pressing oil over the hair.
7. Use a moderately warm comb to press short hair on the temples and back of the neck. ✔

✔ Completed—Learning Objective No. 5

SAFETY PRECAUTIONS FOR HAIR PRESSING

SPECIAL PROBLEMS

PRESSING FINE HAIR

When pressing fine hair, follow the same procedure as for normal hair, being careful not to use a hot pressing comb or too much pressure. To avoid hair breakage, apply less pressure to the hair near the ends. After completely pressing the hair, style it.

PRESSING SHORT, FINE HAIR

When pressing short, fine hair, extra care must be taken at the hairline. When the hair is extra short, the pressing comb should not be too hot because the hair is fine and will burn easily; a hot comb can also cause accidental burns, which are very painful and can cause scars. In the event of an accidental burn, immediately apply 1% gentian violet jelly to the burn.

PRESSING COARSE HAIR

When pressing coarse hair, apply enough pressure so that the hair remains straightened.

PRESSING TINTED, LIGHTENED, OR GRAY HAIR

Tinted, lightened, or gray hair requires special care in hair pressing. Lightened or tinted hair might require conditioning treatments, depending on the extent to which it has been damaged. To obtain good results, use a moderately heated pressing comb applied with light pressure.

◆ NOTE: Avoid excessive heat on tinted, lightened, or gray hair as discoloration or breakage can occur.

REVIEW QUESTIONS

THERMAL HAIR STRAIGHTENING (HAIR PRESSING)

1. What is another name for hair pressing?
2. What is the purpose of hair pressing?
3. Name the types of hair presses.
4. Under what circumstances should hair not be pressed?
5. How is an accidental scalp burn treated?
6. How do you test implements for your pressing service?
7. What types of hair require moderate heat?

THE ARTISTRY OF ARTIFICIAL HAIR

15

LEARNING OBJECTIVES

AFTER COMPLETING THIS CHAPTER, YOU SHOULD BE ABLE TO:

1. List the reasons people wear wigs.
2. Identify the different types of wigs, extensions, and hairpieces.
3. Demonstrate the procedure for taking wig measurements.
4. Describe the method used when ordering wigs.
5. Demonstrate the procedures for blocking a wig and fitting a wig.
6. Demonstrate the procedure for cleaning a wig.
7. Demonstrate the procedure for shaping, setting, and styling a wig.
8. Demonstrate the procedure for coloring a wig.
9. Describe the various types of hairpieces and their uses.
10. List the safety precautions to be followed in handling wigs.

INTRODUCTION

Throughout history, people have used wigs to beautify their appearance. The ancient Egyptians first wore wigs in 4000 B.C. for a very practical reason: to protect their hair from the sun. The wearing of wigs spread from Asia and Europe to America, where their use has become increasingly popular.

The use of wigs and hairpieces in hairstyling worldwide is a significant and exciting part of the beauty industry. The sale, styling, and servicing of artificial hair can be a source of increased salon income.

To offer the best possible service, the stylist must learn the following:

1. How wigs and hairpieces can improve the client's appearance.
2. How wigs and hairpieces are made and fitted.
3. How to select and style wigs and hairpieces to best benefit the client.
4. How to clean and service wigs and hairpieces.

WHY PEOPLE WEAR WIGS

People wear wigs for several reasons:

1. Personal choice—to cover up baldness due to heredity, and sparse or damaged hair.
2. Medical—to cover hair loss due to a health problem. Wigs have become popular hair replacements for use by people who have had hair loss due to illness, injury, or shock to the nervous system. Both men and women use wigs in these instances to replace lost hair and maintain their usual hairstyle.
3. Fashion—for changes in everyday hairstyles, to increase length and volume, and for decorative purposes and special occasions.
4. Practicality—for flexibility and ease of style change. For example, black clients might want to wear a straight style without chemically relaxing their hair, and a wig provides the flexibility to do so. ✔

✔ Completed—Learning Objective No. 1

THE REASONS PEOPLE WEAR WIGS

TYPES OF WIGS

Wigs can be made from human hair, synthetic hair (***modacrylic*** is the general term used to describe synthetic wig fibers), animal hair, or a blend of two or three types.

You can use a simple test to tell the difference between human hair and synthetic hair. Cut a small piece of hair from the back of the wig. With a lighted match, burn this hair and observe the following:

1. Human hair burns slowly and gives off a strong odor.
2. Synthetic hair burns quickly and gives off little or no odor. You can feel small, hard beads in the burnt ash of synthetic hair.

HUMAN HAIR WIGS

The quality of a wig depends largely on whether it is constructed by hand or by machine. Expensive, custom-made wigs are hand knotted into a fine mesh foundation. (See Figs. 15.1, 15.2) In cheaper wigs, hair is sewn by machine into a net cap in circular rows. (See Figs. 15.3–15.5)

The quality of a wig also depends on the kind of hair it contains (human or synthetic), and how it is fitted to the client's measurements.

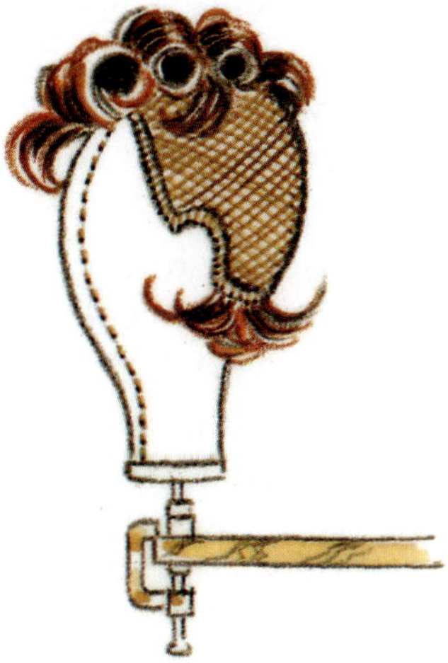

15.1—Hand-knotted wig.

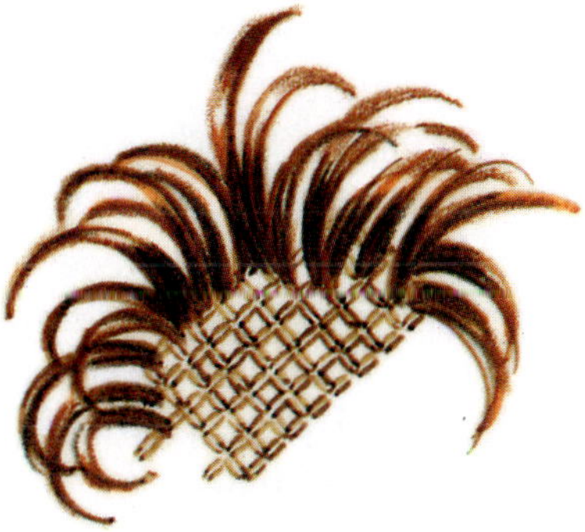

15.2—Hair crocheted and hand knotted into mesh foundation.

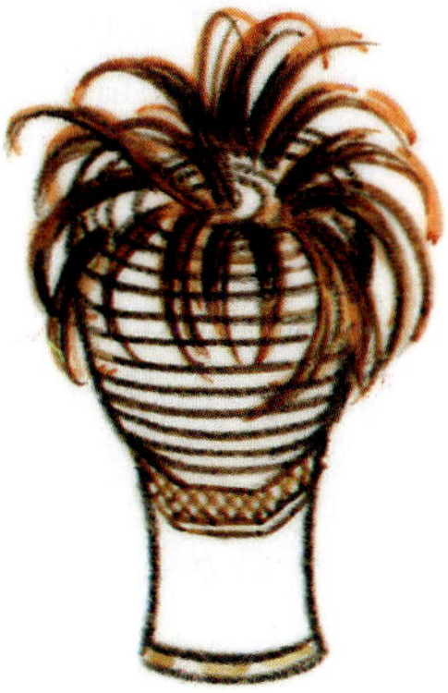

15.3—Weft wig (top view).

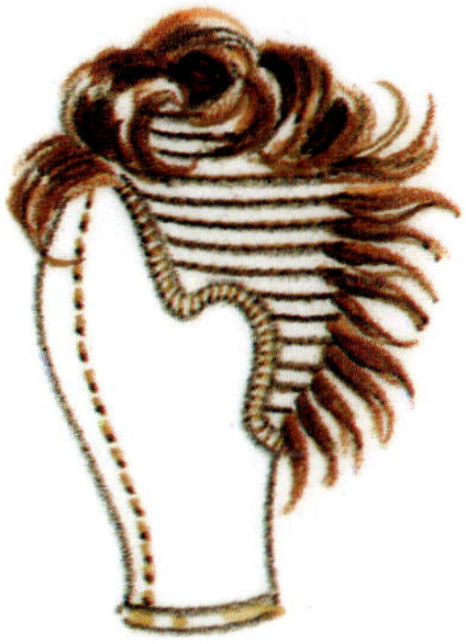

15.4—Weft wig (side view).

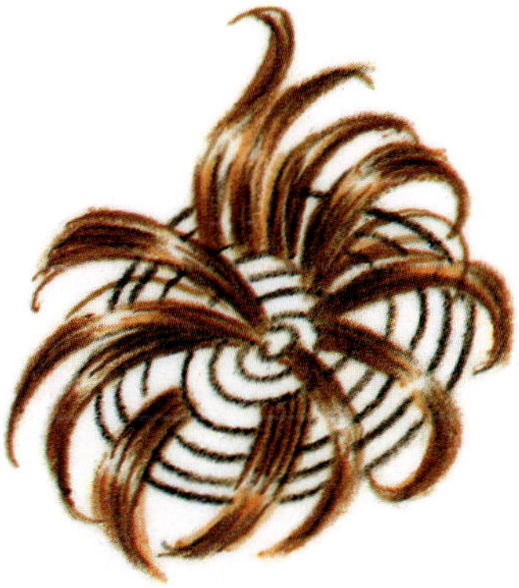

15.5—Hair sewn by machine into net cap or weft in circular rows.

SYNTHETIC WIGS AND HAIRPIECES

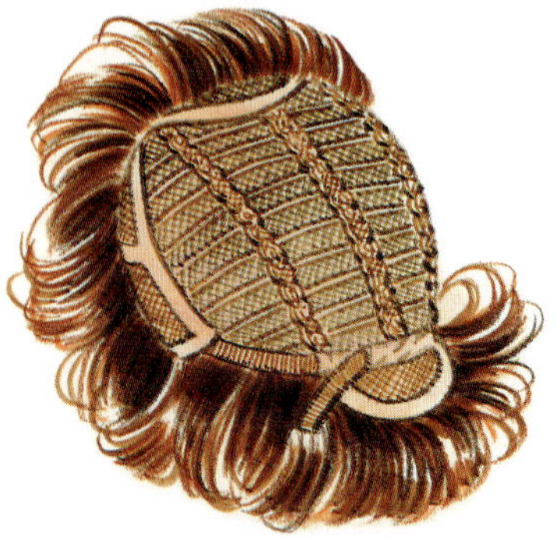

15.6—Synthetic, handmade stretch wig.

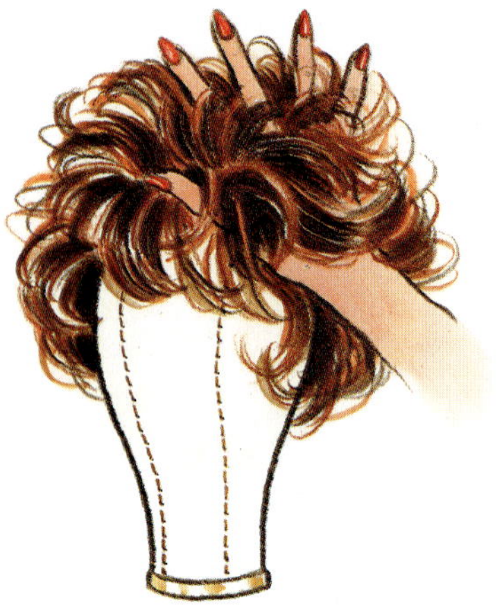

15.7—No-cap wig.

The manufacture of synthetic fibers has greatly improved. Modacrylic fibers, such as dynel, kanekalon, venicelon, and others, have eliminated most of the disadvantages of synthetic hair. Synthetic hair now closely resembles human hair in texture, resiliency, porosity, pliability, durability, sheen, and feel. These fibers can retain curl well, are nonflammable, and do not oxidize and change color in sunlight. In fact, some synthetic fibers appear so much like human hair that it is difficult to distinguish between them.

The many advantages of synthetic hair have led manufacturers to accept its use in wigs and hairpieces. Synthetically produced hair costs less than human hair and its supply is unlimited. It is also easier for the cosmetologist to use since synthetic hair is rolled on spools. Manufacturers weave synthetic wigs and hairpieces from long threads drawn from these spools.

You can find handmade synthetic stretch wigs, machine-made synthetic stretch wigs, and handmade synthetic fitted wigs. (See Fig. 15.6) You must carefully select any type of wig for quality, proper fit, and good workmanship in order to satisfy your clients in terms of wear, comfort, and style.

Also available is the ***no-cap wig,*** composed of rows of wefting sewn to elastic bands. No-cap wigs are lighter and cooler to wear than other types of wigs. (See Fig. 15.7)

Wig caps and hairpieces can be made of cotton, synthetic and cotton, all synthetic, or reinforced elastic. Hairpieces are generally made with a synthetic base that does not shrink when shampooed. Synthetic hairpieces come in wiglets, demi-wigs, braids, chignons, cascades, and falls.

HAIR EXTENSIONS

Hair extensions are permanent additions of hair that can make hair look longer, add thickness and volume, or vary an existing hairstyle. Extensions can be made from either human or synthetic hair, and can be affixed by gluing, fusing, or braiding the additional hair.

MEN'S WIGS

Many men now use wigs or toupees to compensate for hair loss. A toupee has adhesive applied to the base of the hairpiece so that the hairpiece sticks to the scalp.

To make men's hair appear fuller, many clients are using hair extensions. These extensions are interwoven or braided onto the existing hair, giving sparse areas the appearance of added thickness.

Once added, the extensions are styled to complement the client's hair type and facial features. ✔

✔ Completed—Learning Objective No. 2

TYPES OF WIGS

TAKING WIG MEASUREMENTS

To ensure a comfortable and secure fit, you must accurately measure the client's head. First, brush the hair down smoothly and pin it as flatly and tightly to the scalp as possible. Then, keeping close to the head without pressure, measure the head with a tape measure.

PROCEDURE

1. Measure the circumference of the head. Place the tape completely around the head, starting at the hairline at the middle of the forehead; place the tape above the ears, around the back of the head, and return to the starting point. (See Fig. 15.8)
2. Measure from the hairline at the middle of the forehead, over the top, to the nape of the neck. Bend the head back and measure to the point where the wig will ride on the base of the skull at the nape. (See Fig. 15.9)

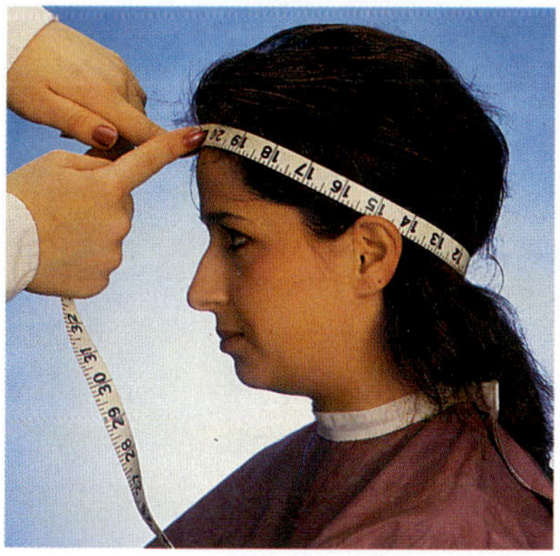

15.8—Measure circumference of head.

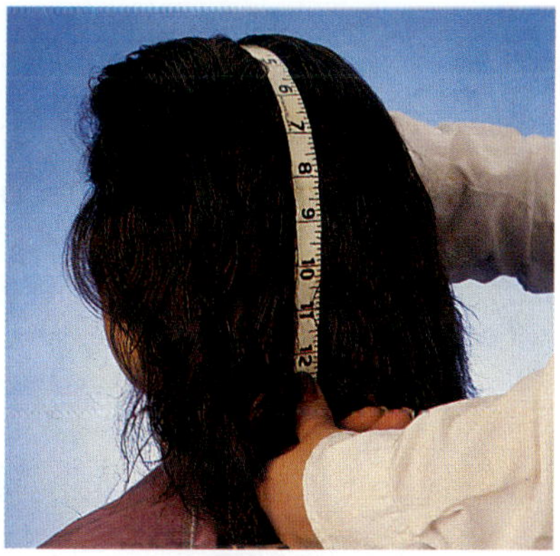

15.9—Measure from hairline at middle of forehead to nape.

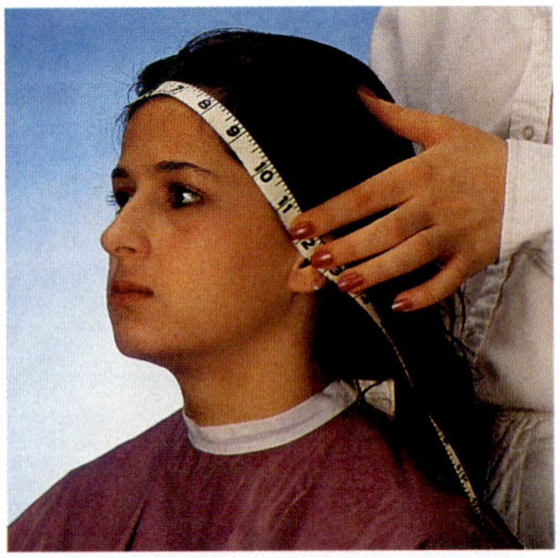

15.10—Measure across forehead.

3. Measure from ear to ear, across the forehead. (See Fig. 15.10)
4. Measure from ear to ear, over the top of the head. (See Fig. 15.11)
5. Place the tape across the crown and measure from temple to temple. (See Fig. 15.12)
6. Measure the width of the napeline, across the nape of the neck. (See Fig. 15.13)

◆ NOTE: Always check to make certain your measurements are accurate. ✔

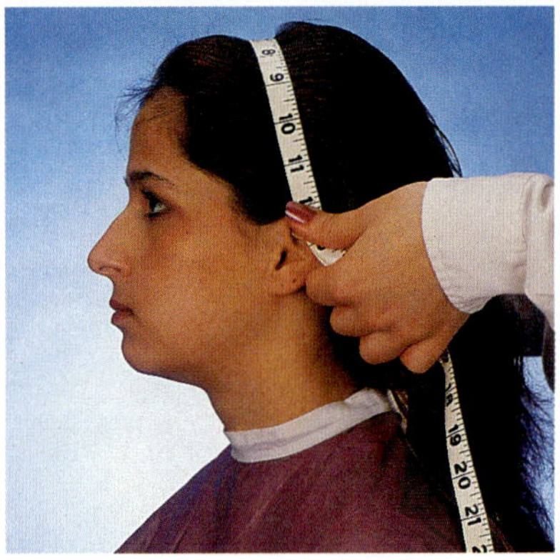

15.11—Measure top of head.

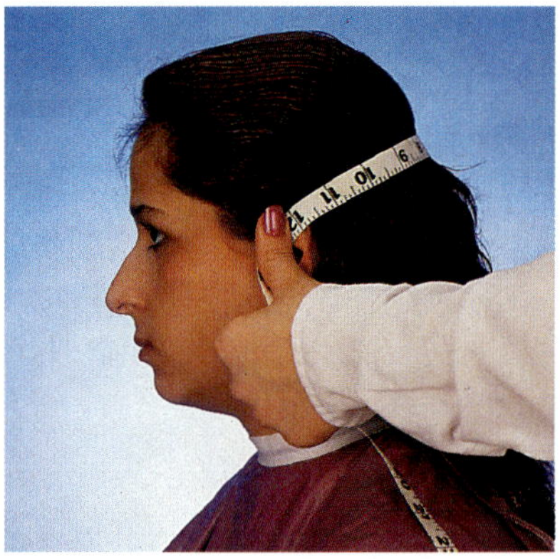

15.12—Measure from temple to temple.

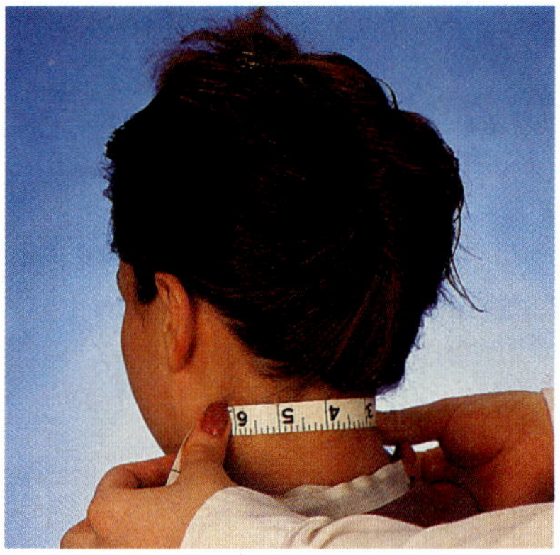

15.13—Measure width of napeline.

✔ Completed—Learning Objective No. 3

TAKING WIG MEASUREMENTS

ORDERING THE WIG

When ordering the wig, keep a written record of the client's head measurements and forward a copy to the wig dealer or manufacturer. Also specify what you desire as to:

1. Hair shade. If necessary, submit samples of the client's hair to the manufacturer. When you submit hair samples, you should use hair that has been freshly shampooed, tinted, or rinsed.
2. Quality of hair.
3. Length of hair.
4. Type of hair part and pattern. ✔

✔ Completed—Learning Objective No. 4

ORDERING WIGS

BLOCKING THE WIG

A block is a head-shaped form usually made of canvas-covered cork or styrofoam, to which a wig is secured for fitting, cleaning, and styling. Use properly protected canvas blocks for all professional wig services, because they stand up under continuous pinning and rough handling. T-pins ("T" shaped pins) are used to attach a hairpiece to a block. There are six sizes of canvas blocks available: 20", 20½", 21", 21½", 22", and 22½" (50, 51.25, 52.5, 53.75, 55, and 56.25 cm). A swivel clamp is used for better block control.

Good blocking gives you professional results when shaping, setting, and combing out a wig. It also reduces the possibility of disturbing the comb-out when you remove the T-pins.

Fit the wig comfortably on the right size block. Do not stretch a wig onto a block that is too big or let it hang too loosely on a block that is too small. If you stretch and pin a wig, it can expand if you wet the cap; when you hang a wig too loosely, it can shrink if you wet the cap (if made of cotton).

Mount the wig on the correct head size block and pin as follows:

1. At the center of the forehead.
2. At each side of the temple. (See Fig. 15.14)
3. At the center of the nape.
4. At each corner of the nape. (See Fig. 15.15)
   (These illustrations show the proper placement of T-pins.)

Styrofoam blocks are used for storing or displaying the wig.

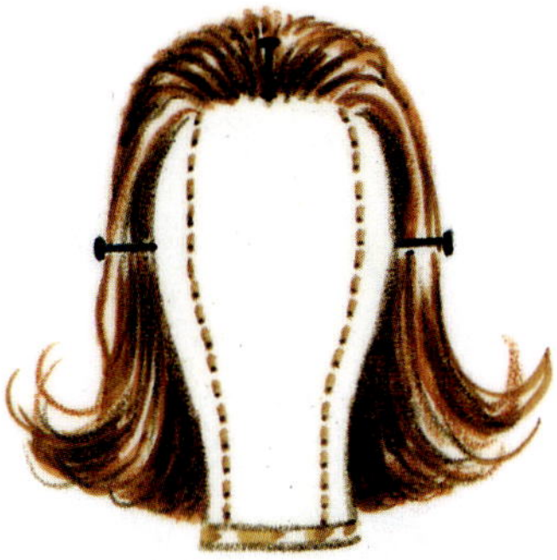

15.14—Place one T-pin at center of forehead and one at each side.

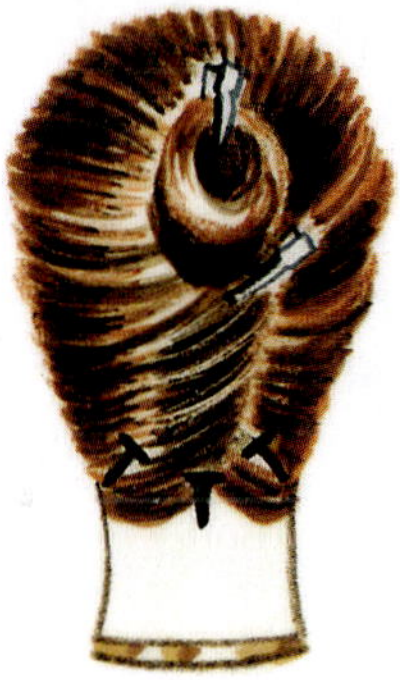

15.15—Place one T-pin at center of nape and one at each corner.

FITTING THE WIG

After the wig has been made according to specific measurements, you might have to adjust it to fit your client's head comfortably.

ADJUSTING THE WIG TO A LARGER SIZE

If the wig is too tight, you might have to stretch it. Turn the wig inside out and wet its foundation with hot water. Stretch the wig carefully (without ripping) onto a larger size block and pin it securely. Then allow the wig to dry naturally. (This process may have to be repeated more than once if the wig has to be enlarged more than one size.)

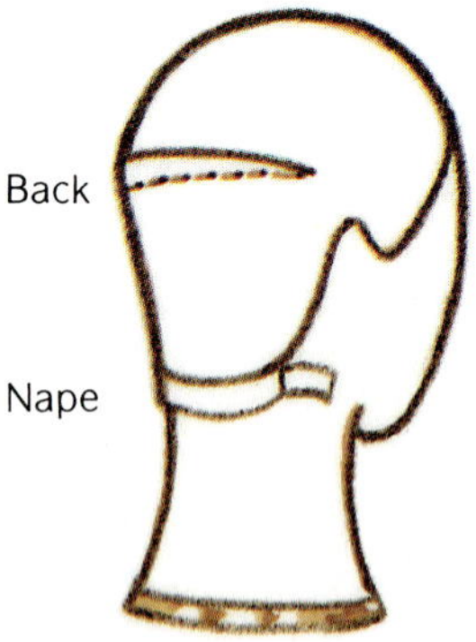

15.16—Horizontal tuck.

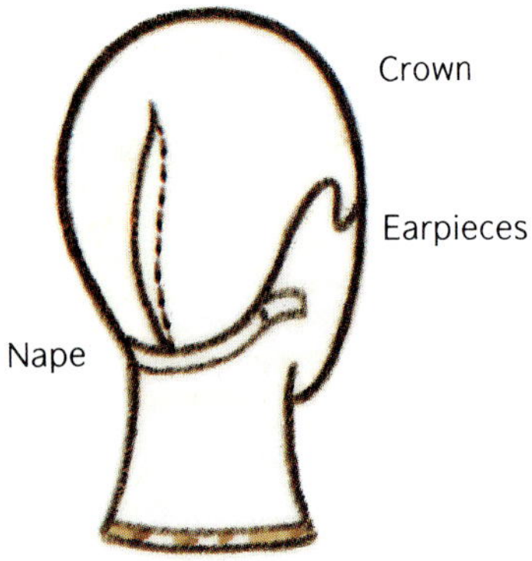

15.17—Vertical tuck.

ADJUSTING THE WIG TO A SMALLER SIZE

If the wig is too loose, you must adjust it to fit properly.

Tucking

You can sew tucks to improve the fit of a wig that is too big.

1. ***Horizontal tucks*** shorten the wig from front to nape. They are made across the back of the wig to remove excess bulk, and shorten the length of the crown area of the wig. (See Fig. 15.16)
2. ***Vertical tucks*** remove width at the back of the wig from ear to ear. (See Fig. 15.17)

Check the cap fit after each tuck. Too much tucking can cause the wig to ride up and create new fitting problems.

Check both earpieces to be certain they are directly across from each other and do not touch the ears. If the wig touches the ear, make a small horizontal tuck over the ear to raise the wig. If the wig rubs or touches the side of the ear, make a small vertical tuck behind the ear to pull the wig back and eliminate the problem.

If a wig is too long from forehead to nape, make a tuck approximately ¼″ (.625 cm) deep on the weft. Always sew a tuck toward the crown, never away from it, or hair will stand away from the wig when you comb it out. When tacking a tuck, be certain that you take out as much hair as possible before you complete the stitching process. The same applies if a wig is too large from the crown to the ear and it leans on the client's ears. You can correct this by stitching horizontally along the wefting.

◆ NOTE: When you adjust a ventilated or hand-tied wig, you should sew the tucks on the inside of the foundation. However, when you adjust a machine-made or wefted wig, you can sew horizontal tucks either inside or outside the wig.

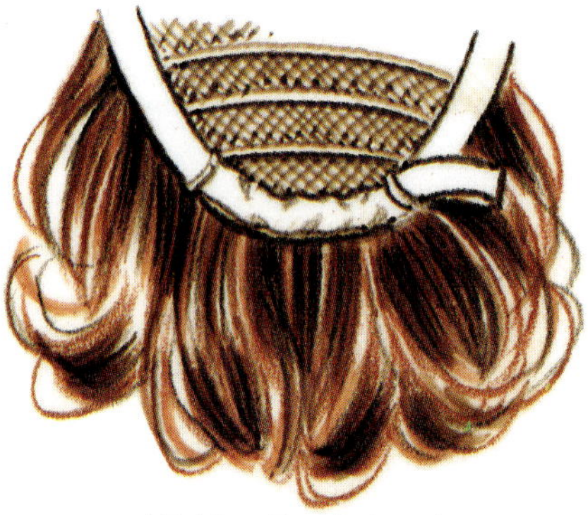

15.18—Elastic band.

THE ELASTIC BAND

In the final step of the wig adjustment process, you must adjust the elastic band at the back of the wig. Pull the elastic band at the back of the wig to make the wig fit evenly and snugly at the back of the head and then fasten it. Some stylists favor pinning the ends of the elastic band with a small safety pin to allow for more convenience when making later adjustments or replacements. The elastic band does require periodic adjustment or replacement, because these bands stretch or deteriorate when exposed to body heat and cleaning fluids over a period of time. Other stylists believe that the band should be stitched securely and the stitches broken when adjustment or replacement is needed. (Fig. 15.18) ✔

✔ Completed—Learning Objective No. 5

BLOCKING AND FITTING WIGS

CLEANING WIGS

HUMAN HAIR WIGS

You should clean a human hair wig every 2 to 4 weeks, depending on how often it is worn or when you are ready to restyle it, using a nonflammable liquid cleanser. Refer to the manufacturer's suggestions and cleaning instructions.

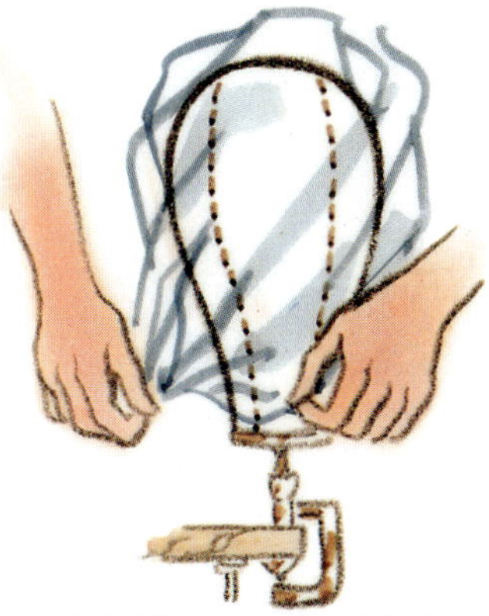
15.19—Covering block.

Procedure

1. Cover the block with a plastic cover to protect the canvas. (See Fig. 15.19)
2. Block the wig. Remove back-combing, if necessary. Direct the hair off the hairline. Brush the hair to loosen dirt and hair spray.
3. Before you take the wig off the block to clean it, mark the size of the wig on the block so you can keep the wig the same size after you have finished cleaning it. You do this by placing a T-pin into the block on an angle next to the edge of the cap and directly in front of the six T-pins securing the wig. (See Figs. 15.20, 15.21) Remove the wig and proceed with the cleaning.

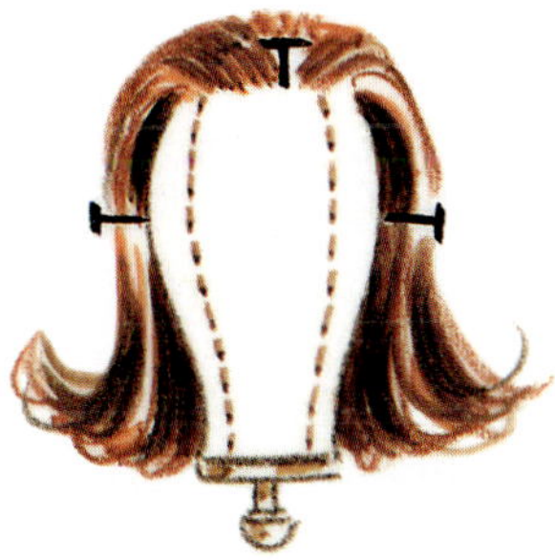
15.20—Front view.

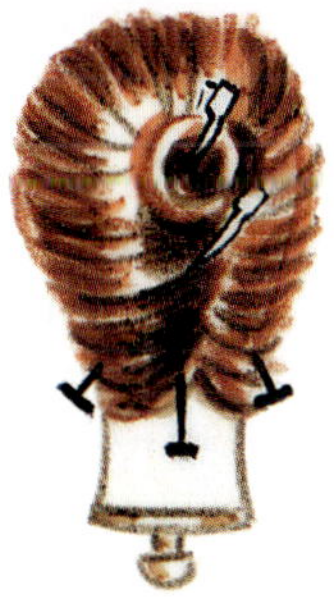
15.21—Back view.

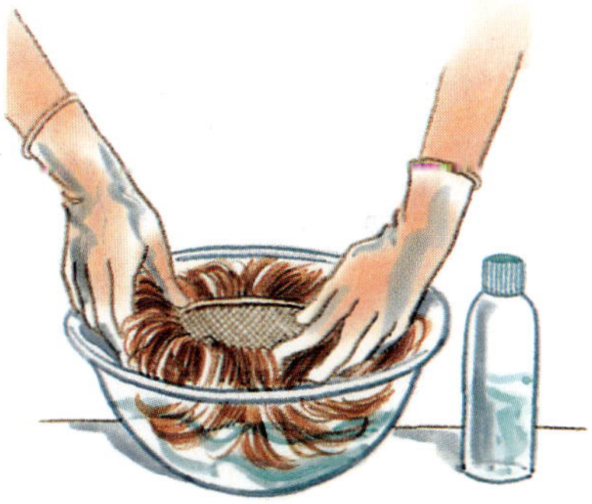
15.22—Wash wig with nonflammable liquid cleanser.

4. Wear rubber gloves to protect your hands. Saturate the wig in 3 ounces (90 ml) of nonflammable liquid cleanser in a large glass or porcelain bowl. With the hair side down, dip the wig up and down until it is clean. (See Fig. 15.22)

   Alternate method: *Swirl the wig around in the liquid cleanser. If necessary, clean the edges and inside foundation with a cotton ball or toothbrush.*

5. Gently shake the wig to remove excess fluid. Place the wet wig immediately on the canvas block. Stretch the wig lightly and pin it securely to the block. (See Fig. 15.23)
6. When the wig is dry, set and style it.

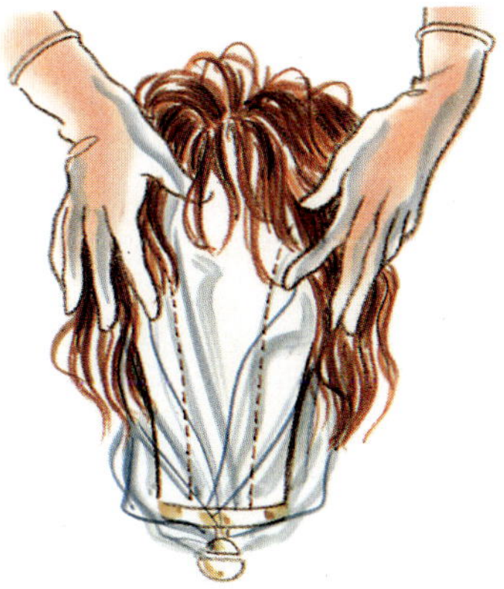
15.23—Placing wig on block.

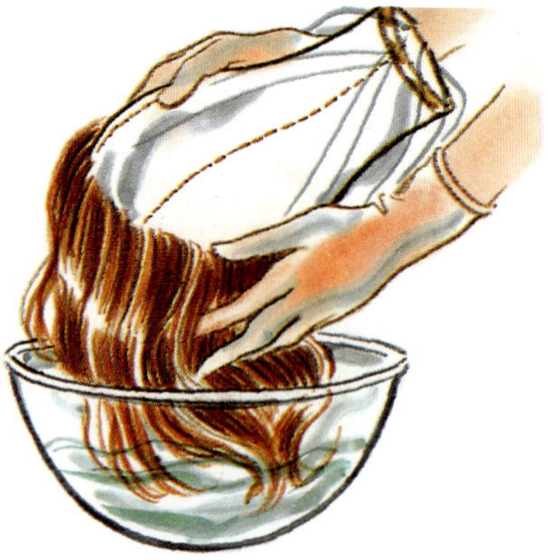
15.24—Saturate wig and work solution through hair.

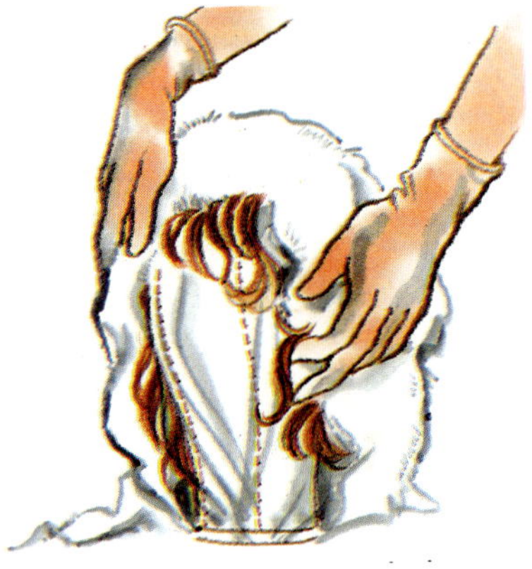
15.25—Towel dry hair.

HAND-TIED WIGS

Since hand-tied wigs have a more delicate structure than machine-made wigs and cost much more, you should clean them on a block.

Procedure

1. Cover the canvas block with plastic to protect the canvas.
2. Clean the edges and inside foundation with a cotton ball or toothbrush.
3. Block the wig.
4. Saturate the wig in a large glass or plastic bowl containing liquid cleaner. (See Fig. 15.24)
5. Soak the wig for 3 to 4 minutes.
6. Comb the cleaning solution through the length of hair with a wide-tooth comb.
7. Work the solution into the entire wig.
8. Carefully towel blot. (See Fig. 15.25)
9. Allow to dry naturally on the block for about ½ hour.
10. Give a conditioning treatment, if necessary.
11. Set and style the wig.

SYNTHETIC WIGS

Synthetic wigs and hairpieces need not be cleaned as often as human hair wigs. Synthetic fibers are nonabsorbent (lack porosity) and do not attract dust and dirt.

Clean and style synthetic wigs and hairpieces about every 3 months, depending on the amount of wear and styling. Use tepid or cool water to clean the wig; hot water takes the curl out of synthetic wigs. Do not comb or brush while wet.

Procedure

1. Cover the block with plastic to protect the canvas.
2. Mount the wig on the block and outline the size (as described earlier).
3. Brush the wig free of tangles and spray before cleaning.
4. Fill a container with mild shampoo or a specially formulated cleaner, according to the manufacturer's directions. Use tepid or cool water.
5. Remove the wig from the block. Swish the wig through cleaning solution for a few minutes. Rinse thoroughly in cool water.
6. Use a small brush or cotton to clean the mesh foundation.
7. Squeeze out excess water and towel blot. (Do not wring or twist wig.)
8. T-pin the wig on the proper size block and let dry naturally.

9. Do not brush a synthetic wig when it is wet; this can take out the curl.
10. Do not expose a synthetic wig to the excess heat of a hairdryer. This concentrated heat can cause the synthetic hair strands to stick together and lose their curl.
11. When the wig dries completely, brush out the hair and spray with conditioner to add luster.

◆ NOTE: If you must reduce drying time, place the wig in a cool dryer using only the fan. Since most synthetic wigs are pre-styled, they require no further styling.

CONDITIONING THE WIG

A wig differs from natural human hair in that it does not have its own supply of natural oils for self-lubrication. Since wig cleaners usually dry the hair excessively, use a conditioning treatment after each cleaning to keep the wig hair from drying and looking dull. This also keeps the wig in good condition. (See Fig. 15.26)

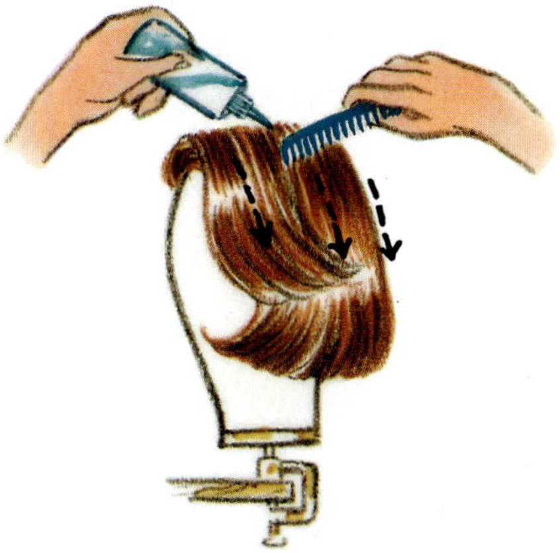

15.26—Condition wig after cleaning.

Procedure

1. Cover the block with plastic and block the wig properly.
2. Apply conditioner. Distribute the conditioner evenly on clean, damp hair using a wide-tooth comb. Rinse conditioner out of hair according to product's instructions.
3. Set and style the wig. ✔

✔ Completed—Learning Objective No. 6

CLEANING WIGS

SHAPING WIGS

HUMAN HAIR WIGS

You can shape (cut) a wig in the same way you cut natural hair on the head. However, you must consider the fact that a wig holds about twice as much hair as a human head. Thus, if you do not thin and taper the wig properly, it will look bulky and artificial. You can thin the wig with either a razor or thinning shears. Concentrate on removing bulk from the top hairline, in back of the ears, and around the face. You do not usually have to thin these areas on natural hair.

Cut as close to the wig foundation as possible, without damaging the cap itself. Thin hair close to the cap to remove additional bulk and to make sure you have not left hair spurs that will stick out when you style the wig later. Special care must be taken so that knots on the hand-knotted wig remain tight. Take equal care to not cut any of the wefts or sewing threads on the wefted wig. When you cut a wig, keep in mind that the hair will not grow back to cover an error in judgment. Proceed cautiously. Although it is more convenient to shape the wig on a canvas block, it is a good

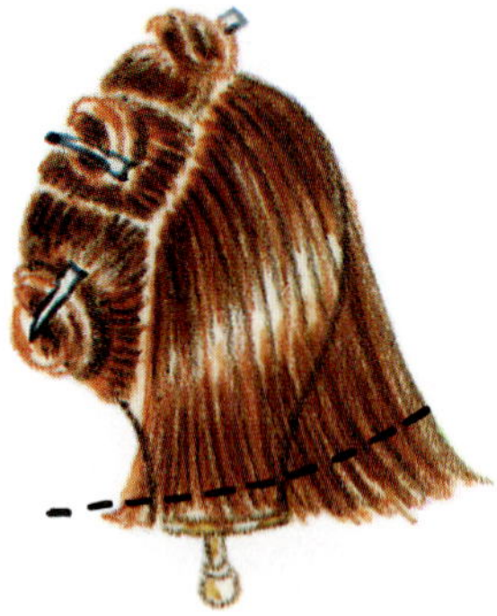

15.27—Part off a 2" (5 cm) guideline and cut to desired length.

idea to cut the wig while it is on the client's head in order to suit the client's natural hair and facial features. Thus, you might find that the best technique is to cut a guideline on the client's head and then transfer the wig to the block. This ensures that the wig is being cut to the proper length. Then, you can move the wig to the block, secure it firmly, and avoid slippage during the rest of the shaping process. When you place the wig on the canvas block to cut it, set it carefully at the correct hairline distance and continue cutting the remaining hair evenly. Continue the shaping process, section by section, until the entire wig has been shaped. (Figs. 15.27–15.33)

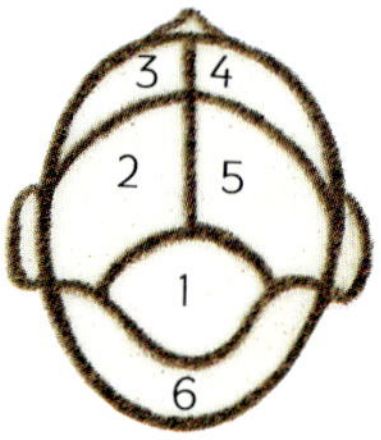

15.28—Top front.

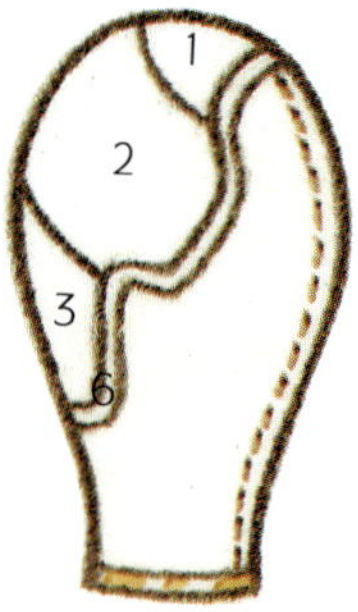

15.29—Right side.

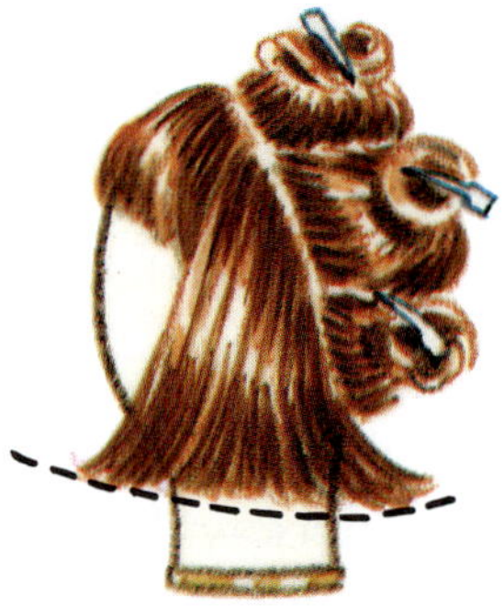

15.30—Left side of head. This illustrates a completely cut guideline.

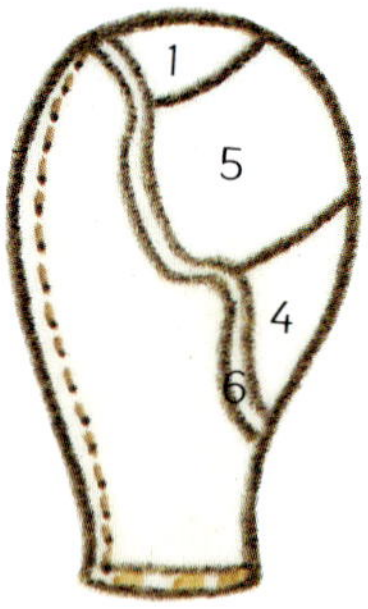

15.31—Left side.

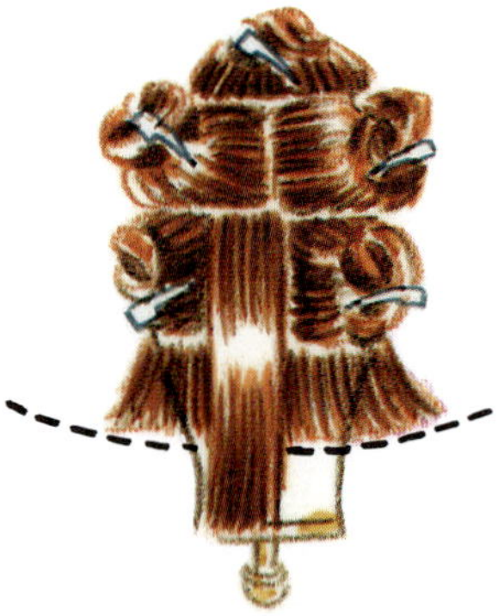

15.32—Back of head. Let down center back hair. Cut to the same length as guideline.

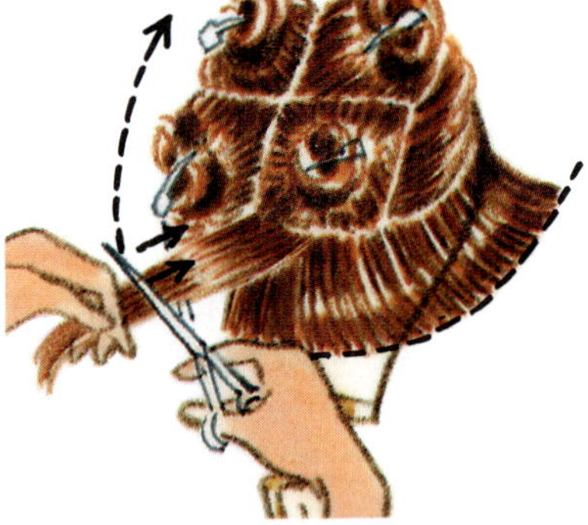

15.33—Back of head. Pick up a strand of the guideline. With hands arched at a 45° (.785 rad.) angle, cut into longer hair. Proceed with a sweeping upward motion.

SYNTHETIC HAIR WIGS

Always cut synthetic wigs when dry, because the fibers can stretch out of shape if pulled when wet. Use only scissors and thinning shears on synthetic fiber or on a mixture of synthetic and human hair. Because synthetic fibers do not have the resiliency or flexibility of human hair, they can dull a razor badly. As a result, a razor can cause permanent damage to the wig.

SETTING AND STYLING WIGS

Setting wig hair resembles setting hair on the human head, except for hairline coverage and the need for a tight curl at the nape area. You must also consider the added fullness of the client's hair, plus the hair and foundation of the wig when setting and styling the wig. Wigs are always set and styled on the blocking. (Figs. 15.34, 15.35)

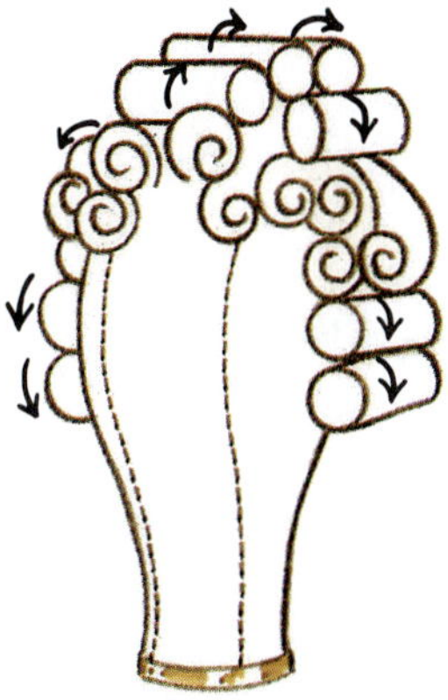

15.34—Setting on block.

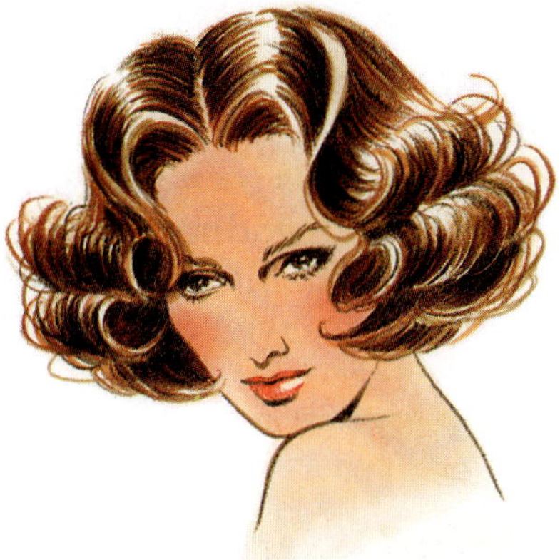

15.35—Finished style.

Pin curls replace rollers in the front hairline, temple, and nape to keep the style close to the head. (Fig. 15.36) Use T-pins instead of clippies or bobby pins to hold both rollers and curls more securely. Set, dry, and style hair in the usual manner. (Fig. 15.37)

Cutting and styling synthetic wigs differs from cutting and styling human hair wigs in the following ways:

You may only tease or back comb wigs at the base of their fibers. Otherwise, you will damage the fibers that should be kept perfectly smooth at the wig surface. Damage to the hair shaft (by thinning) leaves you with a frizzy, fuzzy-looking wig.

Synthetic wigs are pre-cut into definite styles by their manufacturers. If the client desires a change, a good quality synthetic wig can be combed into different styles by a skilled stylist. These comb-out styles are all based on the basic pre-cut factory-created style. However, a stylist must be guided by the client's wishes.

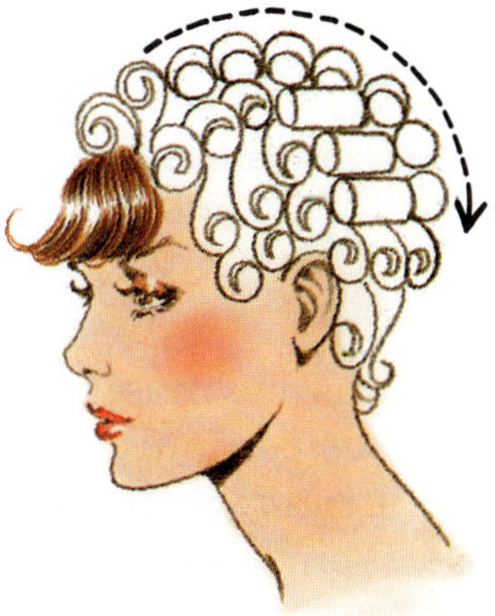

15.36—How the setting would look on the head.

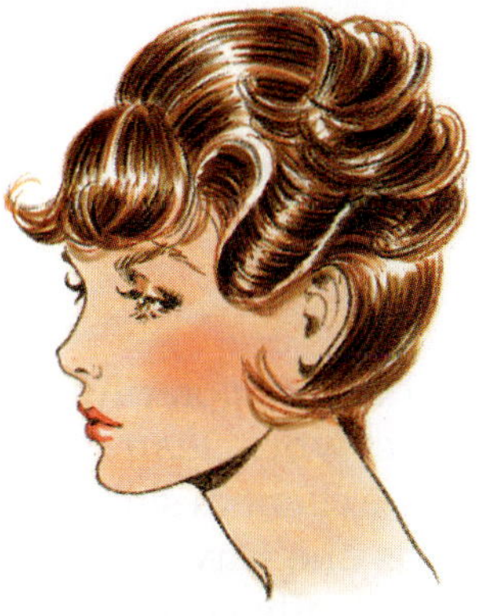

15.37—Finished style.

PUTTING ON AND TAKING OFF A WIG

A simple but very important procedure is the way you remove a wig from a block and place it on the client's head. (Fig. 15.38) (It is a good idea to show the client the proper way to put on and take off the wig.)

COMBING CLIENT'S HAIR INTO A WIG

Depending on the style, set the client's hair that is to be blended with the wig in pin curls. When the wig is ready to be combined with the client's own hair, secure the wig starting either at the top or bottom depending on where you set the pin curls. When the wig is comfortably adjusted, comb and blend the client's hair into the style of the wig. (Fig. 15.39)

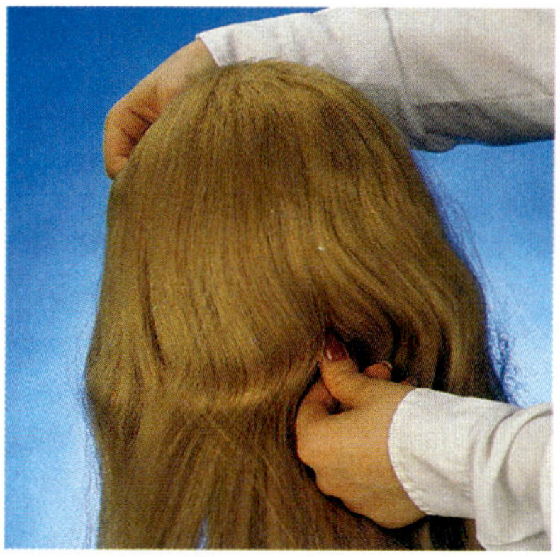

15.38—Place wig on front of client's head. While holding wig securely on top, glide it back to nape. Pull securely over sides, front, and back.

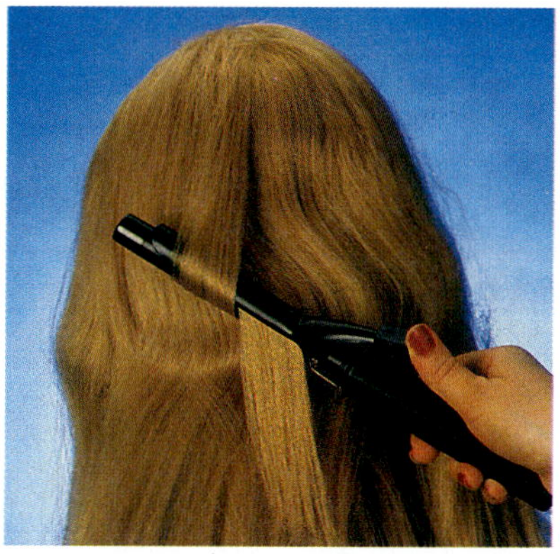

15.39—Recomb, adjust, and style to suit client.

✔ Completed—Learning Objective No. 7

SHAPING, SETTING, AND STYLING WIGS

REMOVING A WIG

To remove a wig, place only your thumb under the cap at the nape. ***Do not put your fingers into the hair.*** Have the client bend down his or her head. Then, slide the wig off. ✔

WIG COLORING

COLOR RINSES

Color rinses temporarily color human hair wigs and must be reapplied whenever you clean the hair. Color rinses can only darken the hair; if the client desires a lighter color, a different wig must be worn.

Here is one way to apply a color rinse. (Your instructor's method may be equally correct.)

Procedure

1. Pin the wig securely on a plastic-covered block.
2. Dampen the clean hair, using a spray applicator bottle.
3. If you are unsure about which color to use, strand test the color rinse on the back of the wig.
4. Spray hair with the color rinse. Distribute it evenly with a downward motion, using a small brush and wide-tooth comb. (See Fig. 15.40)
5. Apply setting lotion in the usual manner. (See Fig. 15.41)
6. Set, dry, (see Fig. 15.42) and comb out the hair to the desired style.

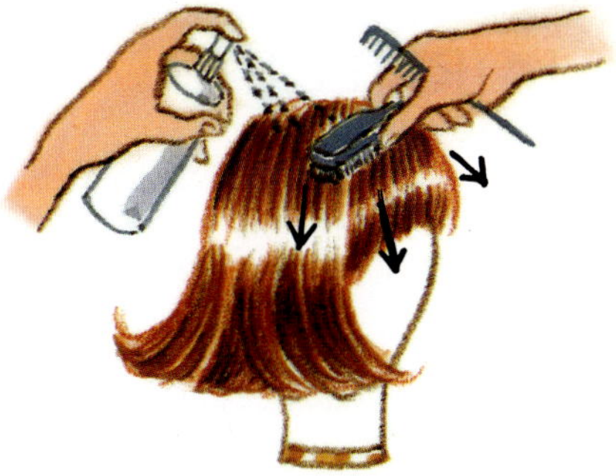

15.40—Spray hair with color rinse.

◆ NOTE: In addition to color rinses, you can color human hair wigs with a semi-permanent tint. However, you should never attempt to lighten (bleach) any wig or hairpiece.

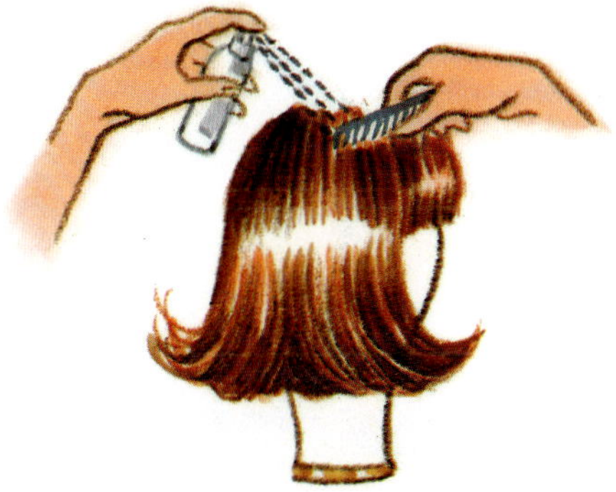

15.41—Apply setting lotion.

SEMI-PERMANENT TINTS

Semi-permanent tints are referred to as 6-week tints. They are self-penetrating and require no peroxide. They do not change the basic structure of the hair.

Here is one way to apply semi-permanent tints to machine-made wigs:

Procedure

1. Mount the wig on the appropriate plastic-covered block and outline the size with T-pins.
2. Remove all teasing, tangles, and snarls.
3. Clean the wig and comb the hair smooth.
4. Remove the wig from the block.
5. Immerse the wig in a glass bowl of hot water and semi-permanent tint solution.
6. Leave it completely immersed for 10 minutes.
7. Remove it and rinse with cold water.
8. Apply conditioner.
9. Block, set, dry, and comb out in the usual manner.

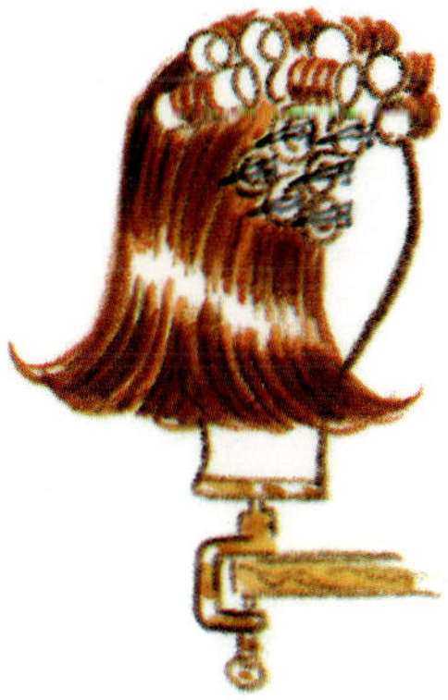

15.42—Set, dry, and comb out.

PERMANENT TINTS

Since 100% human hair wigs and hairpieces have been subjected to extensive processing, applying a permanent tint to this kind of hair can be very risky and will result in uneven coloring. ✔

✔ Completed—Learning Objective No. 8

COLORING WIGS

CAUTION

When tinting wigs, be sure to follow the manufacturer's directions.

HAIRPIECES

You can create a variety of hairstyles with hairpieces, fashioning them for either daytime or evening wear. Hairpieces come in various forms, such as:

1. ***Switches.*** These are long wefts of hair mounted with a loop at the end. They are constructed with one to two stems of hair. Better switches are constructed with three stems to provide greater flexibility in styling and braiding. They can be worked into the hair or braided to create special styling effects. (See Fig. 15.43)
2. ***Wiglets.*** These are hairpieces with a flat base that are used in special areas of the head. They are used primarily to blend with the client's own hair in order to extend the range of hair in a particular section of the head. Wiglets can be worked into the top of the hair in curls or under the hair to give height and body. They can also be used to create special effects. (See Fig. 15.44)
3. ***Bandeau.*** This is a hairpiece that is sewn to a headband. The headband, which is replaceable and comes in different colors, serves as an excellent disguise for the hairline. The bandeau hairpiece is usually worn over the hair and dressed casually. (See Fig. 15.45)
4. ***Fall.*** This is a section of hair, machine wefted on a round base, running across the back of the head and available in various lengths. Falls have a thick, plushy look. *Short falls* range from 12″ to 14″ (30 to 35 cm) in length (see Fig. 15.46); *demi-falls* from 15″ to 20″ (37.5 to 50 cm); and *long falls* from 18″ to 24″ (45 to 60 cm).

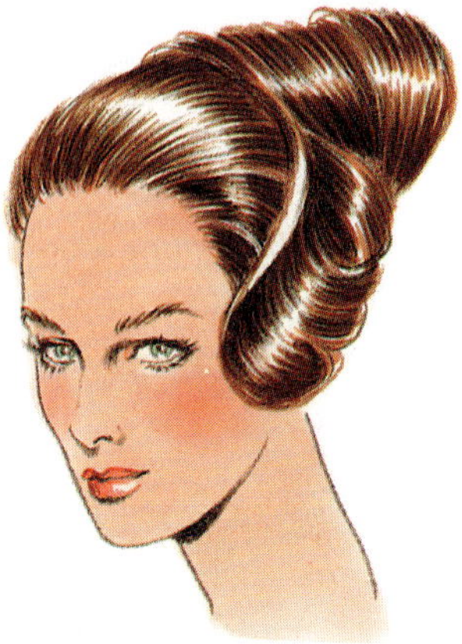

15.43—Switch.

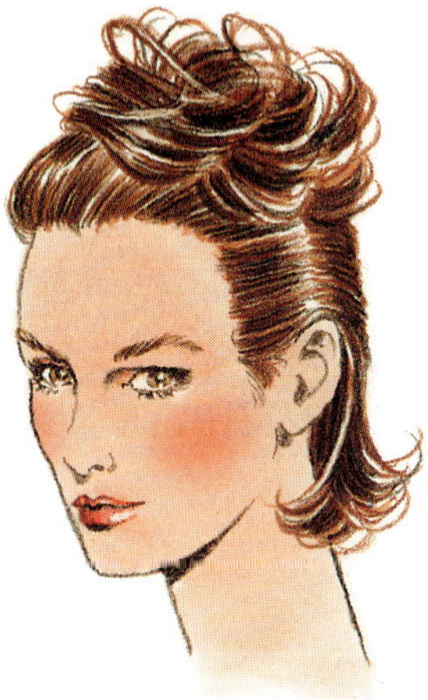

15.44—Wiglet.

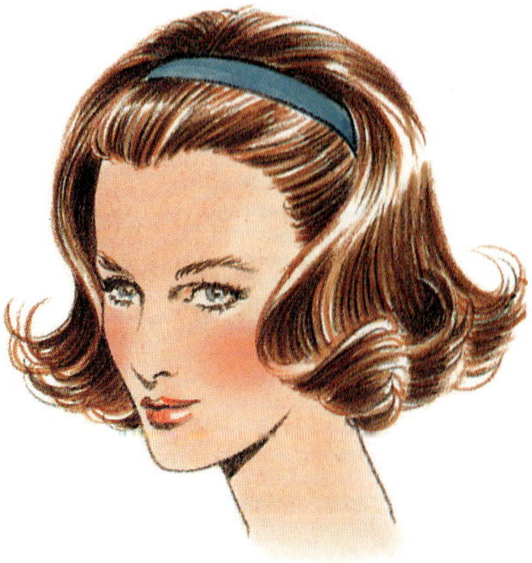

15.45—Bandeau.

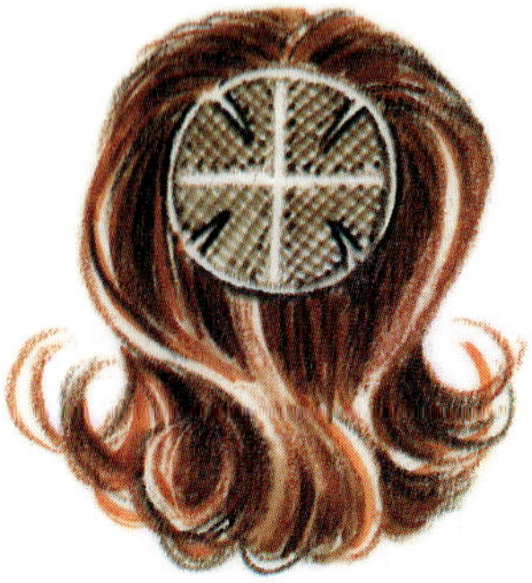

15.46—Short fall.

5. ***Demi-fall*** or ***demi-wig.*** This is a large-base hairpiece designed to fit the shape of the head. The demi-fall or demi-wig generally ranges in length from 15″ to 20″ (37.5 to 50 cm).
6. ***Cascade.*** This is a hairpiece on an oblong base that offers an endless variety of styling possibilities. Cascades can be styled in curls, braids, a pageboy, or used as a filler with the client's own hair. (See Fig. 15.47)
7. ***Braid.*** This is a switch whose strands are woven, interlaced, or entwined. Some are prepared with a thin wire inside so that they can be formed into various shapes. Wireless braids hang loose on the head.
8. ***Chignon.*** This is a knot or coil of hair, created from synthetic hair, that is worn at the nape or crown of the head. A chignon works best when worn in combination with another hairpiece.
9. ***Crown curls.*** These are a group of light curls worn on top of the head.
10. ***Frosting curls.*** These are segments of frosted or blended hair pinned into natural hair to simulate frosted or streaked hair. ✔

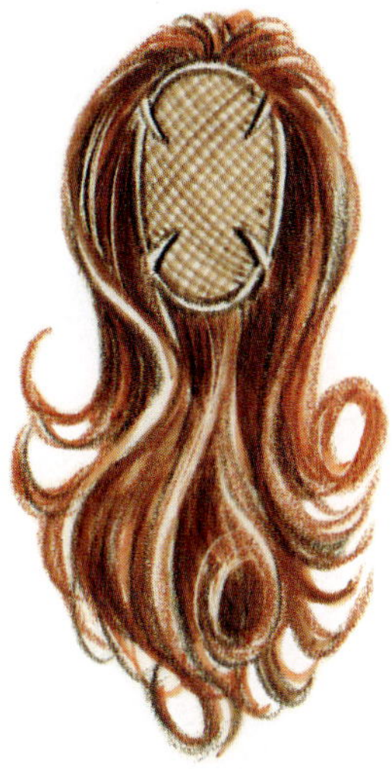

15.47—Cascade.

✔ Completed—Learning Objective No. 9

TYPES OF HAIRPIECES

SAFETY PRECAUTIONS

1. Take great care when combing or brushing wigs to avoid matting.
2. When cleaning a wig or hairpiece, never rub or wring out the fluid.
3. When you shape (cut) a wig or hairpiece, use great care; once the hair has been cut, it cannot grow back.
4. When you comb a freshly set wig, use a wide-tooth comb to help you gain greater control and to avoid damaging the wig's foundation.
5. When you clean or work with a wet wig, always mount it on a block of the same head size as the wig to avoid stretching.
6. Take accurate measurements of the client's head to ensure a comfortable and secure fit.
7. Recondition wigs as often as necessary to prevent dry or brittle hair.
8. If needed, clean wigs before setting and styling.
9. Brush and comb wigs and hairpieces with a downward movement.
10. Never lighten (bleach) a wig or hairpiece.
11. Never give a permanent to a wig or hairpiece. ✔

✔ Completed—Learning Objective No. 10

SAFETY PRECAUTIONS

Question & Answer

HAIR EXTENSIONS FOR FINE HAIR

Q *I have a young client whose hair is very fine all over and quite thin in the crown and down the back. Which extension technique is best for this type of hair?*

A Your client is a good candidate for the "bonding" technique of attaching hair extensions. You must first determine whether or not the person is allergic to any type of adhesive. You must also determine the length of hair needed (or desired) by the client. It is not advisable to bond weft lengths longer than 15 inches. Another point to consider is whether or not your client has an excessively oily scalp, or if she requires hair-conditioning treatments that contain oil, since oil can dislodge bonding adhesive.

Cut the weft pieces into strips approximately two inches wide and attach them randomly throughout the hair. Even if you place them side-by-side, it takes the weight off any one spot. You may also consider combining both methods of attaching bonds if the situation calls for it. For instance, if a client wears a definite side part, a bonded strip just below the part will not be as obvious as a sewn weft. It serves as well to cover the wefts sewn beneath it.

Latex-based adhesive bond is easily removed from the natural hair and the weft extension. It comes out completely, allowing the extension to be readjusted as necessary.

—*From* Milady's Salon Solutions *by Louise Cotter*

REVIEW QUESTIONS

THE ARTISTRY OF ARTIFICIAL HAIR

1. List some of the reasons people wear wigs.
2. Name the different types of wigs, extensions, and hairpieces.
3. What is the purpose of a hair extension?
4. What is the purpose of blocking a wig?
5. How often should a human hair wig be cleaned?
6. Where should a wig be set and styled?
7. What effect does a color rinse have on a human hair wig?

NOTES

NOTES

NOTES

NOTES

NOTES

NOTES

NOTES

NOTES

NOTES

NOTES

NOTES

NOTES

NOTES

NOTES

NOTES

NOTES

NOTES

NOTES